Physical Therapy and Rehabilitation - Research and Clinical Application

Edited by Hideki Nakano

Published in London, United Kingdom

Physical Therapy and Rehabilitation - Research and Clinical Application
http://dx.doi.org/10.5772/intechopen.1008597
Edited by Hideki Nakano

Assistants to Editor: Takato Nishida and Shun Sawai

Contributors
Saima Gul, Ryosuke Yamamoto, Shin Murata, Shun Sawai, Shoya Fujikawa, Takato Nishida, Yusuke Shizuka, Naoki Shimizu, Hideki Nakano, Iván F. Mondragón B., Wilson A. Henández M., Catalina Alvarado-Rojas, Diego Mendez, Jeronimo Rueda, David E. González, Guillermo A. Aguilera, Julian D. Colorado, Yusuke Shizuka, Shun Sawai, Takato Nishida, Shoya Fujikawa, Ryosuke Yamamoto, Naoki Shimizu, Hideki Nakano, Takato Nishida, Shin Murata, Shun Sawai, Shoya Fujikawa, Ryosuke Yamamoto, Yusuke Shizuka, Naoki Shimizu, Hideki Nakano, Shoya Fujikawa, Shin Murata, Shun Sawai, Takato Nishida, Ryosuke Yamamoto, Yusuke Shizuka, Naoki Shimizu, Hideki Nakano, Chijindu-Orji Iseh-Ntah, Stefka Stoilova, Hiromi Nakamura-Thomas, Peter Bredu-Darkwa, Ichiro Yamamoto, Yuri Fujiwara

First published in London, United Kingdom, 2026 by IntechOpen
IntechOpen is the global imprint of INTECHOPEN LIMITED, registered in England and Wales, registration number: 11086078, 167-169 Great Portland Street, London, W1W 5PF, United Kingdom

For EU product safety concerns: IN TECH d.o.o., Prolaz Marije Krucifikse Kozulić 3, 51000 Rijeka, Croatia, info@intechopen.com or visit our website at intechopen.com.

British Library Cataloguing-in-Publication Data
A catalogue record for this book is available from the British Library

Physical Therapy and Rehabilitation - Research and Clinical Application
Edited by Hideki Nakano
p. cm.
Print ISBN 978-1-83635-082-8
Online ISBN 978-1-83635-081-1
eBook (PDF) ISBN 978-1-83635-083-5

Meet the editor

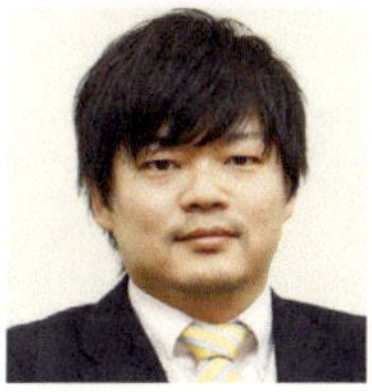

Dr. Hideki Nakano is a Physical Therapist and Associate Professor at the Neurorehabilitation Laboratory, Graduate School of Health Sciences, Kyoto Tachibana University, Japan. He received his Ph.D. in Health Science from Kio University, Japan. He previously served as a JSPS Research Fellow at the Neurorehabilitation Research Center, Kio University, Japan, and the Queensland Brain Institute, University of Queensland, Australia. He specializes in neuroscience, neurophysiology, and rehabilitation science, conducting research using non-invasive methods for measuring and stimulating brain function, including electroencephalography (EEG), transcranial magnetic stimulation (TMS), and transcranial electrical stimulation (tES). His current primary research interest is developing rehabilitation evaluation and treatment methods that utilize neuroimaging and neuromodulation of brain function for healthy older adults and patients with neurological disorders.

Contents

Preface

Rehabilitation is a cornerstone of modern healthcare, enabling individuals to regain function, sustain independence, and participate meaningfully in everyday life. As clinical needs become more complex and the evidence base expands, physical therapy and rehabilitation increasingly require an integrated view, one that connects mechanistic understanding with practical assessment, effective intervention, and patient-centered outcomes. This edited volume, *Physical Therapy and Rehabilitation – Research and Clinical Application*, was developed to offer such a perspective, bringing together contributions that span foundational concepts, emerging technologies, and real-world clinical considerations.

The book is organized into four sections that reflect major domains of contemporary rehabilitation practice and research. Section 1, *Neurological Rehabilitation and Neurotechnology*, highlights how advances in neuroscience and engineering are reshaping neurological rehabilitation. Topics include neurophysiological perspectives that inform exercise-based therapy, clinically meaningful assessment approaches, and technology-enabled rehabilitation strategies that can enhance engagement and support recovery. Collectively, these contributions underscore the importance of linking mechanisms to practice while maintaining a clear focus on functional improvement.

Section 2, *Aging, Frailty, and Postural Control*, addresses the challenges associated with aging societies worldwide. Rehabilitation professionals encounter complex interactions among motor control, cognition, balance, and mobility that influence fall risk, independence, and quality of life. This section considers changes across the lifespan, the conceptual and practical challenges of evaluating frailty-related conditions, and contemporary approaches to assessing postural control. The emphasis is placed on clinical relevance, how to interpret assessment findings and use them to guide prevention and intervention strategies.

Section 3, *Musculoskeletal Rehabilitation and Integrative Care*, focuses on common musculoskeletal issues and chronic conditions that affect movement and participation. It presents perspectives on intervention selection, therapeutic approaches used in clinical practice, and integrative care frameworks that recognize the multidimensional needs of individuals living with long-term musculoskeletal disorders. The goal is to support evidence-informed decision-making while acknowledging patient preferences and real-world constraints.

Finally, Section 4, *Participation, Communication, and Patient-Centered Outcomes*, centers on the broader aims of rehabilitation: enabling meaningful activity, supporting communication and social participation, and evaluating outcomes that matter to patients and families. This section emphasizes how rehabilitation extends beyond impairment-level change and highlights the value of outcome measurement, community living considerations, and the lived experience of disability and recovery.

This volume is intended for physical therapists, rehabilitation clinicians, researchers, educators, and advanced trainees seeking a structured overview of current topics across the rehabilitation continuum. While each contribution reflects a distinct focus, the shared aim is consistent: to strengthen the bridge between research knowledge and clinical application, and to support rehabilitation that is both scientifically grounded and genuinely patient-centered.

I want to express my sincere gratitude to all contributing authors for their expertise, professionalism, and commitment to advancing rehabilitation practice and research. Appreciation is also extended to the editorial and production teams who supported the development of this volume. In addition, I would like to acknowledge the valuable assistance provided by the Assistants to the Editor, Takato Nishida (Seijoh University, Japan) and Shun Sawai (Kyoto Tachibana University, Japan), whose support contributed significantly to the editorial process.

Hideki Nakano, Ph.D.
Associate Professor,
Neurorehabilitation Laboratory,
Graduate School of Health Sciences,
Kyoto Tachibana University,
Kyoto, Japan

Section 1

Neurological Rehabilitation and Neurotechnology

Chapter 1

Exercise Therapies and Their Neurophysiological Basis

Saima Gul

Abstract

Exercise therapy is a structured, evidence-based approach to physical activity aimed at improving health outcomes, rehabilitating injuries, and enhancing neurological functions. Various forms of physical activity, including aerobic exercise, strength training, and motor rehabilitation, influence brain networks, improving cognitive function and motor control. These therapies are widely used in neurological rehabilitation for conditions such as stroke, Parkinson's disease, and multiple sclerosis. The neurophysiological basis of exercise therapy revolves around its effects on the central and peripheral nervous systems, modulating brain plasticity, neurogenesis, neurotransmitter activity, and neurotrophic factors. Mechanisms such as increased blood flow, synaptic plasticity, and neurotrophic factor release contribute to their benefits. Understanding the neurophysiological basis of exercise therapies provides insights into optimizing treatment strategies for neurological and mental health disorders, promoting overall brain health and recovery. This chapter will open up the integration of exercise therapies with neurorehabilitation, explore different exercise therapies and their neural impact on neurological and psychological conditions, discuss neurophysiological foundations of exercises, describe how exercise affects the nervous system, provide direction on designing neurophysiologically informed exercise programs, and highlight the future direction and emerging trends of these exercise therapies.

Keywords: neuroplasticity, exercise therapy, neurotransmitter regulation, motor rehabilitation, brain health

1. Introduction

Exercise therapies signify systematically planned and prescribed physical activities aimed at restoring, maintaining, and improving physical and functional capacities in individuals with acute or chronic conditions. Differentiated from general physical activity, exercise therapy is goal-directed, individualized, and embedded within therapeutic frameworks, often guided by clinical reasoning to target specific impairments, activity limitations, or participation restrictions.

In neurorehabilitation, exercise therapies have acquired increasing attention for their role in endorsing brain health and enhancing functional recovery. Their aims are to enhance recovery and functional outcomes in individuals with neurological impairments through interventions that control the plastic potential of the central and peripheral nervous systems. Among the diverse therapeutic strategies endeavored, exercise therapies have emerged as a central pillar due to their profound influence on neuromuscular function, neuroplasticity, cardiovascular fitness, and psychosocial well-being [1]. Exercise therapies in rehabilitation encompass a broad range of physical activities, from structured aerobic and resistance training to task-specific, repetitive motor practice designed to retrain lost or impaired functions.

1.1 Historical context and evolution of exercise therapy in neurorehabilitation

The use of physical activity to enhance motor recovery in individuals with neurological disorders has deep historical roots, but it gained scientific grip in the twentieth century, remarkably after World War II, when the rising need to rehabilitate soldiers with neurological disorders, like traumatic brain and spinal cord injuries, headed to the development of more structured and systematic interventions [2]. Early rehabilitation approaches primarily involved passive modalities and compensation techniques, such as range of motion exercises and basic mobility drills. However, a significant shift occurred in the latter half of the century, catalyzed by advances in neuroscience and motor control theories. Concepts like the Bobath approach and proprioceptive neuromuscular facilitation (PNF) introduced the importance of sensorimotor integration and active patient involvement [3].

As research on neuroplasticity emerged, it became evident that the brain could reorganize and adapt following injury. This understanding prompted a transition to activity-based, task-specific therapies that actively engage patients in meaningful movement [4]. The integration of high-intensity training and enriched environments became central to modern neurorehabilitation. Experimental and clinical studies further demonstrated that exercise not only improves motor function but also induces neurobiological changes, such as synaptic plasticity, angiogenesis, and neurogenesis, particularly in critical areas like the motor cortex and hippocampus [5, 6]. These findings have solidified the role of exercise therapy as a dynamic and essential tool in promoting recovery and enhancing the functional capacity of individuals with neurological impairments.

2. Neurophysiological foundations of exercise

2.1 Mechanisms of action: How exercise affects the nervous system

Exercise, traditionally recognized for its benefits to musculoskeletal strength, cardiovascular endurance, and psychological well-being, is now increasingly appreciated for its profound influence on the nervous system. Recent advances in neuroscience and rehabilitation have revealed that physical activity triggers a wide array of neurophysiological processes that contribute to both brain health and functional recovery. Additionally, these physical exercises exert profound effects on the brain, not only through mechanical and metabolic changes but also *via* complex neurochemical and structural adaptations. These mechanisms include neuroplasticity, neurogenesis, modulation of neurotransmitters, and the expression of neurotrophic factors, especially brain-derived neurotrophic factor (BDNF). Together, they create a dynamic environment that supports neural adaptation, cognitive function, emotional regulation, and motor control. Exercise-induced neuroplasticity enhances the brain's capacity to reorganize and form new neural connections, which is critical in learning and recovery following injury. Neurogenesis, primarily observed in the hippocampus, contributes to memory and mood regulation. Additionally, exercise modulates key neurotransmitters, such as dopamine, serotonin, and norepinephrine, which are integral to motivation, attention, and emotional balance. The upregulation of neurotrophic factors like BDNF plays a central role in supporting neuronal growth, survival, and synaptic plasticity. These effects are particularly relevant in clinical and therapeutic settings, including stroke rehabilitation, management of neurodegenerative conditions, and treatment of mood disorders. Understanding these core mechanisms underscores the role of exercise as a powerful non-pharmacological intervention capable of inducing meaningful neurophysiological changes. This chapter delves into these mechanisms and explores how movement-based therapies can be optimized to support neural health and rehabilitation outcomes.

2.2 Neuroplasticity and neurogenesis: Structural adaptations to exercise

Neuroplasticity and neurogenesis signify the brain's remarkable capacity to adapt structurally and functionally in response to internal and external stimuli, including exercise. Once believed to be largely static in adulthood, the brain is now discerned to be capable of extensive reorganization and regeneration, especially under the influence of physical activity. These adaptations are central to cognitive enhancement, emotional regulation, and rehabilitation following neurological injury [7].

Neuroplasticity incorporates a range of mechanisms through which the nervous system modifies its structure and connectivity. *Synaptic plasticity* is one of its critical forms, which involves changes in the strength and number of synapses. Underlying synaptic plasticity, long-term potentiation (LTP) is a key process, which strengthens communication between neurons and serves as a foundational mechanism for learning and memory. Exercise-based therapies, like aerobic and skill-based exercises, have been shown to enhance LTP-like processes, especially in the hippocampus, a brain region essential for memory formation [8].

One more attribute of neuroplasticity is *cortical remapping,* where areas of the brain reorganize and assume new functions in response to training or injury. For instance, motor rehabilitation exercises can lead to reorganization within the primary motor cortex, promoting better motor control and recovery in individuals with neurological damage such as stroke [6]. This cortical adaptability is particularly relevant in the context of physical therapy and motor learning, where targeted exercise interventions can drive functional improvements through neuroanatomical change.

Myelin plasticity is a further critical yet often overlooked form of neuroplasticity. Myelin, the fatty sheath surrounding axons, facilitates efficient nerve conduction. Evidence shows that physical activity can stimulate oligodendrocyte proliferation and new myelin formation, enhancing neural efficiency and speed of transmission [9]. This form of plasticity supports improved motor learning and coordination, especially during skill acquisition and recovery.

Besides these plastic changes, *neurogenesis* (the birth of new neurons) also contributes significantly to brain adaptability. Earlier thought to occur only during development, neurogenesis has been firmly established as an ongoing process in the adult brain, particularly within the hippocampal dentate gyrus. Aerobic exercise is a potent promoter of neurogenesis, increasing the proliferation and survival of neural progenitor cells. Rodent studies have shown that voluntary running enhances hippocampal neurogenesis, with associated improvements in spatial memory and stress resilience [7, 10]. Human studies validate these findings, linking physical fitness to increased hippocampal volume and improved cognitive performance, especially in aging populations [11].

Concurrently, these structural brain adaptations illustrate how exercise acts as a neurobiological catalyst, reorganizing cortical maps, enhancing synaptic strength, generating new neurons, and increasing myelination. These changes support not only better learning and memory but also emotional regulation and functional recovery from neurological disorders. The implications are profound, particularly in rehabilitation settings, where exercise-based interventions can harness neuroplasticity and neurogenesis to optimize outcomes. As such, physical activity should be considered not only a tool for physical health but also a central component of brain health and recovery.

2.3 Neurotransmitters and brain health: Chemical mediators of exercise effects

Neurotransmitters are the brain's chemical messengers, playing an essential role in regulating pain perception, mood, arousal, motor control, and attention. They are integral to the communication between neurons and significantly influence brain health. Developing evidence has emphasized the profound effects of physical exercise on these neurotransmitter systems, underscoring exercise as a powerful modulator of brain function and mental well-being.

Dopamine, one of the key neurotransmitters affected by exercise, is essential for reward processing, movement, attention, and motivation. Exercise enhances dopaminergic activity by increasing dopamine synthesis, release, and receptor sensitivity. This is especially relevant in neurological conditions, such as Parkinson's disease, where degeneration of dopamine-producing neurons leads to motor deficits. Regular physical activity can improve motor function and slow disease progression by supporting dopaminergic signaling in the brain [12]. In addition, increased dopamine availability contributes to enhanced emotional regulation and cognitive performance.

Another of the most well-known neurotransmitters influenced by exercise is *serotonin*, which plays a crucial role in anxiety regulation, mood stabilization, and emotional processing. Physical activity elevates serotonin levels by increasing the availability of its precursor, tryptophan, and by increasing receptor sensitivity. These changes are associated with reduced symptoms of depression and anxiety, and improved overall mood [13]. This serotonergic modulation through exercise parallels some mechanisms of antidepressant medications, suggesting that exercise can serve as a complementary or alternative treatment in mood disorders.

Catecholamine, specifically *norepinephrine*, involved in alertness and stress regulation, also sees increased levels following exercise [14]. This neurotransmitter is particularly active in the prefrontal cortex, where it supports arousal, attention, and working memory. Through these mechanisms, physical activity has been shown to enhance cognitive functions, particularly decision-making and executive function, while also promoting better stress management [14]. These benefits make exercise a valuable adjunct to behavioral and cognitive therapies.

Additionally, a vital neurotransmitter modulated by physical activity is *gamma-aminobutyric acid (GABA)*, the brain's primary inhibitory neurotransmitter. GABA helps maintain the balance between inhibition and excitation in the brain's neural circuits. Exercise lifts GABAergic activity, reducing neural over-excitation and promoting relaxation and stress resilience. This is especially beneficial in conditions like epilepsy and anxiety, where inhibitory control is often compromised [15]. Enhanced GABA function contributes to emotional regulation and improved mental clarity following exercise.

DOI: http://dx.doi.org/10.5772/intechopen.1011545

In addition, *endorphins* and *endocannabinoids* are naturally occurring compounds with opioid- and cannabinoid-like effects. Evidence shows that these compounds are released during moderate to intense physical activity. These substances are basic players in the "runner's high" phenomenon, characterized by feelings of euphoria, reduced pain perception, and stress relief. Endocannabinoids influence cannabinoid receptors to modulate pain and mood, while endorphins act on the body's opioid receptors. These neurochemicals also suppress the hypothalamic-pituitary-adrenal (HPA) axis response to stress, further promoting a sense of calm and emotional stability [16].

Together, these neurotransmitter systems illuminate the multi-faceted effects of exercise on brain function. By enhancing serotonergic, GABAergic, dopaminergic, noradrenergic, and endorphinergic pathways, physical activity not only brings about immediate psychological benefits but also supports long-term neuroplastic changes. These changes underlie improved emotional regulation, cognitive performance, and motor control. Moreover, they play a critical role in rehabilitation and neuroprotection, providing a non-pharmacological strategy to enhance mental health and prevent neurodegenerative decline.

2.4 Neurotrophic factors: Molecular drivers of brain health

Exercise is a powerful modulator of brain function, not only enhancing cerebral blood flow and oxygenation but also triggering a cascade of molecular events that promote brain plasticity. At the forefront of these molecular changes are neurotrophic factors, proteins that support the development, survival, and function of neurons. Among them, brain-derived neurotrophic factor (BDNF) is the most studied and is known to play a key role in how physical activity benefits the brain. However, several other molecules, including vascular endothelial growth factor (VEGF), insulin-like growth factor 1 (IGF-1), and fibronectin type III domain-containing protein 5 (FNDC5)/irisin, work along with BDNF to mediate the cognitive and emotional enhancements linked to regular exercise [17].

2.4.1 Brain-derived neurotrophic factor (BDNF)

BDNF is a significant member of the neurotrophic family that plays a key role in neuronal survival, synaptic plasticity, and cognitive function. It acts primarily through its receptor, tropomyosin receptor kinase B (TrkB), to activate several intracellular signaling pathways, including *MAPK/ERK*, which stimulates gene transcription associated with neural growth and differentiation; *PI3K/Akt*, which promotes cell survival and offers neuroprotective effects; and *PLC-γ*, which enhances synaptic transmission and plasticity.

Exercises like aerobic and cognitively engaging activities performed at moderate-to-high-intensity, strongly elevate both peripheral and central BDNF levels. This rise in BDNF has been consistently associated with improved memory, learning, mood regulation, and protection against age-related cognitive decline and neurodegeneration. Studies, for instance, those by Szuhany et al. [18] have shown that regular exercise significantly boosts BDNF levels, supporting its critical role in brain health. Additionally, the type, intensity, and duration of exercise are keynote modulators of BDNF responsiveness, with longer and more vigorous sessions showing more profound effects [19].

2.4.2 Insulin-like growth factor 1 (IGF-1)

IGF-1 is another potent neurotrophic agent influenced by physical activity. Produced in greater quantities during and after exercise, IGF-1 can cross the blood-brain barrier and is instrumental in promoting neurogenesis, particularly within the hippocampus, a brain region critical for learning and memory. IGF-1 works synergistically with BDNF, amplifying its effects on synaptic plasticity and neural connectivity. Research emphasizes how exercise-induced IGF-1 not only contributes to neuronal growth but also enhances angiogenesis [20], further supporting brain health through improved vascular supply.

2.4.3 Vascular endothelial growth factor (VEGF)

Previously vascular endothelial growth factor (VEGF) known for its role in promoting angiogenesis. In the brain, VEGF helps improve cerebral perfusion, ensuring an adequate supply of oxygen and nutrients to neurons, particularly during heightened metabolic demands, such as those encountered during learning or adaptation. Exercise considerably upregulates VEGF, which, in turn, supports the metabolic and structural needs of neurons undergoing plastic changes. Studies have demonstrated that improved vascularization plays a key role in maintaining neuronal health and facilitating the delivery of other neurotrophic factors [17].

2.4.4 Fibronectin type III domain-containing protein 5 (FNDC5)/irisin

Muscle-brain signaling pathway involves FNDC5, a protein expressed in skeletal muscle during physical activity. This protein is cleaved to produce irisin (**Figure 1**), a hormone that enters the bloodstream and subsequently the brain, where it stimulates the expression of BDNF, especially in the hippocampus. This finding, first elucidated by Wrann et al. [21], underscores the systemic nature of exercise-induced neuroplasticity, where peripheral muscular activity can directly influence central nervous system function and structure.

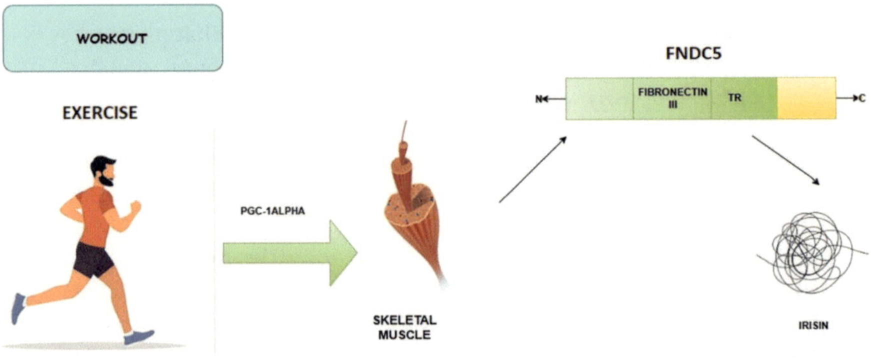

Figure 1.
How exercise produces irisin: Irisin is a hormone produced during exercise. As a result of exercise, PGC-1α, a protein in muscles, becomes active. PGC-1α triggers the production of one more protein, FNDC5. FNDC5 contains an N-terminal (a signal sequence); fibronectin III (important for structure); a TR (part that anchors in the transmembrane region); and a C-terminal tail (part in the cytosolic region). FNDC5 is then cut in a process called proteolytic cleavage, which releases irisin.

Collectively, these neurotrophic factors highlight the intricate and multidimensional relationship between physical activity and brain health. Exercise serves as a potent biological stimulus that not only improves cardiovascular fitness but also initiates molecular events crucial for memory, learning, long-term cognitive resilience, and emotional regulation. By enhancing the production and activity of IGF-1, irisin, BDNF, and VEGF, regular physical activity promotes a brain environment favorable to growth, adaptation, and repair. Intrinsically, understanding and leveraging these molecular mechanisms can substantially inform therapeutic strategies aimed at mitigating neurodegenerative disorders and enhancing mental well-being.

2.5 Sensorimotor integration and exercise

Sensorimotor integration is the brain's ability to process sensory stimuli in multiple areas of the cerebral cortex (association areas) and combine this sensory input with motor output to produce smooth, coordinated movement [22]. Exercise, specifically sensorimotor training, for instance, proprioceptive, balance, and coordination exercises, enhances the central nervous system's capacity to process multimodal sensory feedback. This leads to improved motor control and functional performance. Neurophysiological adaptations play a vital role in this process. Spinal cord modulation occurs through repetitive training, which refines reflex pathways and enhances reciprocal inhibition. The cerebellum, essential for coordinating movement, adapts by updating motor commands based on sensory feedback and prediction errors, a process heightened with task-specific practice. Furthermore, the somatosensory cortex undergoes reorganization, mainly after injury or immobilization, restoring accurate body maps *via* active movement and sensory stimulation. Exercise similarly increases the efficiency of sensorimotor loops connecting the cerebellum, spinal cord, and sensory cortex. Evidence from somatosensory evoked potentials (SEPs) demonstrates enhanced neural responsiveness subsequent sensorimotor training, which supports better motor precision and learning. Together, these adaptations highlight the importance of exercise in optimizing sensorimotor function and enhancing neuroplasticity in both healthy and impaired individuals.

2.6 Motor control and corticospinal adaptation

Motor control is controlled by complex hierarchical and parallel processes involving the brain, brainstem, spinal cord, and peripheral effectors. Central to voluntary movement, the corticospinal tract (CST) undergoes significant adjustment in response to exercise. Skill-based and resistance training increase motor unit recruitment and synchronization, leading to enhanced muscle strength and coordination [23]. These improvements reflect both structural and functional plasticity within the CST. Functional MRI studies have shown increased motor cortex activation after strength and skill acquisition, suggesting that cortical representations are reshaped by training [24]. Exercise also boosts corticospinal excitability, evidenced by heightened motor evoked potentials (MEPs) elicited through transcranial magnetic stimulation. Furthermore, repetitive motor training strengthens synaptic connections at spinal motoneurons, enhancing neuromuscular efficiency. Task-specific training reduces co-contraction and promotes smoother, more efficient movement patterns. Bilateral coordination activities additionally foster transcallosal communication, improving interhemispheric connectivity, which is particularly beneficial in neurorehabilitation contexts such as poststroke recovery [25]. Together, these corticospinal adaptations underline the dynamic nature of motor control and its modulation through targeted exercise interventions.

2.7 Autonomic nervous system (ANS) regulation and exercise

Exercise plays a dynamic role in regulating the autonomic nervous system (ANS) by balancing sympathetic and parasympathetic activity. Chronic training enhances parasympathetic tone, whereas acute physical activity increases sympathetic output to meet cardiovascular demands. This shift is evident in increased baroreflex sensitivity, reduced resting heart rate, and improved heart rate variability (HRV) [26]. These adjustments signify greater autonomic flexibility and improved stress regulation.

Neurophysiologically, regular exercise reduces allostatic load by dampening the hypothalamic-pituitary-adrenal (HPA) axis, thereby protecting the central nervous system from chronic stress effects [27]. Furthermore, enhanced ANS function fosters neurovisceral integration so strengthening connections between the prefrontal cortex and limbic system, and leading to better emotional regulation, affective processing, and cognitive control [28].

This autonomic modulation is vital not only for cardiovascular efficiency but also for emotional and immune resilience. Individuals with autonomic dysfunction, such as those with fibromyalgia or postural orthostatic tachycardia syndrome (POTS), often benefit from graded exercise programs that restore autonomic balance and improve overall well-being [29]. Thus, exercise serves as a key modulator of neurophysiological and systemic health through its impact on the ANS.

3. Different exercise therapies and their neural impact

Exercise therapy encompasses a wide range of physical activities designed to improve function, restore mobility, and enhance overall health. From a neurophysiological perspective, these interventions influence the nervous system at multiple levels, from synaptic plasticity and neurotransmitter regulation to structural brain changes and motor control adaptations (**Figure 2**). Understanding the different types of exercise therapies and their specific neural mechanisms is essential for clinical application in neuromuscular rehabilitation, neuroplasticity facilitation, and cognitive enhancement.

3.1 Aerobic (endurance) exercise

Aerobic exercises, for instance, walking, cycling, and swimming, involve rhythmic and sustained movement of large muscle groups. Such activities have been extensively studied for their impact on brain function and structure. Aerobic exercise enhances cerebral blood flow, promotes angiogenesis, and stimulates the release of neurotrophic factors, particularly brain-derived neurotrophic factor (BDNF). BDNF supports neurogenesis, especially in the hippocampus, which is critical for learning and memory [8]. Regular aerobic activity has also been associated with increased cortical thickness, improved white matter integrity, and enhanced functional connectivity in key brain networks [30].

Aerobic training reduces neuroinflammation and oxidative stress, contributing to neuroprotection in aging populations and individuals with neurodegenerative disorders such as Alzheimer's and Parkinson's diseases [31]. Additionally, it modulates neurotransmitter systems, including increased dopamine and serotonin availability, thereby enhancing mood and cognitive flexibility.

DOI: http://dx.doi.org/10.5772/intechopen.1011545

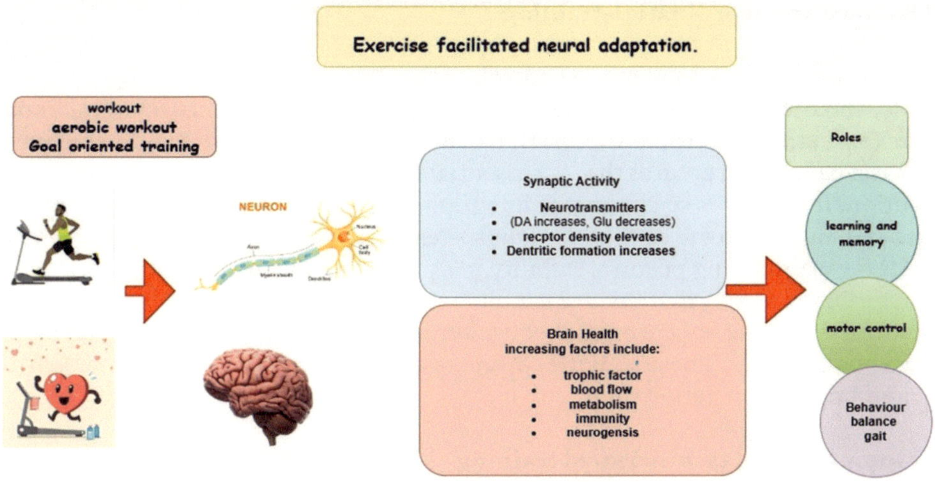

Figure 2.
How exercise supports brain health: Exercises can help the brain by promoting excitation-inhibition balance of DA-Glu neurotransmitters, and by strengthening the connections between nerve cells (synapses). It also boosts brain health by promoting the expression of neurotrophic and anti-inflammatory factors. These changes improve movement, learning, memory, and overall behavior.

3.2 Resistance (strength) training

Resistance training includes exercises that improve muscle strength and endurance through load-bearing activities, for example, weightlifting, resistance band workouts, and body-weight exercises. Resistance training positively influences neuroplasticity through hormonal pathways, especially by increasing levels of insulin-like growth factor-1 (IGF-1), which has neurotrophic and neuroprotective properties [32]. IGF-1 facilitates neuronal growth and synaptic plasticity, particularly in motor areas and the hippocampus.

Research shows that strength training improves executive function, working memory, and processing speed in older adults [33]. Resistance exercise also contributes to motor unit recruitment refinement and increases corticospinal excitability, promoting improved motor control and muscle activation patterns.

3.3 Flexibility and mobility exercises

Flexibility training, including stretching, yoga, and tai chi, aims to enhance the range of motion and reduce muscle stiffness. While often underestimated in terms of neural benefit, these practices have significant effects on the nervous system. Mobility exercises influence proprioceptive feedback and sensorimotor integration. Activities like yoga and tai chi incorporate slow, deliberate movements, breathing control, and focused attention, which stimulate the parasympathetic nervous system and enhance vagal tone [34].

These exercises have been shown to increase gray matter volume in brain regions related to interoception and self-regulation, including the insula and anterior cingulate cortex [35]. Additionally, they promote stress reduction *via* downregulation of the hypothalamic-pituitary-adrenal (HPA) axis and lower cortisol levels, improving emotional regulation and cognitive clarity.

3.4 Balance and coordination training

Exercises focusing on postural control, such as proprioceptive training, balance boards, and dual-task exercises, are critical for populations with neurological impairments (e.g., stroke, multiple sclerosis). Balance training stimulates the cerebellum and basal ganglia, structures that are essential for motor planning, timing, and execution. It augments sensorimotor integration by improving afferent feedback from joints and muscles to the central nervous system. This sensory reweighting process is crucial for maintaining postural stability in dynamic environments [36].

Coordination drills that involve simultaneous upper and lower limb movements or crossing the midline improve interhemispheric communication, especially through the corpus callosum. These activities promote cortical reorganization, motor learning, and improved reaction time.

3.5 Motor skill and task-oriented training

Task-oriented exercises involve repetitive practice of functional tasks (e.g., reaching, grasping, walking), often used in neurorehabilitation. Motor learning principles, like specificity, repetition, and feedback, guide this type of training. These exercises engage motor cortices, the premotor area, and supplementary motor areas, reinforcing neural pathways through use-dependent plasticity. Functional magnetic resonance imaging (fMRI) studies reveal increased activation in sensorimotor networks after motor training [6].

Repetitive task practice enhances synaptic efficacy and cortical map reorganization. It also promotes the recruitment of adjacent or contralesional brain areas in response to injury, particularly in stroke recovery. The involvement of attentional and reward systems also modulates dopamine release, enhancing motivation and learning [1].

3.6 High-intensity interval training (HIIT)

HIIT involves short bursts of intense activity interspersed with periods of rest or low-intensity exercise. While traditionally associated with cardiovascular fitness, HIIT has emerging evidence in the field of cognitive and neural health. HIIT promotes rapid increases in BDNF and catecholamines (e.g., dopamine, norepinephrine), facilitating synaptic plasticity and cognitive arousal [37]. Acute bouts of HIIT improve attention, processing speed, and executive function, potentially due to enhanced perfusion and arousal of the prefrontal cortex.

Moreover, HIIT may stimulate hippocampal neurogenesis and improve insulin sensitivity, both of which contribute to better brain health and reduced cognitive decline.

3.7 Neuromotor and sensorimotor integration training

These trainings include exercises that combine sensory stimuli with motor responses, like tactile stimulation, vestibular rehabilitation, and neurodevelopmental treatment (NDT). These methods are frequently used in pediatric and neurorehabilitation settings.

Vestibular training engages brainstem nuclei, the cerebellum, and the parietal cortex to improve spatial orientation and postural reflexes [38]. Sensorimotor training fosters neuroplasticity through enhanced sensory discrimination and integration.

Tactile and proprioceptive inputs shape somatosensory cortical maps, facilitating improved motor control and spatial awareness.

Through multisensory engagement and repetition, these approaches can help reorganize cortical areas affected by injury or disease and support functional recovery in both children and adults.

4. Exercise in neurological conditions

Traumatic brain injury (TBI), stroke, multiple sclerosis (MS), Parkinson's disease (PD), and spinal cord injury (SCI) are often associated with a spectrum of functional impairments, including sensory dysfunctions, motor deficits, cognitive limitations, and altered autonomic responses. Exercise, as a therapeutic modality, has gained significant attention in neurorehabilitation due to its capacity to improve motor learning, neuroplastic changes, and enhance functional outcomes. Evidence suggests that targeted, task-specific, and intensity-graded exercise can influence the underlying neurophysiological mechanisms that support recovery and adaptation in neurological populations [1, 39].

The clinical application of exercise therapies in neurological rehabilitation has evolved notably, with growing practical support for their effectiveness. Evidence-based practice (EBP) emphasizes integrating patient preferences, clinical expertise, and the best available research evidence to guide health care decisions. In neurorehabilitation, applying exercise therapies using an evidence-based framework enhances treatment efficacy, individualizes care, and optimizes functional recovery.

Several studies demonstrated the efficacy of exercise in improving neurological outcomes. Resistance training, aerobic exercise, and task-specific motor interventions have shown benefits in multiple neurological disorders, including stroke, PD, and MS.

4.1 Clinical application and evidence-based practice

4.1.1 Stroke

Evidence indicates that early mobilization and progressive task-oriented exercise enhance neuroplasticity and improve functional outcomes poststroke. Poststroke rehabilitation heavily relies on exercise to regain motor control, balance, and functional independence. A Cochrane review by Saunders et al. [40] found that physical rehabilitation involving repetitive task training significantly improved walking speed, upper limb function, and daily activities in stroke survivors. Task-specific training, such as constraint-induced movement therapy (CIMT), treadmill training with body-weight support, and robotic-assisted movements, promotes cortical reorganization and enhances voluntary control [41]. High-intensity interval training (HIIT) has also been shown to improve cardiovascular fitness and walking capacity in chronic stroke survivors [42]. Aerobic exercise also increases cerebral perfusion and promotes angiogenesis, contributing to better recovery [43]. Aerobic exercise poststroke not only enhances physical function but also improves mood, cognition, and overall quality of life.

4.1.2 Parkinson's disease

Exercise interventions for PD have been shown to reduce motor symptoms and improve gait, balance, and quality of life. Exercise in PD focuses on alleviating bradykinesia, rigidity, postural instability, and gait disturbances. Regular physical activity, including aerobic training, resistance training, and balance exercises, improves motor symptoms and slows functional decline [44]. Importantly, evidence supports the role of forced-exercise paradigms, where individuals exercise at a rate higher than their voluntary pace, which is effective in enhancing motor outcomes and possibly influencing dopaminergic function in the basal ganglia [45]. A meta-analysis by Shen et al. [46] confirmed that aerobic and resistance exercises lead to significant improvements in Unified Parkinson's Disease Rating Scale (UPDRS) scores. The mechanisms likely involve enhanced dopaminergic signaling and improved synaptic plasticity. Dance therapy, tai chi, and boxing programs have also demonstrated benefits in balance, coordination, and cognitive functioning [47].

4.1.3 Multiple sclerosis

Exercise in MS has historically been approached with caution due to fatigue and thermosensitivity. However, modern research supports that appropriately tailored exercise programs can improve strength, endurance, mobility, and fatigue levels without exacerbating symptoms [48]. Resistance training and aerobic conditioning are both effective, while aquatic therapy provides a low-impact, thermoregulated environment conducive to improved movement and pain relief. In individuals with MS, regular exercise has been shown to reduce fatigue, improve walking ability, and enhance mood. A randomized controlled trial (RCT) by Sandroff et al. [49] showed that aerobic training resulted in increased hippocampal volume and improved memory performance, suggesting that exercise also benefits cognitive function in MS through neuroprotective mechanisms.

4.1.4 Spinal cord injury

In individuals with incomplete SCI, locomotor training using treadmills with body-weight support, robotic exoskeletons, and functional electrical stimulation (FES) can activate central pattern generators and facilitate stepping movements [50]. For complete SCI, upper body aerobic exercise and resistance training enhance cardiovascular health and upper limb function. Emerging evidence also supports the role of epidural stimulation and activity-based therapies in promoting volitional movement in certain cases of chronic SCI.

4.1.5 Traumatic brain injury

Exercise post-TBI is cautiously approached due to potential cognitive deficits, vestibular dysfunction, and post-concussive symptoms. Once medically steady, individuals benefit from progressive aerobic exercise, which improves executive function, attention, and emotional regulation [51]. Task-specific activities, balance training, and dual-task exercises are essential to restore functional independence and community participation.

4.2 Determining exercise parameters: FITT principles

Designing an exercise program for neurological patients requires careful consideration of the Frequency, Intensity, Time, and Type (FITT) principles. Adapting these parameters to the patient's condition and functional level is essential for safety and

DOI: http://dx.doi.org/10.5772/intechopen.1011545

effectiveness. Studies normally recommend 3–5 sessions per week for moderate-intensity aerobic exercise as the set *frequency*, and 2–3 times per week for resistance training [52]. Moderate to vigorous *intensity*, evaluated by heart rate or perceived exertion, is frequently needed to stimulate neuroplastic adaptations. However, intensity must be adjusted in cases of fatigue or autonomic dysfunction. *Time* for sessions of at least 20–30 minutes has been associated with cognitive and motor improvements, though shorter sessions may be used initially and progressed over time. The *type* of exercise should match the therapeutic goals: for instance, gait training for mobility, strength training for muscle activation, or dual-task exercises for cognitive-motor integration.

4.3 Barriers to implementation

Regardless of the proven benefits, several barriers may hinder the clinical application of exercise therapies in neurorehabilitation settings: *Physical limitations:* Neurological impairments, for example, spasticity, ataxia, and fatigue, can limit participation. Clinicians must adapt exercises to minimize fall risk and accommodate deficits. *Cognitive and emotional barriers*: Depression, apathy, and cognitive dysfunction can reduce motivation and adherence. Multidisciplinary support and motivational interviewing can help address these issues. *Logistical constraints*: Inadequate access to rehabilitation facilities, transportation issues, and cost can impede consistent participation. Home-based exercise programs and telerehabilitation offer feasible alternatives. *Clinician knowledge and training*: Various therapists may lack confidence in prescribing high-intensity or neuro-specific exercises. Continued professional development and integration of neuroscience principles into clinical training are essential.

5. Exercise and mental health: Neurophysiological connections

For a long time, it has been known that exercise has physical health benefits, but increasing attention is now being paid to its potent role in enhancing mental health. Increasing evidence supports the idea that physical activity exerts significant neurophysiological effects that influence cognition, emotional regulation, mood, and psychological resilience. These effects are mediated by complex interactions involving neurotrophic factors, neurotransmitters, hormonal responses, and brain network connectivity. Understanding these underlying mechanisms is essential for integrating exercise into treatment plans for individuals with mental health disorders, such as anxiety, depression, and cognitive impairment.

5.1 Mental health disorders and the brain

Mental health disorders, for instance, depression and anxiety, are associated with dysregulation in several neurobiological systems, such as *neurotransmitter imbalance* (involving serotonin, dopamine, norepinephrine, and gamma-aminobutyric acid (GABA)); *HPA axis hyperactivity* (leading to elevated cortisol levels and impaired stress response); *reduced neurogenesis and hippocampal volume* (especially in depression); and *decreased connectivity and activity in the prefrontal cortex*, affecting emotional regulation and decision-making.

Interventions that positively influence these systems can help alleviate symptoms and improve overall psychological well-being. Exercise has emerged as a low-cost, accessible, and effective approach with minimal side effects.

5.2 Neurochemical and hormonal effects of exercise

5.2.1 Neurotransmitter regulation

Exercise stimulates the synthesis and release of several neurotransmitters involved in mood regulation. *Serotonin (5-HT),* ("feel-good" neurotransmitter), serotonin levels increase with aerobic exercise, enhancing mood and emotional stability [13]. Physical activity also increases *dopamine* availability in the striatum and prefrontal cortex, improving motivation, reward processing, and attention [53]. Exercise-induced elevations in *norepinephrine* contribute to heightened alertness and stress resilience. Exercise also modulates *GABA*ergic and *glutamate*rgic signaling, helping balance excitatory and inhibitory activity in the brain [54].

5.2.2 Hypothalamic-pituitary-adrenal (HPA) axis regulation

Chronic stress is a key contributor to mood disorders, and it dysregulates the HPA axis. Exercise acts as a mild stressor that, over time, helps recalibrate the stress response system. Regular physical activity reduces baseline cortisol levels and improves cortisol reactivity, contributing to better stress management and emotional control [55].

5.3 Neuroplasticity and brain-derived neurotrophic factor (BDNF)

BDNF plays a pivotal role in synaptic plasticity, learning, and memory, and its levels are consistently found to be low in individuals with depression. Exercise has been shown to elevate peripheral and central BDNF levels, particularly in the hippocampus and prefrontal cortex [17]. This neurotrophic support facilitates: *neurogenesis*, especially in the dentate gyrus of the hippocampus; *dendritic branching and synaptogenesis*; enhancing neural connectivity; and *cognitive improvements*, including memory, executive function, and processing speed. BDNF's role as a mediator between physical activity and brain function supports the idea that exercise can act as a biological treatment for mood and cognitive disorders.

5.4 Brain structural and functional changes

Neuroimaging studies provide compelling evidence that exercise induces structural and functional changes in the brain. Long-term aerobic exercise is associated with *hippocampal growth*, countering atrophy observed in depression and aging [11]. *Enhanced connectivity in the default mode network (DMN)*: this network, which is hyperactive in depression, is modulated by exercise, leading to reduced rumination and improved focus [56]. *Improved prefrontal cortex function*: strengthened top-down regulation from the prefrontal cortex aids in emotional control and stress management.

Functional MRI studies also show increased activation in brain regions involved in emotion regulation, attention, and reward processing after exercise interventions.

5.5 Exercise and specific mental health conditions

Exercise is now recognized as an effective intervention for mild to moderate *depression*. Numerous randomized controlled trials and meta-analyses support its use as a standalone or adjunct treatment. A systematic review by Schuch et al. [57] concluded that exercise has a large antidepressant effect, comparable to that of

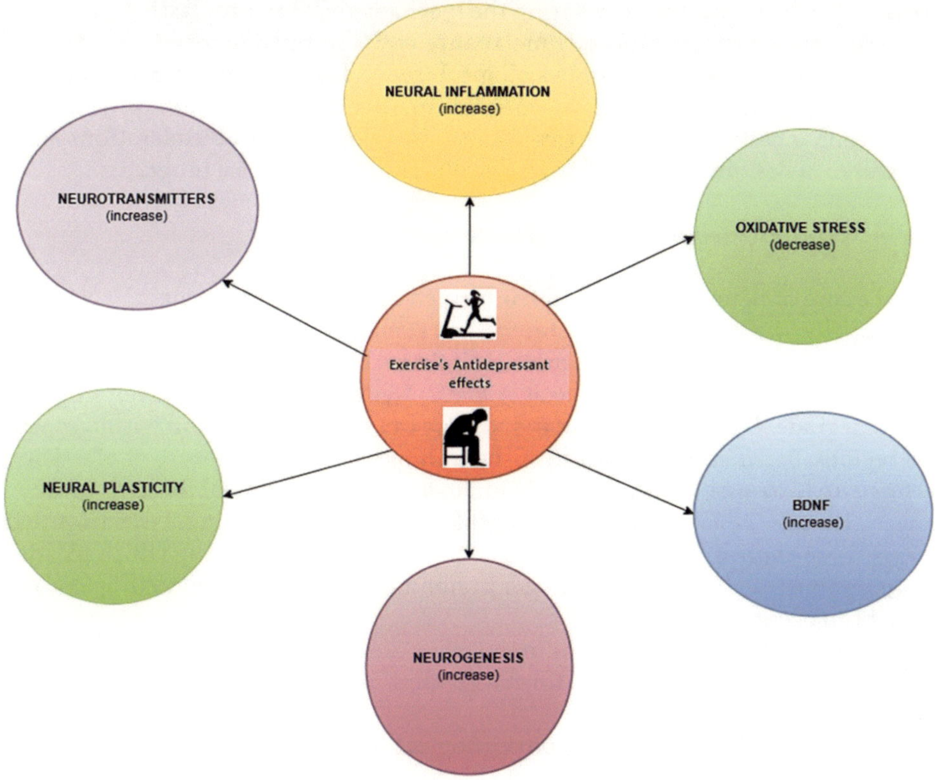

Figure 3.
Processes behind exercise-induced antidepressant effects: Exercise exerts antidepressant effects by inhibiting oxidative stress, ↓ing neuroinflammation, ↑ing neurotransmitter levels, and enhancing BDNF levels, neurogenesis, and synaptic plasticity.

pharmacotherapy in many cases. These mechanisms include: improved monoamine regulation; increased BDNF and neurogenesis; distraction from negative thoughts; and enhanced self-efficacy and social interaction in group settings.

Regular exercise reduces both trait and state *anxiety*, possibly by desensitizing the body's stress response systems and enhancing parasympathetic tone. A meta-analysis by Stubbs et al. [58] found that aerobic exercise significantly reduced symptoms in individuals with generalized anxiety disorder and panic disorder.

Exercise has protective effects against age-related *cognitive decline and dementia*. Moderate to vigorous physical activity improves executive function and memory, and delays the progression of Alzheimer's disease through improved cerebrovascular function and neurotrophic support [59]. On the basis of this research evidence, together it suggests that exercise may help reduce depression by affecting several brain processes, such as oxidative stress, neurotransmitters, neuroplasticity, neurotrophic factors, neurogenesis, and neuroinflammation (**Figure 3**).

6. Designing neurophysiologically informed exercise programs

Designing exercise programs for individuals with neurological disorders requires an understanding that goes beyond traditional musculoskeletal principles. With the increasing body of research elucidating the mechanisms of neuroplasticity, neurogenesis, and synaptic adaptation, clinicians are now equipped to formulate exercise prescriptions grounded in neurophysiological principles. Such programs aim not only to restore motor function but also to optimize brain reorganization, improve cognition, and enhance overall neurological health. Here are the key considerations and frameworks in designing neurophysiologically informed exercise programs.

6.1 Principles of neuroplasticity in exercise prescription

At the core of neurophysiologically informed exercise programs lies the concept of *neuroplasticity*, the brain's ability to reorganize itself by forming new neural connections in response to learning or an injury [1]. Several principles underpin the use of exercise to drive neuroplasticity: *Use it or lose it:* Neural circuits not actively engaged begin to degrade. *Use it and improve it:* Exercise can enhance function within specific brain regions. *Specificity:* The nature of the training dictates the nature of plasticity. *Repetition and intensity:* Repeated, high-intensity activity is crucial for long-term changes. *Salience:* Tasks must be meaningful to the individual to induce lasting neural changes. *Time matters:* There are critical windows post-injury during which plasticity is more responsive. *Age matters:* Younger brains are more plastic, but neurogenesis and learning can occur at any age [1].

These principles guide clinicians in selecting exercises that are functional, appropriately dosed, and individualized for the greatest neurological impact.

6.2 Exercise modalities and neurophysiological impact

Aerobic activity has a potent impact on the central nervous system. It increases cerebral blood flow, upregulates neurotrophic factors like BDNF, and enhances hippocampal neurogenesis [11]. These changes contribute to improvements in memory, mood, and executive function. Moderate-intensity aerobic exercise (60–75% HRmax), 3–5 times per week for 30–45 minutes, is often recommended for promoting cognitive and neuroplastic changes [60].

While traditionally associated with musculoskeletal adaptations, resistance training also has significant neurophysiological benefits. It promotes synaptic efficacy and motor unit recruitment and can improve motor control and reaction time. 2–3 sessions per week focusing on major muscle groups with progressive overload, ideally integrated with balance and coordination tasks for neural engagement [61].

Task-specific training, such as constraint-induced movement therapy or locomotor training, utilizes *Hebbian learning principles*, where repeated, coordinated activity strengthens synaptic connections. Motor learning exercises should be goal-oriented, progressively challenging, and feedback-rich to optimize motor cortex reorganization [62].

6.3 Integrating cognitive and sensory stimulation

Cognition and sensory processing are closely tied to motor output. Designing exercise programs that integrate dual-task components (e.g., walking while solving arithmetic problems) can stimulate frontal-striatal circuits involved in attention and working memory, enhancing cortical engagement.

Moreover, exercises that incorporate visual, auditory, or somatosensory feedback, like using mirrors, vibration, or cueing, can enhance sensory integration and refine motor output through sensorimotor plasticity [63].

6.4 Progression and dose optimization

Just as in traditional rehabilitation, exercise programs must follow the principles of overload and progression. However, in neurological populations, dose-response relationships may differ due to fatigue, medication effects, and cognitive impairments. For instance: at least 3–5 days per week for aerobic activity; 2–3 days for resistance training; monitored using HR, RPE, or the talk test; tailored for safety in populations with autonomic dysfunction; sessions of at least 30 minutes are effective, with modifications for tolerance; chosen based on goals—gait training for mobility, resistance for strength, balance for fall prevention, etc.

Programs must also account for neurological fatigue, using interval training or rest periods to avoid overtraining and neuroinflammatory responses.

6.5 Incorporating technology and feedback systems

Modern rehabilitation incorporates biofeedback, virtual reality, and neurofeedback to guide and refine performance. These tools engage the brain's reward systems and enhance error correction, critical for motor relearning [64].

6.6 Psychosocial and motivational considerations

Patient engagement is crucial for neuroplasticity. Programs should be salient, aligning with the individual's goals and interests. Motivational interviewing, goal setting, and self-efficacy strategies improve adherence and activate dopaminergic pathways critical for learning and reward [65].

Involving caregivers, providing social support, and ensuring culturally relevant practices further enhance participation, especially in long-term management.

7. Future directions and emerging trends

As the field of neurorehabilitation evolves, so too does our understanding of how exercise therapies influence the brain. New technologies, enhanced mechanistic insights, and personalized medicine are driving innovation in neurophysiologically informed rehabilitation. This section highlights the most promising directions and emerging trends in exercise therapies that hold the potential to revolutionize neurological care.

7.1 Personalized and precision rehabilitation

The future of neurorehabilitation lies in precision medicine, tailoring interventions to individual characteristics such as genetics, neural biomarkers, cognitive profiles, and behavioral traits. Research suggests that genetic polymorphisms, such as BDNF Val66Met, can influence a person's neuroplastic response to exercise [66]. Personalized exercise prescriptions may 1 day be based on these genetic and molecular markers, improving outcomes and reducing variability in treatment response.

Advanced imaging and electrophysiological techniques, such as functional MRI (fMRI), EEG, and transcranial magnetic stimulation (TMS), can be used to assess cortical excitability, brain connectivity, and plasticity potential, thereby guiding individualized interventions [67].

7.2 Integration of artificial intelligence and machine learning

Artificial intelligence (AI) and machine learning (ML) are increasingly being incorporated into exercise and rehabilitation platforms. These technologies can: predict patient recovery trajectories; optimize training parameters; monitor adherence and performance; and provide real-time feedback using wearable sensors. For instance, ML algorithms can analyze kinematic and physiological data collected from wearable devices during gait training, allowing for the dynamic adjustment of intensity and task complexity [68]. AI-driven virtual coaches and robotic systems are emerging to support long-term adherence in home-based exercise programs.

7.3 Neurotechnologies and brain-computer interfaces

Brain-computer interfaces (BCIs) represent a revolutionary approach to exercise-based neurorehabilitation. BCIs allow patients to control external devices (e.g., robotic limbs, virtual avatars) through real-time decoding of brain signals. This direct engagement of neural circuits enhances neuroplasticity through closed-loop feedback, particularly useful in patients with severe motor impairments [69].

Coupling BCIs with functional electrical stimulation (FES) or robot-assisted gait training can further promote motor recovery by synchronizing intention with action. These interventions are being actively researched in populations with stroke, spinal cord injury, and cerebral palsy.

7.4 Virtual and augmented reality (VR/AR)

The use of immersive technologies, particularly VR and AR, is rapidly growing in neurological rehabilitation. These tools provide engaging, multisensory environments that stimulate cognitive and motor systems simultaneously, promoting sensorimotor integration and task-specific learning [64].

Virtual environments can be tailored for specific goals, e.g., balance training in Parkinson's disease or upper limb rehabilitation in stroke, and often include gamification to improve adherence and motivation. Augmented reality overlays real-time digital information on physical environments, aiding in movement correction and feedback.

7.5 Telerehabilitation and mobile health (mHealth)

The rise of telerehabilitation and mobile health technologies has revolutionized access to exercise-based therapy, particularly in underserved or remote populations. These platforms allow real-time video supervision, remote monitoring, and data collection through smartphone applications and wearable devices [70].

Exercise prescription and progression can now be delivered virtually with feedback loops that incorporate data from motion sensors, heart rate monitors, and GPS. This expansion supports continuity of care and long-term adherence, especially for chronic neurological conditions such as multiple sclerosis and Parkinson's disease.

7.6 Combined cognitive and physical training

There is growing recognition of the cognitive benefits of physical exercise, and emerging programs now integrate dual-task training, simultaneously challenging the motor and cognitive domains. This strategy is especially relevant for older adults and those with neurodegenerative conditions, where cognitive-motor interactions are critical for function and safety [71].

Neuroscientific research supports that simultaneous cognitive and physical tasks activate prefrontal and parietal networks, enhancing attention, executive control, and working memory. This dual-targeting approach is likely to be further developed through interactive technologies and cognitive gaming.

7.7 Epigenetics and molecular profiling

The field of epigenetics offers exciting insights into how exercise influences gene expression without altering DNA sequences. Regular physical activity modulates epigenetic markers, such as DNA methylation and histone acetylation, affecting the expression of genes involved in plasticity, inflammation, and metabolism [72].

Future therapies may use molecular profiling to identify individuals who would benefit most from specific types of exercise, and to monitor treatment efficacy at a cellular level. This approach supports the development of biomarker-driven interventions in neurorehabilitation.

7.8 Immune and inflammatory modulation through exercise

Emerging evidence suggests that exercise modulates the immune system and neuroinflammation, key components in many neurological disorders, including multiple sclerosis, Alzheimer's disease, and depression. Exercise reduces pro-inflammatory cytokines (e.g., IL-6, TNF-α) and increases anti-inflammatory mediators and neuroprotective factors like IGF-1 and VEGF [73].

The anti-inflammatory effect of regular moderate exercise may help slow disease progression, reduce relapse rates, and improve mental health outcomes. Future programs may be dosed specifically to optimize immune modulation based on disease phenotype.

7.9 Cross-disciplinary collaborations and systems neuroscience

The future of exercise-based neurorehabilitation depends on cross-disciplinary collaboration between physiotherapists, neuroscientists, bioengineers, and data scientists. A systems neuroscience approach is increasingly being adopted—looking at motor behavior as an emergent property of multiple interacting systems (nervous, musculoskeletal, cognitive, etc.).

This integrative view is supported by computational models that simulate motor learning and neuroplasticity, enabling more precise predictions of recovery and response to intervention [74]. Such models can guide clinicians in selecting optimal strategies for different patient profiles.

7.10 Promoting lifelong brain health

Finally, there is a growing shift toward using exercise not only as a rehabilitation tool but also as a preventive strategy to maintain brain health across the lifespan. Public health campaigns and clinical guidelines are beginning to recognize exercise as a form of "neurotherapy" capable of reducing dementia risk, improving mental well-being, and enhancing cognitive reserve.

Programs like "Exercise is Medicine" are gaining traction globally, advocating for the prescription of physical activity as a primary intervention for both neurological and psychiatric conditions [75]. Promoting lifelong movement habits may ultimately reduce healthcare burdens and improve quality of life across populations.

The future of neurophysiologically based exercise therapy is bright and rapidly evolving. Advances in technology, neuroscience, genetics, and data analytics are paving the way for more personalized, effective, and accessible rehabilitation strategies. As these trends continue to develop, they promise to redefine how clinicians assess, prescribe, and monitor exercise interventions, with the ultimate goal of enhancing neuroplasticity, restoring function, and improving the lives of individuals with neurological disorders.

8. Conclusion

Exercise therapies have emerged as a cornerstone in neurorehabilitation, grounded in robust neurophysiological principles. The interaction between physical activity and the nervous system encompasses a dynamic interplay of neuroplasticity, neurogenesis, synaptic modulation, and neurochemical regulation. This chapter outlined the core mechanisms by which exercise exerts its effects on brain and spinal cord function, and reviewed how specific modes of exercise, such as aerobic training, resistance exercises, task-specific motor practice, and dual-task paradigms, contribute to neurological recovery.

At the cellular and molecular levels, exercise stimulates the release of neurotrophic factors, such as brain-derived neurotrophic factor (BDNF), insulin-like growth factor 1 (IGF-1), and vascular endothelial growth factor (VEGF), all of which play pivotal roles in synaptogenesis, angiogenesis, and neuronal survival [5, 30]. Functional neuroimaging studies demonstrate that exercise modifies brain network connectivity, enhances cortical excitability, and supports executive function, especially in populations affected by stroke, Parkinson's disease (PD), multiple sclerosis (MS), and age-related cognitive decline [76].

Moreover, different types of exercise interventions elicit unique patterns of neurophysiological response. Aerobic exercise enhances global cerebral perfusion and supports hippocampal volume preservation, resistance training strengthens motor unit recruitment and corticospinal excitability, and motor learning-based therapies engage use-dependent plasticity essential for task re-acquisition [36, 39]. The dose, intensity, and timing of exercise relative to neurological insult, such as in poststroke rehabilitation, are increasingly understood as critical variables that influence neurorecovery.

Exercise therapies, when rooted in neurophysiological principles, have the power to transform neurological rehabilitation. Understanding how physical activity shapes the nervous system enables clinicians to design more targeted, effective, and individualized interventions. By leveraging current evidence and embracing future innovations, healthcare professionals can optimize recovery, improve function, and enhance quality of life for individuals with neurological disorders.

The neurophysiological basis of exercise therapy carries significant clinical implications, particularly for the design, timing, and progression of intervention strategies in neurological rehabilitation.

One of the most consistent findings in both animal and human studies is that early initiation of task-specific training facilitates optimal recovery by capitalizing on the critical period of heightened neuroplasticity following neural injury [1]. Clinicians

DOI: http://dx.doi.org/10.5772/intechopen.1011545

should strive to begin motor-based therapies as early as medically feasible, ensuring that activities are functionally relevant and progressively challenging.

Therapists must prioritize repetitive, goal-directed, and feedback-driven movements to strengthen cortical reorganization and motor learning pathways. This is especially crucial in stroke rehabilitation, where maladaptive plasticity may occur in the absence of skilled therapy.

Author details

Saima Gul
Department of Rehabilitation Sciences, Shifa Tameer e Millat University, Islamabad, Pakistan

*Address all correspondence to: saimagul.ahs@stmu.edu.pk

References

[1] Kleim JA, Jones TA. Principles of experience-dependent neural plasticity: Implications for rehabilitation after brain damage. Journal of Speech, Language, and Hearing Research: JSLHR. 2008;**51**(1):S225-S239

[2] Sung YB, Lee DH. Descriptive study on rehabilitation treatment methods for improving upper limb function in stroke patients. International Journal of Advanced Nursing Education and Research. 30 Aug 2020;**5**(2):19-28

[3] Smith M. Neurological rehabilitation: Optimizing motor performance. Physiotherapy Canada. 2015;**67**(2):215-216

[4] Nudo RJ. Recovery after brain injury: Mechanisms and principles. Frontiers in Human Neuroscience. 2013;7:887

[5] Cotman CW, Berchtold NC, Christie LA. Exercise builds brain health: Key roles of growth factor cascades and inflammation. Trends in Neurosciences. 2007;**30**(9):464-472

[6] Nudo RJ. Mechanisms for recovery of motor function following cortical damage. Current Opinion in Neurobiology. 2006;**16**(6):638-644

[7] van Praag H, Kempermann G, Gage FH. Running increases cell proliferation and neurogenesis in the adult mouse dentate gyrus. Nature Neuroscience. 1999;**2**(3):266-270

[8] Cotman CW, Berchtold NC. Exercise: A behavioral intervention to enhance brain health and plasticity. Trends in Neurosciences. 2002;**25**(6):295-301

[9] Fields RD. White matter in learning, cognition and psychiatric disorders. Trends in Neurosciences. 2008;**31**(7):361-370

[10] Lee MC, Inoue K, Okamoto M, Liu YF, Matsui T, Yook JS, et al. Voluntary resistance running induces increased hippocampal neurogenesis in rats comparable to load-free running. Neuroscience Letters. 2013;**537**:6-10

[11] Erickson KI, Voss MW, Prakash RS, Basak C, Szabo A, Chaddock L, et al. Exercise training increases size of hippocampus and improves memory. Proceedings of the National Academy of Sciences of the United States of America. 2011;**108**(7):3017-3022

[12] Fisher BE, Li Q, Nacca A, Salem GJ, Song J, Yip J, et al. Treadmill exercise elevates striatal dopamine D2 receptor binding potential in patients with early Parkinson's disease. Neuroreport. 2013;**24**(10):509-514

[13] Meeusen R, De Meirleir K. Exercise and brain neurotransmission. Sports Medicine (Auckland, N.Z.). 1995;**20**(3):160-188

[14] McMorris T, Tomporowski PD, Audiffren M, editors. Exercise and Cognitive Function. Hoboken, NJ: Wiley; 2009. 377 p

[15] Smith PJ, Blumenthal JA, Hoffman BM, Cooper H, Strauman TA, Welsh-Bohmer K, et al. Aerobic exercise and neurocognitive performance: A meta-analytic review of randomized controlled trials. Psychosomatic Medicine. 2010;**72**(3):239-252

[16] Dietrich A, McDaniel WF. Endocannabinoids and exercise. British Journal of Sports Medicine. 2004;**38**(5):536-541

[17] Gustafsson T, Knutsson A, Puntschart A, Kaijser L, Nordqvist ACS,

Sundberg CJ, et al. Increased expression of vascular endothelial growth factor in human skeletal muscle in response to short-term one-legged exercise training. Pflügers Archiv. 2002;**444**(6):752-759

[18] Szuhany KL, Bugatti M, Otto MW. A meta-analytic review of the effects of exercise on brain-derived neurotrophic factor. Journal of Psychiatric Research. 2015;**60**:56-64

[19] Knaepen K, Goekint M, Heyman EM, Meeusen R. Neuroplasticity - Exercise-induced response of peripheral brain-derived neurotrophic factor: A systematic review of experimental studies in human subjects. Sports Medicine (Auckland, N.Z.). 2010;**40**(9):765-801

[20] Trejo JL, Carro E, Torres-Aleman I. Circulating insulin-like growth factor I mediates exercise-induced increases in the number of new neurons in the adult hippocampus. Journal of Neuroscience: The Official Journal of the Society for Neuroscience. 2001;**21**(5):1628-1634

[21] Wrann CD, White JP, Salogiannnis J, Laznik-Bogoslavski D, Wu J, Ma D, et al. Exercise induces hippocampal BDNF through a PGC-1α/FNDC5 pathway. Cell Metabolism. 2013;**18**(5):649-659

[22] Matur Z, Öge AE. Sensorimotor integration during motor learning: Transcranial magnetic stimulation studies. Noro Psikiyatri Arsivi. Dec 2017;**54**(4):358-363. DOI: 10.5152/npa.2016.18056

[23] Aagaard P, Simonsen EB, Andersen JL, Magnusson P, Dyhre-Poulsen P. Increased rate of force development and neural drive of human skeletal muscle following resistance training. Journal of Applied Physiology. 2002;**93**(4):1318-1326

[24] Karni A, Meyer G, Jezzard P, Adams MM, Turner R, Ungerleider LG. Functional MRI evidence for adult motor cortex plasticity during motor skill learning. Nature. 1995;**377**(6545):155-158

[25] Stinear CM, Byblow WD, Ackerley SJ, Barber PA, Smith MC. Predicting recovery potential for individual stroke patients increases rehabilitation efficiency. Stroke. 2017;**48**(4):1011-1019

[26] Buchheit M, Gindre C. Cardiac parasympathetic regulation: Respective associations with cardiorespiratory fitness and training load. American Journal of Physiology-Heart and Circulatory Physiology. 2006;**291**(1):H451-H458

[27] Hillman CH, Erickson KI, Kramer AF. Be smart, exercise your heart: Exercise effects on brain and cognition. Nature Reviews Neuroscience. 2008;**9**(1):58-65

[28] Thayer JF, Ahs F, Fredrikson M, Sollers JJ, Wager TD. A meta-analysis of heart rate variability and neuroimaging studies: Implications for heart rate variability as a marker of stress and health. Neuroscience and Biobehavioral Reviews. 2012;**36**(2):747-756

[29] Carter JB, Banister EW, Blaber AP. Effect of endurance exercise on autonomic control of heart rate. Sports Medicine (Auckland, N.Z.). 2003;**33**(1):33-46

[30] Voss MW, Vivar C, Kramer AF, van Praag H. Bridging animal and human models of exercise-induced brain plasticity. Trends in Cognitive Sciences. 2013;**17**(10):525-544

[31] Kirk-Sanchez NJ, McGough EL. Physical exercise and cognitive performance in the elderly: Current perspectives. Clinical Interventions in Aging. 2014;**9**:51-62

[32] Cassilhas RC, Viana VAR, Grassmann V, Santos RT, Santos RF, Tufik S, et al. The impact of resistance exercise on the cognitive function of the elderly. Medicine and Science in Sports and Exercise. 2007;**39**(8):1401-1407

[33] Liu-Ambrose T, Nagamatsu LS, Voss MW, Khan KM, Handy TC. Resistance training and functional plasticity of the aging brain: A 12-month randomized controlled trial. Neurobiology of Aging. 2012;**33**(8):1690-1698

[34] Gerritsen RJS, Band GPH. Breath of life: The respiratory vagal stimulation model of contemplative activity. Frontiers in Human Neuroscience. 2018;**12**:397

[35] Villemure C, Čeko M, Cotton VA, Bushnell MC. Neuroprotective effects of yoga practice: Age-, experience-, and frequency-dependent plasticity. Frontiers in Human Neuroscience. 2015;**9**:281

[36] Taubert M, Draganski B, Anwander A, Müller K, Horstmann A, Villringer A, et al. Dynamic properties of human brain structure: Learning-related changes in cortical areas and associated fiber connections. Journal of Neuroscience: The Official Journal of the Society for Neuroscience. 2010;**30**(35):11670-11677

[37] Saucedo Marquez CM, Vanaudenaerde B, Troosters T, Wenderoth N. High-intensity interval training evokes larger serum BDNF levels compared with intense continuous exercise. Journal of Applied Physiology (Bethesda, MD: 1985). 2015;**119**(12):1363-1373

[38] Han BI, Song HS, Kim JS. Vestibular rehabilitation therapy: Review of indications, mechanisms, and key exercises. Journal of Clinical Neurology (Seoul Korea). 2011;**7**(4):184-196

[39] Mang CS, Campbell KL, Ross CJD, Boyd LA. Promoting neuroplasticity for motor rehabilitation after stroke: Considering the effects of aerobic exercise and genetic variation on brain-derived neurotrophic factor. Physical Therapy. 2013;**93**(12):1707-1716

[40] Saunders DH, Sanderson M, Hayes S, Johnson L, Kramer S, Carter DD, et al. Physical fitness training for stroke patients. Cochrane Database of Systematic Reviews. 2020;**3**(3):CD003316

[41] Langhorne P, Bernhardt J, Kwakkel G. Stroke rehabilitation. The Lancet. 2011;**377**(9778):1693-1702

[42] Saunders DH, Sanderson M, Hayes S, Kilrane M, Greig CA, Brazzelli M, et al. Physical fitness training for stroke patients. Cochrane Database of Systematic Reviews. 2016;**3**(3):CD003316

[43] Billinger SA, Arena R, Bernhardt J, Eng JJ, Franklin BA, Johnson CM, et al. Physical activity and exercise recommendations for stroke survivors: A statement for healthcare professionals from the American Heart Association/ American Stroke Association. Stroke. 2014;**45**(8):2532-2553

[44] Goodwin VA, Richards SH, Taylor RS, Taylor AH, Campbell JL. The effectiveness of exercise interventions for people with Parkinson's disease: A systematic review and meta-analysis. Movement Disorders: Official Journal of the Movement Disorder Society. 2008;**23**(5):631-640

[45] Ridgel AL, Vitek JL, Alberts JL. Forced, not voluntary, exercise improves motor function in Parkinson's disease patients. Neurorehabilitation and Neural Repair. 2009;**23**(6):600-608

[46] Shen X, Wong-Yu ISK, Mak MKY. Effects of exercise on falls, balance,

and gait ability in Parkinson's disease: A meta-analysis. Neurorehabilitation and Neural Repair. 2016;**30**(6):512-527

[47] Earhart GM. Dance as therapy for individuals with Parkinson disease. European Journal of Physical and Rehabilitation Medicine. 2009;**45**(2):231-238

[48] Latimer-Cheung AE, Pilutti LA, Hicks AL, Martin Ginis KA, Fenuta AM, MacKibbon KA, et al. Effects of exercise training on fitness, mobility, fatigue, and health-related quality of life among adults with multiple sclerosis: A systematic review to inform guideline development. Archives of Physical Medicine and Rehabilitation. 2013;**94**(9):1800-1828.e3

[49] Du L, Xi H, Zhang S, Zhou Y, Tao X, Lv Y, et al. Effects of exercise in people with multiple sclerosis: A systematic review and meta-analysis. Frontiers in Public Health. 2024;**12**:1387658

[50] Harkema S, Gerasimenko Y, Hodes J, Burdick J, Angeli C, Chen Y, et al. Effect of epidural stimulation of the lumbosacral spinal cord on voluntary movement, standing, and assisted stepping after motor complete paraplegia: A case study. Lancet (London, England). 2011;**377**(9781):1938-1947

[51] Snowden T, Morrison J, Boerstra M, Eyolfson E, Acosta C, Grafe E, et al. Brain changes: Aerobic exercise for traumatic brain injury rehabilitation. Frontiers in Human Neuroscience. 2023;**17**:1307507

[52] Gomes-Osman J, Cabral DF, Morris TP, McInerney K, Cahalin LP, Rundek T, et al. Exercise for cognitive brain health in aging: A systematic review for an evaluation of dose. Neurology: Clinical Practice. 2018;**8**(3):257-265

[53] Robertson CL, Ishibashi K, Chudzynski J, Mooney LJ, Rawson RA, Dolezal BA, et al. Effect of exercise training on striatal dopamine D2/D3 receptors in methamphetamine users during behavioral treatment. Neuropsychopharmacology: Official Publication of the American College of Neuropsychopharmacology. 2016;**41**(6):1629-1636

[54] Mikkelsen K, Stojanovska L, Polenakovic M, Bosevski M, Apostolopoulos V. Exercise and mental health. Maturitas. 2017;**106**:48-56

[55] Rethorst CD, Trivedi MH. Evidence-based recommendations for the prescription of exercise for major depressive disorder. Journal of Psychiatric Practice. 2013;**19**(3):204-212

[56] Saris IMJ, Penninx BWJH, Dinga R, van Tol MJ, Veltman DJ, van der Wee NJA, et al. Default mode network connectivity and social dysfunction in major depressive disorder. Scientific Reports. 2020;**10**(1):194

[57] Schuch FB, Vancampfort D, Richards J, Rosenbaum S, Ward PB, Stubbs B. Exercise as a treatment for depression: A meta-analysis adjusting for publication bias. Journal of Psychiatric Research. 2016;**77**:42-51

[58] Stubbs B, Vancampfort D, Rosenbaum S, Firth J, Cosco T, Veronese N, et al. An examination of the anxiolytic effects of exercise for people with anxiety and stress-related disorders: A meta-analysis. Psychiatry Research. 2017;**249**:102-108

[59] Bherer L, Erickson KI, Liu-Ambrose T. A review of the effects of physical activity and exercise on cognitive and brain functions in older adults. Journal of Aging Research. 2013;**2013**:657508

[60] Ratey JJ, Loehr JE. The positive impact of physical activity on cognition during adulthood: A review of underlying mechanisms, evidence and recommendations. Reviews in the Neurosciences. 2011;**22**(2):171-185

[61] Liu-Ambrose T, Donaldson MG. Exercise and cognition in older adults: Is there a role for resistance training programmes? British Journal of Sports Medicine. 2009;**43**(1):25-27

[62] Winstein CJ, Stein J, Arena R, Bates B, Cherney LR, Cramer SC, et al. Guidelines for adult stroke rehabilitation and recovery: A guideline for healthcare professionals from the American Heart Association/American Stroke Association. Stroke. 2016;**47**(6):e98-e169

[63] Sugiyama T, Liew SL. The effects of sensory manipulations on motor behavior: From basic science to clinical rehabilitation. Journal of Motor Behavior. 2017;**49**(1):67-77

[64] Laver KE, Lange B, George S, Deutsch JE, Saposnik G, Crotty M. Virtual reality for stroke rehabilitation. Cochrane Database of Systematic Reviews. 2017;**11**(11):CD008349

[65] Sleight AG, Gerber LH, Marshall TF, Livinski A, Alfano CM, Harrington S, et al. A systematic review of functional outcomes in cancer rehabilitation research. Archives of Physical Medicine and Rehabilitation. 2022;**103**(9):1807-1826

[66] Kleim JA, Chan S, Pringle E, Schallert K, Procaccio V, Jimenez R, et al. BDNF val66met polymorphism is associated with modified experience-dependent plasticity in human motor cortex. Nature Neuroscience. 2006;**9**(6):735-737

[67] Thickbroom GW. Transcranial magnetic stimulation and synaptic plasticity: Experimental framework and human models. Experimental Brain Research. 2007;**180**(4):583-593

[68] Khera P, Kumar N. Role of machine learning in gait analysis: A review. Journal of Medical Engineering & Technology. 2020;**44**(8):441-467

[69] Ang KK, Guan C, Phua KS, Wang C, Zhou L, Tang KY, et al. Brain-computer interface-based robotic end effector system for wrist and hand rehabilitation: Results of a three-armed randomized controlled trial for chronic stroke. Frontiers in Neuroengineering. 2014;**7**:30

[70] Kairy D, Lehoux P, Vincent C, Visintin M. A systematic review of clinical outcomes, clinical process, healthcare utilization and costs associated with telerehabilitation. Disability and Rehabilitation. 2009;**31**(6):427-447

[71] Herold F, Hamacher D, Schega L, Müller NG. Thinking while moving or moving while thinking – Concepts of motor-cognitive training for cognitive performance enhancement. Frontiers in Aging Neuroscience. 2018;**10**:228

[72] Denham J, O'Brien BJ, Charchar FJ. Telomere length maintenance and cardio-metabolic disease prevention through exercise training. Sports Medicine (Auckland, N.Z.). 2016;**46**(9):1213-1237

[73] Pedersen BK. Physical activity and muscle-brain crosstalk. Nature Reviews Endocrinology. 2019;**15**(7):383-392

[74] Reinkensmeyer DJ, Burdet E, Casadio M, Krakauer JW, Kwakkel G, Lang CE, et al. Computational neurorehabilitation: Modeling plasticity and learning to predict recovery. Journal of NeuroEngineering and Rehabilitation. 2016;**13**(1):42

[75] Löllgen H, Böckenhoff A, Knapp G. Physical activity and all-cause mortality:

An updated meta-analysis with different intensity categories. International Journal of Sports Medicine. 2009;**30**(3):213-224

[76] Petzinger GM, Fisher BE, McEwen S, Beeler JA, Walsh JP, Jakowec MW. Exercise-enhanced neuroplasticity targeting motor and cognitive circuitry in Parkinson's disease. Lancet Neurology. 2013;**12**(7):716-726

Chapter 2

Clinical Applications of Brain Structural Assessment for Post-Stroke Balance Function and Walking Ability

Ryosuke Yamamoto, Shin Murata, Shun Sawai, Shoya Fujikawa, Takato Nishida, Yusuke Shizuka, Naoki Shimizu and Hideki Nakano

Abstract

Difficulties with maintaining posture and walking after stroke substantially restrict independence in daily activities and reduce overall well-being. For this reason, a multidimensional evaluation of balance and gait function is fundamental in the therapeutic settings. Understanding how alterations in brain anatomy relate to post-stroke balance and walking capacity remains a key challenge. Recent progress in neuroimaging analysis has provided new insights into how the extent of damage to connective fiber pathways corresponds to balance control and gait performance in individuals with stroke. This chapter summarizes contemporary evidence and advanced imaging methodologies for exploring neural structures linked to postural and locomotor abilities and considers their relevance for clinical rehabilitation practice.

Keywords: stroke, standing balance, walking ability, brain structure, brain image analysis, rehabilitation

1. Introduction

Stroke is one of the leading causes of death and disability worldwide and a major contributor to conditions requiring care, particularly among older adults [1]. Impairment of walking ability and standing balance following stroke is a core issue that severely limits the activities of daily living (ADL), is linked to an elevated risk of falls, and results in a substantial decline in quality of life (QOL). These motor impairments not only compromise patients' physical and psychological independence but also contribute to increased societal costs, including greater physical and emotional burdens on caregivers and elevated long-term medical and nursing care expenses [2]. In today's rapidly aging society, the development of rehabilitation strategies focused on supporting independence and preventing falls after stroke is a critical component of building sustainable health and care systems. Rehabilitation for patients with stroke is therefore essential, and improvement of standing balance and walking ability is paramount for promoting independence. However, effective rehabilitation necessitates a precise understanding of the underlying causes of each patient's motor impairment and the creation of individualized, optimized intervention plans. Central to this is the quantitative assessment of structural brain changes resulting from injury and their relationship to motor function [3]. Recent advancements in brain imaging techniques, including diffusion tensor imaging (DTI) and voxel-based lesion-symptom mapping (VLSM), have enabled visualization of the effects of white matter fiber bundle damage on standing balance and walking ability [4]. Damage to key neural pathways, such as the corticospinal tract and the superior longitudinal fasciculus (SLF), has been shown to impair stability during standing and walking. Research continues to explore the relationship between these structures and motor function. This chapter examines the brain structural changes associated with walking function and balance control following stroke, introduces brain imaging methods for visualizing and quantifying these changes, and discusses their clinical application. Potential future directions in rehabilitation are also considered.

2. Changes in standing balance and brain structure in stroke patients

This section explores the relationship between standing balance and brain structural changes following stroke.

Postural balance is a highly integrated and complex motor control function that relies on coordinated activity across multiple brain regions, including the cerebellum, vestibular cortex, parietal lobes, and premotor areas. Research has shown that patients with stroke may experience dysfunction in the vestibular and posterior parietal cortices—regions responsible for integrating visual, somatosensory, and vestibular inputs—resulting in disrupted sensory fusion and impaired postural control mechanisms [5]. Damage to the corticospinal tracts, which mediate voluntary movement, and to the superior longitudinal fasciculus, which facilitates sensory motor integration, can further compromise standing balance. These fiber bundles form part of a neural network essential for motor planning, sensory feedback, and attentional control, and they play a central role in the selection of balance strategies and immediate postural responses [6]. With the advancement of techniques such as DTI and disconnection mapping, researchers have begun to quantitatively visualize the association between white matter architecture and standing balance function [7]. Studies have reported that impaired structural connectivity correlates with reduced dynamic balance, with patients who have lower SLF fractional anisotropy (FA) values exhibiting significantly diminished postural stability scores [6]. These findings indicate that balance is not governed solely by motor output but is supported by multidimensional control systems involving broad brain network integration. Consequently, comprehensive assessment of overall structural connectivity—not just localized damage—is vital for clinical evaluation and prognosis of standing balance in patients with stroke. Advanced neuroimaging tools, including DTI and disconnection mapping, may provide key insights into how brain structure relates to function and contribute to the development of next-generation rehabilitation strategies.

3. Walking ability and brain structure changes in patients with stroke

This section discusses how structural alterations in the brain relate to walking performance in stroke survivors.

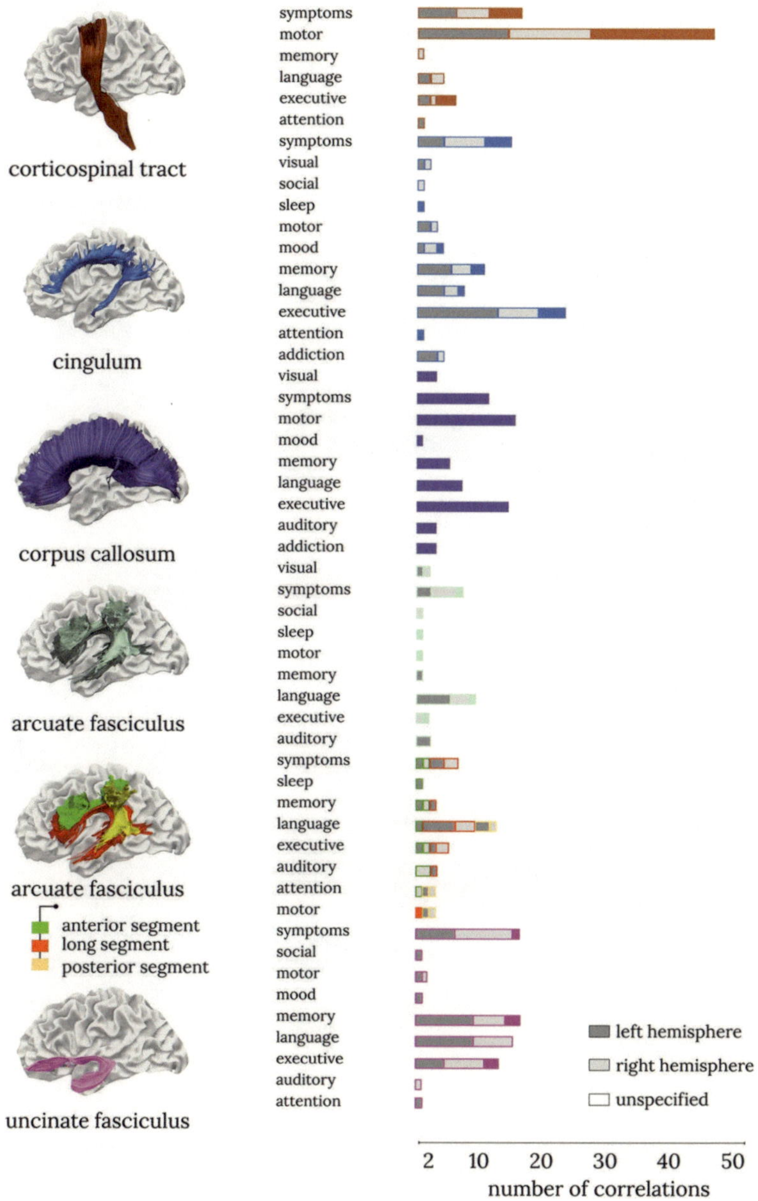

Figure 1.
Diagram showing specificity of neural pathways and regional correlations [4]. This figure illustrates that distinct white matter pathways exhibit varying degrees of association with cognitive, behavioral, and clinical domains, suggesting that pathway specificity often aligns with the diversity of their projections. While the corticospinal tracts show strong links to motor performance, other connectional routes traditionally regarded as non-motor also demonstrate the meaningful involvement, indicating that the functional scope of certain neural pathways remains broader than previously understood.

Walking is a highly complex motor behavior established through the coordinated function of multiple neural systems, including motor control, sensory input, spatial cognition, and attention [8]. Gait impairment following stroke is particularly severe due to reduced voluntary movement caused by damage to the corticospinal tract,

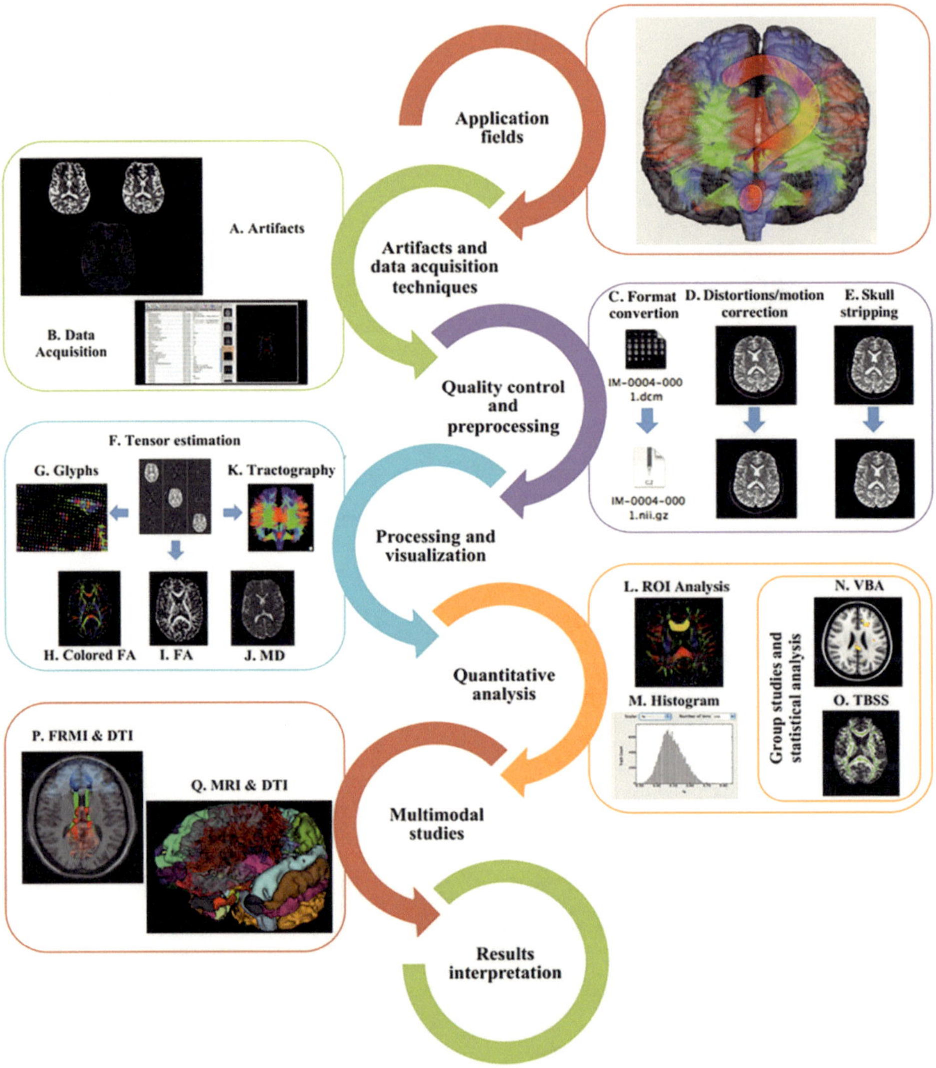

Figure 2.
Typical DTI workflow [13]. This diagram summarizes a general process for diffusion tensor imaging (DTI). The workflow starts by defining research aims and clarifying where the technique is most applicable. Particular attention should be given to image noise or spatial distortion (A) and to configuring acquisition parameters that align with study objectives (B). After data collection, images undergo verification and early preparation, which typically involve steps such as format conversion (C), correction of geometric distortion (D), and removal of extracerebral tissue (E). Tensor estimation (F) then produces directional diffusion information that can be depicted in several formats: orientation glyphs (G); diffusion-based maps, including color-encoded FA (H), FA (I), and MD (J); or reconstructed tracts (K). Analytic strategies may include region-focused mapping (L), histogram evaluation (M), voxel-wise comparisons (N), and tract-based spatial statistics (O). These diffusion findings may further be aligned with functional (P) and anatomical (Q) MRI datasets to support multimodal interpretation. Understanding the outcomes demands careful reflection on both methodological rigor and the biological mechanisms involved.

DOI: http://dx.doi.org/10.5772/intechopen.1013623

with motor paralysis of the lower limbs directly and significantly impacting walking independence [9]. Additionally, injury to the frontoparietal network connecting the frontal and parietal lobes impairs higher motor functions, such as attention distribution during ambulation and adaptive coordination of steps, making balance maintenance difficult, especially under cognitively demanding conditions [10]. Recent DTI studies have begun to identify quantitative associations between alterations in white matter fiber bundles and walking ability. For instance, decreased FA values in the corpus callosum, internal capsule, corticospinal tracts, and superior longitudinal fasciculus have been linked to slower walking speed and diminished balance function [11, 12]. These findings suggest that structural assessment *via* neuroimaging may

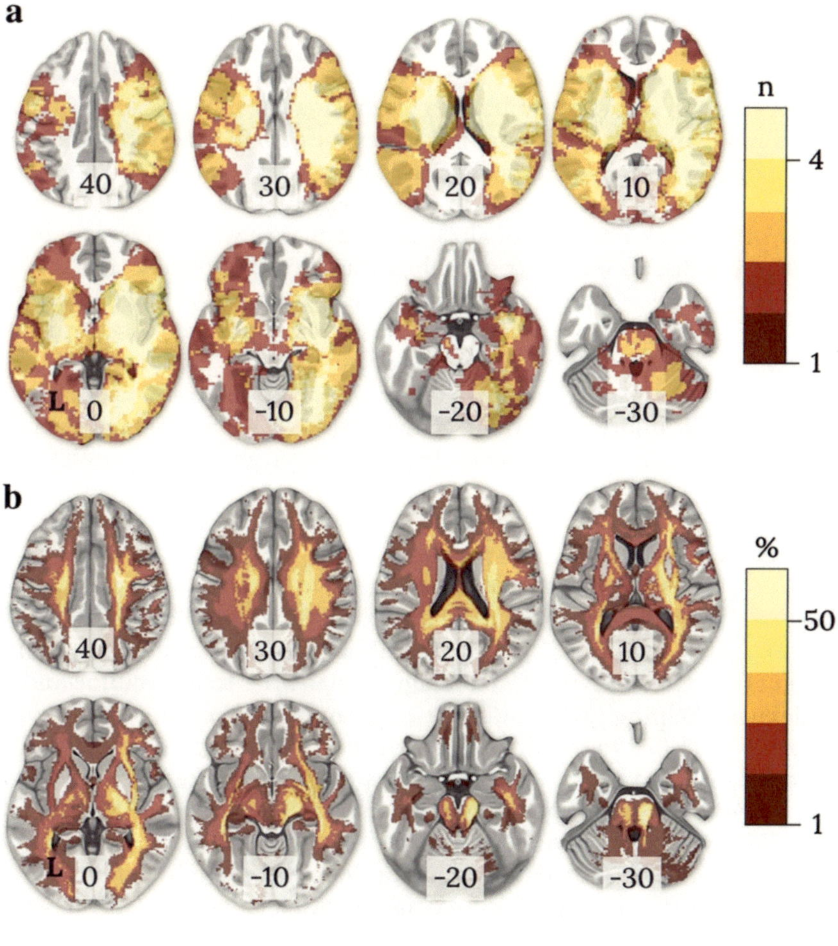

Figure 3.
Diagram showing results of white matter fiber bundle damage characterization using Disconnectome components from the BCBtoolkit [14]. The dataset included 62 individuals whose lesion and disconnection patterns appeared in both hemispheres, showing a right-sided predominance (67%). Each axial slice is annotated with its z—coordinate in neurological orientation, where the image's left corresponds to the left hemisphere. The color gradient conveys the extent of lesion convergence and the likelihood of fiber interruption. L, left hemisphere, n, case count. Right subcortical territories accounted for most of the lesions (n = 27; remaining regions, n < 15), encompassing deep nuclei and limbic structures such as the thalamus, putamen, caudate, pallidum, hippocampus, amygdala, nucleus accumbent, insular cortex, and cingulate or par hippocampal regions. The disconnection components displayed a similar, though right—dominant, spatial configuration, with the densest overlap within ventral visual routes, the internal capsule, and prefrontal projection areas. Collectively, these reconstructions illustrate ongoing advances in mapping network-level disturbances throughout the brain's connective framework.

serve as a valuable biomarker alongside clinical evaluations to predict gait recovery. After stroke, difficulties in walking stem not only from lesions to the corticospinal tract but also from disrupted connectivity within widespread white matter systems and frontoparietal circuits associated with higher-order cognition. Visualizing the mechanisms of these impairments through brain structure assessment is expected to substantially improve the functional outcome prediction and facilitate the design of individualized, optimized rehabilitation strategies (**Figures 1–3**).

4. Brain structure assessment and brain imaging analysis

This section discusses structural brain assessment in patients with stroke and advanced neuroimaging techniques.

Quantitative assessment of brain structures and the application of imaging analysis are critical in stroke rehabilitation for elucidating mechanisms of motor dysfunction and delivering individualized interventions. Recovery of motor function involves neuroplasticity and the reorganization of extensive brain networks, not only at the lesion site but also in adjacent and remote regions [15]. DTI, together with functional MRI (fMRI), enables visualization and quantitative assessment of fiber tract integrity and disruption. Metrics such as fractional anisotropy (FA) and mean diffusivity (MD) serve as indicators of the extent of microstructural damage [16]. Moreover, advanced analytical tools such as BCBtoolkit and tract-based spatial statistics (TBSS) have facilitated the visualization of individual fiber damage, allowing for precise assessment of the relationship between motor functions—including standing balance and walking ability—and brain structure [14, 17]. Clinical implementation of these methods is expected to support more personalized and effective rehabilitation approaches.

4.1 Indicators of brain structure assessment

Indices used to assess brain structure primarily reflect the condition of the cortex and white matter fibers, both of which are critical to understanding functional impairment after stroke. T1-weighted imaging quantifies lesion volume and gray matter thickness, helping to evaluate cortical atrophy and volume loss, which have been increasingly linked to cognitive function and ADL performance [16]. On the other hand, DTI is a prominent method for evaluating cerebral white matter integrity and employs indices such as FA, MD, axial diffusivity (AD), and radial diffusivity (RD). FA serves as an indicator of fiber orientation, and lower values are typically associated with axonal disruption or demyelination. MD indicates water molecule diffusion and is commonly associated with edema and tissue degeneration. Numerous studies have reported correlations between FA values in the corticospinal tract and motor function recovery, underscoring the tract's role in determining motor paralysis prognosis [9]. Beyond the corticospinal system, several major association and commissural tracts—including the superior longitudinal fasciculus and interhemispheric fibers—have been linked to postural control and locomotor performance. Comprehensive evaluation of these pathways remains essential for understanding balance and gait function [7]. In recent years, three-dimensional neurotractography has enabled visualization of fiber bundles, aiding both clinical explanation and the formulation of tailored intervention strategies by clearly depicting affected areas.

DOI: http://dx.doi.org/10.5772/intechopen.1013623

4.2 Brain image analysis methods

Brain imaging analysis refers to scientific techniques for extracting and evaluating structural information using modalities such as MRI, fMRI, and DTI. In stroke research and rehabilitation, DTI-based visualization of white matter damage has become increasingly prevalent alongside fMRI-based lesion volume assessments [18]. Open-source tools—including BCBtoolkit, MRIcron, and FSL—are now widely used in both research and clinical contexts. These tools support the automatic extraction of lesion sites and their superimposition onto standardized brain templates, facilitating the investigation of structural-functional relationships. TBSS is particularly effective for intergroup comparisons and offers clear visualizations of fiber damage patterns. Disconnectome mapping, which estimates disrupted neural networks based on lesion location, is also gaining traction. It holds promise for personalized medicine by identifying likely disconnections and potential compensatory pathways unique to each patient's injury profile [19]. Moreover, predictive models that integrate machine learning algorithms with brain imaging data are being developed to enhance accuracy in forecasting gait outcomes and rehabilitation efficacy.

4.3 Rehabilitation applications and prospects

Information obtained from brain structure assessments and brain imaging analyses provides crucial support for individualizing rehabilitation strategies. For instance, training intensity can be adjusted based on the extent of corticospinal tract damage, and task-oriented training may be introduced to promote neural network reorganization [20]. In particular, the assessment of white matter fiber bundles using DTI enables the prediction of recovery from motor paralysis and balance disorders, offering a scientific foundation for setting rehabilitation goals tailored to each patient. Moreover, if recovery prognosis can be predicted early through brain imaging, it may inform decisions regarding the timing of home discharge and initiation of care services. Magnetic resonance imaging offers diffusion-based approaches that enable the examination of tissue pathways involved in structural alteration and recovery following ischemic stroke. Using DTI, characteristics of the corticospinal tract (CST) can be quantified through directional water movement, providing insight into axonal alignment and microstructural coherence within the brain. Indices comparing FA values between the affected and unaffected corticospinal tracts are frequently applied as indicators of structural asymmetry in diffusion analyses. Typically, reduced FA along the damaged corticospinal pathway suggests more extensive tract disruption and is often accompanied by progressive Wallerian degeneration of descending axons [21]. Quantitative indicators obtained from neuroimaging can act as surrogate markers to anticipate the trajectory of post-stroke recovery and to recognize individuals who are likely to gain meaningful functional benefit from rehabilitation. Employing such metrics may also guide the development of adaptive therapeutic frameworks that tailor interventions to each person's recovery profile.

Looking ahead, future developments include real-time imaging analysis technologies and the construction of AI-based prognostic models. These innovations are expected to enable "visualized interventions" guided by brain imaging findings and support shared decision-making between patients and healthcare professionals. Furthermore, research integrating brain imaging with simple, non-invasive balance assessment techniques—such as virtual light touch—may lead to the development of novel, innovative assessment indices (**Table 1**).

	SIAS-motor total	BBS	FIM-motor
CST	0.571***	0.418***	0.396***
SLF	0.346**	0.380**	0.417***
ATR	0.302*	0.267*	0.332**
CNG	0.194	0.386**	0.341**
IFOF	0.284*	0.433***	0.451***

*Values show correlation with coefficients with their corresponding probability levels. Statistical thresholds: * $p < 0.05$; ** $p < 0.01$; *** $p < 0.001$. ATR, anterior thalamic radiation; CNG, cingulum bundle; CST, corticospinal tract; IFOF, inferior fronto-occipital fasciculus; SLF, superior longitudinal fasciculus; SIAS, Stroke Impairment Assessment Set [12].*

Table 1.
Correlations between FA values in the lesioned hemisphere and clinical outcome measures [12].

5. Conclusions

This chapter explores how alterations in brain organization relate to post-stroke standing balance and locomotor function, drawing on findings from contemporary studies. Historically, therapeutic approaches addressing motor recovery after stroke have been guided mainly by bedside evaluations and functional rating scales. However, the integration of neuroimaging now allows for more scientifically informed intervention design. Impaired standing balance has been associated with damage to multiple brain regions, including the cerebellum, vestibular cortex, parietal lobe, and premotor cortex. Damage involving major connective pathways—particularly the superior longitudinal fasciculus and corticospinal projections—can interfere with neural coordination systems that maintain upright stability, leading to postural instability and a heightened tendency to fall. These findings help define specific targets for balance training within rehabilitation. Regarding walking ability, effective performance involves not only motor control but also the integration of sensory input, attentional processes, and spatial cognition. Damage to the frontoparietal network and impairment of sensory pathways can significantly compromise gait stability and automation. Advances in brain imaging, including DTI, have begun to clarify the quantitative relationships between brain structures and gait function, facilitating individualized gait recovery predictions and intervention planning. Clinically, structural assessment of white matter using indices such as FA and MD is valuable in formulating rehabilitation strategies. For example, early identification of critical nerve fiber damage associated with gait outcomes enables the focused allocation of limited training resources to patients with the highest need. In addition, combining structural brain imaging with simple functional assessments—such as virtual light touch—may bridge anatomical insights with clinical application.

Comprehensive assessment grounded in brain structure supports personalized rehabilitation and maximizes training outcomes. Future challenges include establishing efficient clinical implementation of these assessment tools and enhancing the evidence base through multicenter collaborative research. In conclusion, the clinical application of brain structure assessment holds significant potential to elevate the quality of stroke rehabilitation and represents a critical advancement toward individualized, evidence-based interventions.

Acknowledgements

This work was supported by JSPS KAKENHI Grant Numbers JP23K10417, JP 25KJ2198.

Conflict of interest

The authors declare no conflict of interest.

Author details

Ryosuke Yamamoto[1,2], Shin Murata[1,3], Shun Sawai[1,4], Shoya Fujikawa[1,5], Takato Nishida[1,6], Yusuke Shizuka[1,5], Naoki Shimizu[1,5] and Hideki Nakano[1,3*]

1 Graduate School of Health Sciences, Kyoto Tachibana University, Kyoto, Japan

2 Department of Rehabilitation, Tesseikai Neurosurgical Hospital, Osaka, Japan

3 Department of Physical Therapy, Faculty of Health Sciences, Kyoto Tachibana University, Kyoto, Japan

4 Japan Society for the Promotion of Science (JSPS), Research Fellow (DC), Japan

5 Department of Rehabilitation, Kyoto Kuno Hospital, Kyoto, Japan

6 Faculty of Rehabilitation and Care, Seijoh University, Aichi, Japan

*Address all correspondence to: nakano-h@tachibana-u.ac.jp

References

[1] GBD 2019 Stroke Collaborators. Global, regional, and national burden of stroke and its risk factors, 1990-2019: A systematic analysis for the Global Burden of Disease Study 2019. Lancet Neurology. 2021;**20**(10):795-820. DOI: 10.1016/S1474-4422(21)00252-0. Epub 2021 Sep 3

[2] Yamamoto R, Murata S, Sawai S, Fujikawa S, Shizuka Y, Maru T, et al. Longitudinal changes in factors associated with walking independence at hospital discharge in patients with stroke: A retrospective study. Journal of Clinical Medicine. 2024;**13**(23):7184. DOI: 10.3390/jcm13237184

[3] Stinear CM, Byblow WD, Ackerley SJ, Barber PA, Smith MC. Predicting recovery potential for individual stroke patients increases rehabilitation efficiency. Stroke. 2017;**48**(4):1011-1019. DOI: 10.1161/STROKEAHA.116.015790. Epub 2017 Mar 9

[4] Forkel SJ, Friedrich P, Thiebaut de Schotten M, Howells H. White matter variability, cognition, and disorders: A systematic review. Brain Structure & Function. 2022;**227**(2):529-544. DOI: 10.1007/s00429-021-02382-w. Epub 2021 Nov 3

[5] Petersen SE, Posner MI. The attention system of the human brain: 20 years after. Annual Review of Neuroscience. 2012;**35**:73-89. DOI: 10.1146/annurev-neuro-062111-150525. Epub 2012 Apr 12

[6] Zampieri C, Leary JB, Shahim P, Damiano D, Ho PS, Pham DL, et al. Associations between white matter integrity and postural control in adults with traumatic brain injury. PLoS One. 2023;**18**(11):e0288727. DOI: 10.1371/journal.pone.0288727

[7] Bhadelia RA, Price LL, Tedesco KL, Scott T, Qiu WQ, Patz S, et al. Diffusion tensor imaging, white matter lesions, the corpus callosum, and gait in the elderly. Stroke. 2009;**40**(12):3816-3820. DOI: 10.1161/STROKEAHA.109.564765. Epub 2009 Oct 1

[8] Petersen TH, Willerslev-Olsen M, Conway BA, Nielsen JB. The motor cortex drives the muscles during walking in human subjects. The Journal of Physiology. 2012;**590**(10):2443-2452. DOI: 10.1113/jphysiol.2012.227397. Epub 2012 Mar 5

[9] Stinear CM, Barber PA, Smale PR, Coxon JP, Fleming MK, Byblow WD. Functional potential in chronic stroke patients depends on corticospinal tract integrity. Brain. 2007;**130**(Pt 1):170-180. DOI: 10.1093/brain/awl333

[10] Debaere F, Swinnen SP, Béatse E, Sunaert S, Van Hecke P, Duysens J. Brain areas involved in interlimb coordination: A distributed network. NeuroImage. 2001;**14**(5):947-958. DOI: 10.1006/nimg.2001.0892

[11] Srivastava S, Bhatia MS, Bhargava SK, Kumari R, Chandra S. A diffusion tensor imaging study using a voxel-based analysis, region-of-interest method to analyze white matter abnormalities in first-episode, treatment-naïve major depressive disorder. The Journal of Neuropsychiatry and Clinical Neurosciences. 2016;**28**(2):131-137. DOI: 10.1176/appi.neuropsych.15050120. Epub 2015 Nov 9

[12] Hirata A, Uchiyama Y, Mochizuki M, Koyama T, Domen K. Brain regions associated with balance function assessed by the Berg Balance Scale in post-stroke patients.

Journal of Physical Therapy Science. 2024;**36**(12):803-809. DOI: 10.1589/jpts.36.803. Epub 2024 Dec 1

[13] Soares JM, Marques P, Alves V, Sousa N. A hitchhiker's guide to diffusion tensor imaging. Frontiers in Neuroscience. 2013;7:31. DOI: 10.3389/fnins.2013.00031

[14] Dulyan L, Talozzi L, Pacella V, Corbetta M, Forkel SJ, Thiebaut de Schotten M. Longitudinal prediction of motor dysfunction after stroke: A disconnectome study. Brain Structure & Function. 2022;**227**(9):3085-3098. DOI: 10.1007/s00429-022-02589-5. Epub 2022 Nov 5

[15] Ward NS, Brown MM, Thompson AJ, Frackowiak RS. Neural correlates of motor recovery after stroke: A longitudinal fMRI study. Brain. 2003;**126**(Pt 11):2476-2496. DOI: 10.1093/brain/awg245. Epub 2003 Aug 22

[16] Beaulieu C. The basis of anisotropic water diffusion in the nervous system - A technical review. NMR in Biomedicine. 2002;**15**(7-8):435-455. DOI: 10.1002/nbm.782

[17] Smith SM, Jenkinson M, Johansen-Berg H, Rueckert D, Nichols TE, Mackay CE, et al. Tract-based spatial statistics: Voxelwise analysis of multi-subject diffusion data. NeuroImage. 2006;**31**(4):1487-1505. DOI: 10.1016/j.neuroimage.2006.02.024. Epub 2006 Apr 19

[18] Grefkes C, Fink GR. Reorganization of cerebral networks after stroke: New insights from neuroimaging with connectivity approaches. Brain. 2011;**134**(Pt 5):1264-1276. DOI: 10.1093/brain/awr033. Epub 2011 Mar 16

[19] Thiebaut de Schotten M, Foulon C, Nachev P. Brain disconnections link structural connectivity with function and behaviour. Nature Communications. 2020;**11**(1):5094. DOI: 10.1038/s41467-020-18920-9

[20] Buma FE, Lindeman E, Ramsey NF, Kwakkel G. Functional neuroimaging studies of early upper limb recovery after stroke: A systematic review of the literature. Neurorehabilitation and Neural Repair. 2010;**24**(7):589-608. DOI: 10.1177/1545968310364058. Epub 2010 May 3

[21] Włodarczyk L, Cichon N, Saluk-Bijak J, Bijak M, Majos A, Miller E. Neuroimaging techniques as potential tools for assessment of angiogenesis and neuroplasticity processes after stroke and their clinical implications for rehabilitation and stroke recovery prognosis. Journal of Clinical Medicine. 2022;**11**(9):2473. DOI: 10.3390/jcm11092473

Chapter 3

Advancements in Hand Function Rehabilitation for Stroke Patients: A Scoping Review of Immersive Virtual, Augmented, and Mixed Reality Technologies and an Application Study

Iván F. Mondragón B., Wilson A. Henández M., Catalina Alvarado-Rojas, Diego Mendez, Jeronimo Rueda, David E. González, Guillermo A. Aguilera and Julian D. Colorado

Abstract

Recent advancements in immersive virtual reality (VR), augmented reality (AR), and mixed reality (MR) technologies have demonstrated promising results in the rehabilitation of hand function in stroke patients. These technologies provide immersive, interactive, and engaging environments that significantly improve traditional rehabilitation methods. This chapter offers an overview of the application of emerging technologies used to enhance conventional and servo-assisted systems in the rehabilitation and recovery of hand functions after a stroke. A scoping review was performed, focusing on immersive applications that combine intervention methods, assessment, evaluation, and engagement analysis based on studies published over the past decade. Our revision explores the various applications and benefits of VR, AR, and MR in creating personalized and adaptive rehabilitation programs. In addition, the chapter describes the integration of mixed reality with a robotic hand exoskeleton for therapy, highlighting innovative approaches to improve patient outcomes and offering insights into future research and development directions in this field.

Keywords: hand function rehabilitation, stroke, immersion, virtual reality (VR), augmented reality (AR), mixed reality (MR), exoskeleton

1. Introduction

Stroke is one of the leading causes of long-term disability worldwide, occurring when blood flow to a part of the brain is interrupted or reduced, depriving brain tissue of oxygen and nutrients. This can result in significant motor impairments, particularly affecting the upper limbs (ULs) and hand function. Impaired hand mobility can severely limit a person's ability to perform daily activities, reducing independence and quality of life (QoL). The World Health Organization's Global Health Estimates report that stroke continues to rank among the top three causes of disability-adjusted life years (DALYs) worldwide [1], with expectations of reaching as high as 89.32 per 100,000 people by 2030 [2]. A frequent consequence of stroke is the impairment of fine motor skills in the hand, since the brain areas that control these actions are commonly impacted.

Diverse intervention strategies are available for the rehabilitation of upper limb functionality in stroke survivors [3, 4], aimed at recovering motor abilities, enhancing coordination, and promoting autonomy. Key methods include task-specific training (TST) or task-oriented therapy (TOT), which focuses on practicing meaningful, goal-directed activities, and constraint-induced movement therapy (CIMT), which encourages use of the affected limb by limiting the unaffected one. Bilateral arm training (BAT) promotes coordination between both limbs, while strength training (ST) and range of motion (ROM) exercises help rebuild muscle power and maintain joint flexibility. These therapies focus on enhancing neuroplasticity, which is the brain's capability to reorganize itself and create new neural pathways. Hand rehabilitation typically involves activities to improve strength, coordination, and dexterity, such as grasp-and-release exercises, stretching, and resistance exercises.

To enhance sensory and neuromuscular function, functional electrical stimulation (FES) and neuromuscular electrical stimulation (NMES) are often used, which apply electrical currents to stimulate muscle contractions and support voluntary movement. Sensory stimulation and somatosensory training aim to improve the brain's ability to process tactile input, which is often impaired after stroke. These interventions are useful as they help re-engage the nervous system and promote cortical reorganization. Mental practice (MP) complements these methods by encouraging patients to mentally rehearse movements, activating motor planning areas even in the absence of physical motion.

Supportive and advanced interventions broaden the range of tools for rehabilitation. Noninvasive brain stimulation (NIBS), such as transcranial magnetic stimulation, is used to modulate cortical excitability and support neuroplasticity. In recent years, innovative technologies such as virtual reality (VR), augmented reality (AR), mixed reality (MR), and robotic and exoskeleton therapy [3, 5] have begun to transform stroke rehabilitation. These tools offer immersive and engaging environments that can simulate real-life tasks and provide instant feedback, enhancing patient motivation and adherence. VR and AR systems can gamify therapy, making repetitive exercises more enjoyable, while MR blends physical and digital elements for interactive training. Robotic exoskeletons and smart gloves help with movement and provide precise measurements of hand function, allowing personalized therapy plans. These technologies not only improve outcomes but also allow remote rehabilitation, expanding access to care for patients in underserved areas.

Virtual reality (VR), augmented reality (AR), and mixed reality (MR) are immersive technologies that redefine the boundaries between the physical and digital worlds [6]. VR involves the use of a completely artificial setting that substitutes the user's natural environment with a digitally created scenario. Such an experience is usually mediated through head-mounted displays (HMDs) or envelope projection walls with stereoscopic capabilities like Cave Automatic Virtual Environment (CAVE) [7]. In addition, they could include spatial audio and haptic feedback to enhance realism. The aim of virtual reality (VR) is to establish a feeling of immersion, making users experience as if they are physically present in the digital environment. In contrast, AR overlays digital content onto the real world, allowing users to perceive and interact with both simultaneously. This is commonly achieved through mobile devices or AR glasses, which superimpose images, sound, text, data, or 3D models onto the user's view of their physical environment [6].

Mixed reality (MR) represents a more advanced integration of real and virtual elements, enabling dynamic interaction between physical and digital objects. Unlike AR, which simply adds virtual layers to the real world, MR allows for contextual awareness and spatial anchoring of virtual content. This means that digital objects can respond to and interact with the physical environment in real time. MR systems often rely on sophisticated sensors and spatial mapping technologies, such as those found in devices like the Microsoft HoloLens. The continuum from VR to AR to MR reflects increasing levels of integration between the virtual and physical realms, with MR occupying the most complex and interactive end of the spectrum.

A crucial differentiation in virtual reality experiences is the distinction between 2D and 3D VR environments. Typically, 2D VR pertains to virtual scenes shown on flat displays like monitors or mobile screens, where the perception of depth is restricted and user interactions are limited to conventional input devices [6]. While users can navigate and observe the virtual space, the experience lacks the spatial immersion characteristic of true VR. In contrast, 3D VR employs stereoscopic displays and motion tracking to create a fully immersive environment. Users can move their heads and bodies to explore the space naturally, and interactions are often facilitated through hand controllers or gesture recognition. This depth and interactivity significantly enhance the realism and engagement of the experience.

The idea of immersion plays a crucial role in evaluating the success of VR, AR, and MR technologies. Immersion describes the extent to which a user experiences a sense of being surrounded by and engaged in a virtual or augmented setting. It is influenced by sensory fidelity (visual, auditory, and haptic realism), interactivity, and the coherence of the virtual world [6]. High levels of immersion, including sensory engagement (visual, auditory, and sometimes haptic feedback), can lead to a psychological state known as "presence," where users temporarily suspend disbelief and accept the virtual environment as real. This state is particularly valuable in applications such as training simulations, therapeutic interventions, and educational tools, where realism, engagement, and interactivity (the ability to manipulate and respond to the environment) are critical to success. Nevertheless, there is a lack of comprehensive evidence illustrating how these technology types enhance engagement and effectiveness in the context of poststroke rehabilitation.

Taking into account the distinction mentioned above, this work focuses solely on 3D or immersive VR applications. Throughout the rest of this chapter, the terms VR, AR, and MR specifically refer to 3D or immersive applications. Therefore, this study explores the integration of VR, AR, and MR technologies with conventional and servo-assisted methods to improve rehabilitation and recovery of hand function after stroke. It examines and contrasts their benefits and potential uses. Additionally, it analyzes the bibliometric data related to this topic to grasp historical and ongoing research trends and pinpoint future research directions to progress in this area. The following research question was formulated:

Main research question:

- What is the current state of research on the use of immersive virtual, augmented, and mixed reality technologies for hand function rehabilitation in stroke patients?

Sub-questions:

- What types of VR, AR, and MR technologies have been used in hand rehabilitation for stroke patients?

- What outcomes have been reported regarding the effectiveness of these technologies?

In order to contribute to this revision, we complement it by illustrating how a mixed reality system is integrated with an exoskeleton in order to improve the rehabilitation capabilities.

2. Methods

A literature review was conducted to synthesize and summarize key findings related to the use of immersive virtual reality (VR), augmented reality (AR), and mixed reality (MR) in poststroke hand function rehabilitation. The review followed the Preferred Reporting Items for Systematic Review and Meta-Analyses Extension for Scoping Reviews (PRISMA-ScR) [8]. This is a standardized methodology for scoping reviews that provides a systematic and transparent framework for thoroughly examining pertinent research within a specific domain. Essential keywords like "rehabilitation," "stroke," "patient," "training," "virtual reality," "augmented reality," and "engagement," along with corresponding synonyms, were deliberately chosen. This selection aimed to encompass phrasing diversity and create a more expansive bibliographic dataset. These terms served to refine the search strategy across the chosen databases. Utilizing these keywords and their synonyms, an extensive search equation was constructed as demonstrated below:

```
   TITLE-ABS-KEY(( "rehabilitation" OR "therapy" OR "recovery" OR
"treatment")
   AND ( "stroke" OR "cerebrovascular accident" OR "cva" OR "brain injury")
   AND ( "hand" OR "upper limb" )
   AND ( "virtual reality" OR "vr" OR "augmented reality" OR "ar"
   OR "mixed reality" )
   AND ( "patient" OR "individual" OR "subject" OR "participant")
   AND ( "exercise" OR "training" OR "activity" OR "intervention")
   AND ( "motor skills" OR "movement" OR "coordination" OR "function"
   OR "dexterity") )
```

A search targeting title, abstract, and keywords was conducted using SCOPUS and Web of Science. These databases were selected because of their extensive interdisciplinary scope. The search was confined to journal articles published in English over the last decade. This period was chosen to encompass the recent evolution of affordable immersive VR and AR technologies and their incorporation into stroke rehabilitation. This search initially resulted in 518 documents from SCOPUS and 436 from WoS. By combining the databases and eliminating duplicate entries, 835 records were preliminarily identified for further screening.

VOSviewer, a tool for generating conceptual maps from the titles and abstracts of scientific papers [9], was used to examine the co-occurrence of terms in the 835 papers fused from SCOPUS and WoS. **Figure 1** presents the keyword network and its co-occurrence among 33 out of the 45 keywords automatically analyzed *via* VOSviewer. The size of circles and labels corresponds to the frequency and strength of keyword occurrences, and the color coding corresponds to the average year of publications correlated with respective keywords. This map highlights the trend in the recent literature investigating poststroke rehabilitation using immersive VR applications. It is evident from the map that the primary themes in the selected articles center on VR, patient, and rehabilitation. A trending topic is the usability of technology and its role in motivating the rehabilitation process.

2.1 Inclusion and exclusion criteria

The evaluation of the relevance and eligibility of the records in the review followed a multistage process, as illustrated in **Figure 2**. Initially, the title, abstract, and

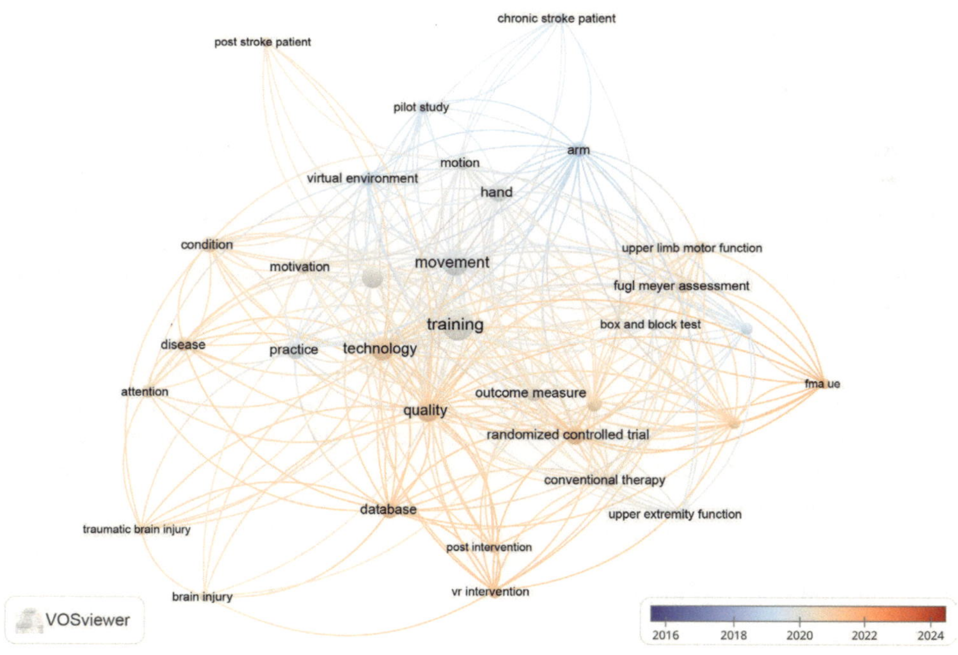

Figure 1.
Concept map showing the relations based on titles and abstracts of fused database papers. The size of circles and labels corresponds to the frequency and strength of keyword occurrences, and the color coding corresponds to the average year of publications correlated with respective keywords. Primary themes in the selected articles center on VR, patient, rehabilitation, and usability.

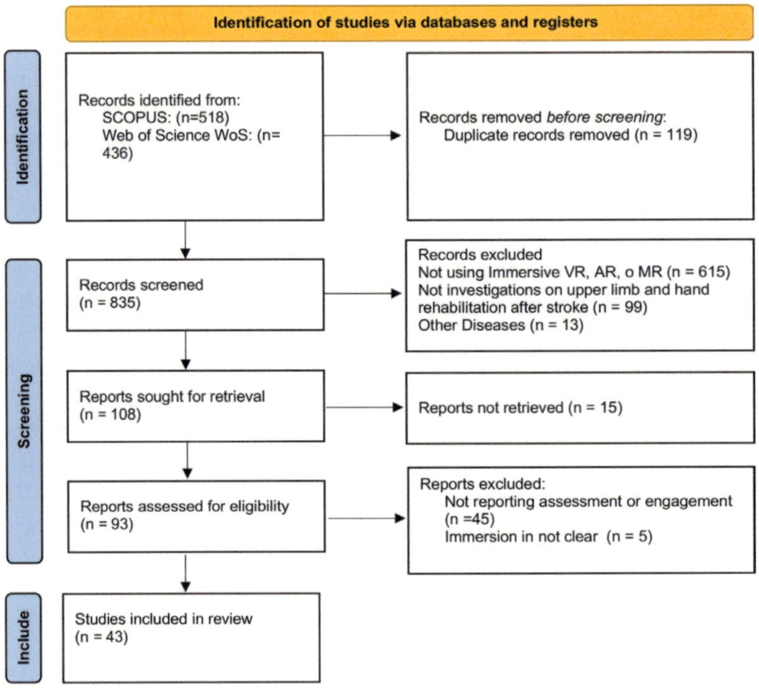

Figure 2.
Summarizing the PRISMA-ScR flow chart for the review process.

keywords of each record were reviewed. Those that appeared relevant were selected for full-text evaluation (93 records). Criteria for inclusion and exclusion were then formulated, and in the preliminary phase, records were deemed eligible for a thorough investigation if their title, abstract, or keywords suggested they offered potential insights into (1) immersive VR, AR, and MR technologies for hand rehabilitation poststroke; (2) the integration of immersive technologies with rehabilitation robotics, gloves, or exoskeletons for poststroke hand rehabilitation; and (3) detailing intervention methods, assessments of effectiveness, or patient engagement analysis concerning the use of immersive technologies in hand rehabilitation. The inclusion criteria, following the guidelines of [10], are shown in **Table 1**.

These studies mainly covered topics including immersive technologies, effectiveness assessment, and engagement scoring, among others. A large portion of the selected documents are randomized controlled trials (RCTs), demonstrating the growing interest in analyzing how these emerging technologies contribute to stroke rehabilitation. Although the primary criterion was to focus on work presenting research findings, a small number of related review articles were taken into account. In instances where overlapping reviews were detected, we methodically identified the most current and thorough review and disregarded those that overlapped with it.

2.2 Data analysis

From every document, the data collected includes the title, publishing name, publication type (such as journal article, review, or book chapter), research domain,

Criteria	Inclusion description	Exclusion description
Population	Adults (18+) who have experienced a stroke and are undergoing hand function rehabilitation.	Studies on non-stroke populations or general upper limb, lower limb, or rehab without arm- and hand-specific focus.
Concept	Use of immersive or 3D VR, AR, and MR technologies for upper limb and hand rehabilitation. Studies reporting on rehabilitation effectiveness, patient engagement, usability, or functional outcomes.	Studies not involving immersive or 3D VR, AR, or MR (e.g., traditional therapy, robotics without immersive tech, screen VR, or AR) or using readily available commercial games. Studies that do not report on engagement, effectiveness, usability, functional outcomes, or technology evaluation.
Context	Journals and books published peer-reviewed articles, clinical trials, pilot studies, feasibility studies, qualitative studies, and mixed methods. Published in English, with publication dates from 2014 to today.	Editorials, opinion pieces, conference abstracts without full text, and congress proceedings.

Table 1.
Inclusion and exclusion criteria.

keywords, technologies utilized (like VR, AR, MR, or robotics), software applications employed, intervention, assessment method, engagement evaluation, and key results.

Records fulfilling one of the following criteria were excluded from further investigation: (1) duplicate record, (2) no apparent investigation of methods for upper limb or hand rehab, (3) works that include lower limb or full-body rehab, and (4) published before 2014.

During a subsequent review stage, the remaining documents underwent a comprehensive full-text evaluation, and items were eliminated according to the following criteria: (1) no English full text available, (2) concentrating solely on technical development without any form of intervention, evaluation (whether for effectiveness or engagement), or method discussion.

Finally, a Microsoft Excel template was designed to retrieve pertinent data from the selected sources of evidence. This template indicates the kind of immersive technology (VR, AR, MR), the integration with rehab robotics or exoskeletons, the type of interventions (CIMT, mirror therapy, motor imagery, task-specific training, mental practice, bilateral training, etc.), the assessment method (FMA, BBT, WMFT, FIM, others), and patient engagement analysis (neuroplasticity, cognition, exergaming, system usability, etc.). This allowed us to chart consistent information on the literature and store it in a systematic manner.

3. Results

Of the 43 selected studies, which were identified as sources of evidence, all were released between 2014 and 2025, with 3 studies appearing in 2025 [11–13], 11 studies from the previous year, 2024 [14–24], 9 studies in 2023 [25–33], and 5 in each of the years 2022 [34–38] and 2021 [39–43], which constitute 75% of the included works. Initially, we examine the types of immersive technology and haptic feedback present in the literature. Subsequently, we concentrate on reviewing various assessment measurement methodologies. Lastly, we explore the engagement evaluation techniques employed.

3.1 Immersive technologies

Head-mounted displays (HMDs) have become the most widely adopted output devices in immersive technologies for rehab in recent years, with 86% of the included studies using them [11–16, 18, 19, 21–23, 25–28, 30–35, 37–55]. They are wearable devices that position one or two small screens directly in front of the user's eyes, often using lenses to create a stereoscopic 3D effect for enhanced depth perception. These devices can be classified by their connectivity and the type of visual interface they use. In terms of connectivity, commercial tethered HMDs (e.g., HTC VIVE, Oculus Rift/Rift S, 56%) rely on external PCs or consoles for high-performance rendering [11, 13, 14, 21, 22, 25–28, 30, 32, 34, 35, 37, 39–42, 48–55] or a custom-made system [56]. Otherwise, standalone HMDs (e.g., Meta (Oculus) Quest series, 19%) are self-contained with onboard processing and sensors [15, 16, 19, 24, 31, 33, 37, 43]. A third category includes mobile-based HMDs, which use a smartphone as both the display and the computing unit [29]. These typically consist of a headset shell with lenses into which the phone is inserted, offering an accessible and affordable entry point into VR (e.g., Samsung Gear VR, Google Cardboard).

Visually, HMDs fall into three main categories: virtual reality HMDs (VR-HMDs), which fully immerse users in digital environments and block out the real world (e.g., PlayStation VR2, Valve Index); video see-through HMDs (VST-HMDs), which use external cameras to capture the real world and display it on internal screens alongside virtual content (e.g., Apple Vision Pro, Meta Quest Pro); and optical see-through HMDs (OST-HMDs), which use transparent lenses or waveguides to overlay digital information directly onto the user's view of the real world (e.g., Microsoft HoloLens 2, Lumus DK-50). Key technical parameters such as resolution, field of view (FOV), refresh rate, and tracking systems (inside-out vs. outside-in) significantly influence the level of immersion, accuracy, and user comfort, making them critical considerations in both consumer and professional applications.

Stationary VR systems offer an alternative to wearable displays by immersing users in virtual environments through fixed installations that include a large screen combined with polarized 3D glasses. The most prominent example is CAVE (Cave Automatic Virtual Environment), where images are projected onto the walls, floor, and sometimes ceiling of a room-sized cube [57]. Users wear 3D glasses and interact with the environment using motion tracking and input devices. Another form includes panoramic projection systems used in simulation centers [20]. These systems are ideal for collaborative experiences that allow multiple users to share the same virtual space. Although they offer high visual fidelity and reduce motion sickness, they are limited by their lack of portability, high cost, and spatial constraints.

Input devices play a crucial role in enabling natural and intuitive interaction with digital environments. These devices include noncontact input or motion detection systems such as the Microsoft Azure Kinect [48] that employ depth detection cameras and AI for full-body motion tracking. Leap Motion Controller [13, 25, 28, 39, 42, 47], which precisely detects detailed hand and finger movements. Time-of-Flight (ToF) sensors [45], Meta Quest 3 Inside-Out Tracking [16], and HTC VIVE Tracker [11, 14], which track body, hand, or finger movements in 3D space without physical contact. Infrared (IR) sensors are also widely used, often embedded in these systems, to detect depth and motion by capturing reflected IR light from the user or surroundings [35]. In addition, handheld controllers [30, 48], data gloves [28], and eye-tracking systems are commonly used to capture gestures, touch, and gaze direction. These input devices enable users to adjust virtual objects, explore settings, and interact with simulations instantly, thereby boosting the sense of presence and engagement in immersive experiences.

Audio output devices are essential to create a convincing immersive experience by simulating spatial soundscapes. These devices range from basic stereo headphones to advanced spatial audio systems that use binaural rendering and head-related transfer functions (HRTFs) to simulate how sound arrives at the ears from different directions. The subcategories include open-back headphones, which offer a more natural soundstage, and closed-back headphones, which provide better isolation. Some HMDs integrate audio systems directly into the headset for convenience. Spatial audio enhances realism, supports directional awareness, and can be used to guide user attention or simulate environmental signals, making it indispensable in VR, AR, and MR applications [57].

Haptic devices provide tactile and kinesthetic feedback, enabling users to “feel” virtual objects and interactions. These devices can be categorized into vibration-based haptics (e.g., game controllers, VR handsets) [14, 21, 23, 30, 37, 40, 48], force-feedback devices (e.g., haptic gloves, exoskeletons) [17, 27, 46, 58], and surface haptics (e.g., touchscreens with variable friction). More advanced technologies include ultrasonic mid-air haptics and electrotactile stimulation, which are still largely experimental. Haptic feedback enhances realism and is particularly valuable in training simulations, such as surgical procedures or mechanical assembly. Nevertheless, obstacles persist in attaining high accuracy and seamless integration with completely immersive VR, AR, and MR systems, alongside enhancements in comfort and cost-effectiveness, particularly for full upper limb haptic systems [58].

Table 2 summarizes a comparison of these devices.

3.2 Effectiveness

Studies have shown that VR, AR, and MR therapies can significantly improve upper limb function. These technologies are commonly used in conjunction with standardized clinical assessments designed to capture different aspects of motor recovery and functional ability, such as the Fugl-Meyer Assessment (FMA) [13, 19–21, 29, 30, 33, 35, 36, 38, 43, 44, 46–48, 50, 51, 55], Box and Block Test (BBT) [12, 19, 22, 46, 53, 54], Nine-Hole Peg Test (NHPT) [12], Barthel Index (BI) and modified BI (MBI) [19, 21, 23, 26, 27, 35, 38, 39, 45, 53–55, 57], and Wolf Motor Function Test (WMFT) [20, 30, 44, 46, 57], among others [3]. Assessments are chosen based on their ability to measure specific domains such as motor control, dexterity, strength, and independence in daily activities.

Motor function is typically assessed using tools like the Fugl-Meyer Assessment for Upper Extremity (FMA-UE), which evaluates movement, coordination, and reflex activity [3]. It is widely regarded as the gold standard for measuring poststroke motor impairment due to its strong psychometric properties. In our revision, 37% of the studies use FMA. The Wolf Motor Function Test (WMFT) (7% of the studies) complements this by focusing on the time and quality of movement during functional tasks, providing insight into how impairments translate into real-world performance. To evaluate dexterity, the Box and Block Test (BBT) (12% of the studies) measures gross manual dexterity, while the Nine-Hole Peg Test (NHPT) (7% of the studies) assesses fine motor coordination and speed, both of which are critical for hand function.

Technology	Main characteristics	Advantages	Disadvantages	Main applications	Usage (VR, AR, MR)	Examples
Head-mounted displays (HMDs)	Worn on head, stereoscopic 3D, tethered/standalone	High immersion, portability, individual user experience	Motion sickness, can be heavy and uncomfortable	Gaming, training, simulations	VR, AR, MR	Tethered HMDs (HTC VIVE, Oculus Rift/Rift S); standalone HMDs (Meta/Oculus Quest series, HoloLens); mobile-based HMDs (Samsung Gear VR, Google Cardboard)
Stationary VR	Fixed position, CAVE systems, large-scale projection, stereoscopic projectors	Group shared VR experience, avoids motion sickness, high resolution	Requires dedicated facilities and software, less portable, expensive	Industrial design, architecture, collaborative simulations	VR	CAVE (BARCO S4, Machdyne Bench, and Corner); stereoscopic projectors (Sony, Barco); active shutter glasses (Volfoni, Sony)
Audio output devices	Stereo headphones, binaural audio, 3D spatial audio	Enhances realism, guides attention	Limited by audio quality, potential discomfort	Spatial awareness, environmental simulation	VR, AR, MR	Stereo Heads, HMDs integrated audio. Spatial audio devices, Music Glove (FlintRehab)
Haptic devices	Tactile feedback, vibration-based, force-feedback	Enhances realism, crucial for training	Cost, complexity, fidelity	Medical training, engineering simulations	VR, MR	Amadeo Trymotion, HandTutor Meditouch, Neofect Smart Glove
Noncontact input	Interpret human movement, gestures, or spatial positioning	Enable seamless, intuitive interaction within virtual environments	Limited precision. Sensitive to environmental factors, not haptic feedback	Medical training, engineering simulations	VR, MR	Leap Motion Controller, Microsoft Kinect, Time-of-Flight (ToF) sensors, Meta Quest 3 Inside-Out Tracking

Table 2.
Comparison of immersive technologies.

To assess how motor impairments affect daily life, tools such as the Barthel Index (BI) and the Modified Barthel Index (MBI) are used by 28% of the included studies to evaluate a patient's ability to perform basic activities of daily living (ADL), such as feeding, dressing, and bathing [3]. These indices are crucial for determining levels of independence and planning for discharge or long-term care. Additional assessments like the Modified Ashworth Scale (MAS) (2%) [36] for spasticity, manual muscle testing for strength, and the national institutes of healt (NIH) Stroke Scale for overall stroke severity provide further context to the upper limb evaluation. Together, these tools form a robust framework for assessing upper extremity function and tailoring rehabilitation to individual needs.

Electromyography (EMG) has also been used by 19% of the studies in conjunction with VR tools for assessing muscle function and neuromuscular health in poststroke rehabilitation of the upper limb. EMG measures the electrical activity produced by skeletal muscles, providing insights into muscle activation patterns, timing, and coordination [14, 26–28, 32, 34]. This information is crucial for understanding the extent of motor impairment and the effectiveness of rehabilitation interventions. EMG can detect abnormal muscle activation, such as co-contractions or spasticity, which are common in stroke patients. By analyzing EMG data, clinicians can tailor rehabilitation programs to target specific muscles and improve motor control. Additionally, EMG can be used to monitor progress over time, allowing for adjustments to therapy based on objective data.

Functional near-infrared spectroscopy (fNIRS) (2 studies) is increasingly used as a noninvasive neuroimaging tool to monitor brain activity during motor recovery tasks [17, 25]. It works by measuring changes in oxygenated and deoxygenated hemoglobin in the cerebral cortex, providing real-time insights into cortical activation patterns during hand movements or rehabilitation exercises.

3.3 Patient engagement

Patient engagement is a critical determinant of success in poststroke rehabilitation, particularly for upper limb recovery, where sustained motivation and active participation are essential for functional improvement. VR and AR have become powerful tools to enhance engagement by transforming repetitive therapeutic exercises into interactive, goal-oriented experiences. They offer dynamic environments that can be tailored to individual needs, thereby increasing adherence and emotional investment in the rehabilitation process. The immersive nature of VR and the contextual increase in AR help bridge the gap between clinical settings and real-world tasks, creating a more meaningful and motivating therapeutic experience. These technologies also improve patient motivation and adherence to rehabilitation programs, which are critical to successful recovery [3].

A key process through which VR and AR aid recovery is neuroplasticity, which refers to the brain's capacity to restructure itself by establishing new neural pathways. Stroke often disrupts motor pathways, and recovery depends on the brain's ability to rewire itself through intensive, task-specific practice. VR/AR-based rehabilitation systems provide a platform for high-frequency, repetitive, and task-oriented training, which are key principles for inducing neuroplastic changes. Six studies (14%) include this concept analysis in their works [12, 13, 22, 27, 35, 46, 55]. These systems can simulate real-life tasks in a controlled, safe environment, allowing patients to practice movements that are functionally relevant. Moreover, real-time feedback and adaptive difficulty levels help reinforce correct motor patterns and maintain the challenge necessary to stimulate cortical reorganization.

Multiple studies confirm that VR-based rehabilitation significantly enhances motor recovery by leveraging the principles of neuroplasticity. For example, in Ref. [51], a scoping review of immersive VR for upper extremity rehabilitation, 85% of the included studies reported measurable improvements in motor function. These improvements were attributed to the high intensity and task-specific nature of VR exercises, which stimulate cortical reorganization. For example, mirror therapy and motor imagery tasks delivered through VR headsets were shown to activate motor-related brain regions, reinforcing neural pathways disrupted by stroke. Furthermore, adaptive difficulty and real-time feedback mechanisms were found to sustain patient motivation and optimize the challenge level, both of which are critical for inducing long-term plastic changes.

Cognitive engagement is another vital aspect of effective rehabilitation. Stroke survivors often experience cognitive deficits alongside motor impairments, including issues with attention, memory, and executive function. VR and AR environments can be designed to simultaneously engage cognitive and motor domains, promoting dual-task training that mirrors the complexity of everyday activities [27, 45]. For instance, a VR task might require a patient to reach for virtual objects while solving simple puzzles or responding to auditory cues, thereby enhancing both motor control and cognitive flexibility. This integrative approach not only improves functional outcomes but also supports the generalization of skills to real-world contexts. For example, Khan et al. [59] found that interventions that incorporated dual-task paradigms, such as reaching tasks combined with memory or attention challenges, demonstrated superior outcomes in both domains compared to motor-only training, suggesting that immersive technologies can support executive function recovery while reinforcing motor skills.

The concept of exergaming (the use of physical activity based on games) has gained traction as a strategy to further increase patient engagement. In VR and AR rehabilitation, exergames transform therapeutic exercises into playful, interactive challenges that reward effort and progress. These games often incorporate elements of competition, achievement, and narrative, which can significantly increase motivation and enjoyment. Importantly, exergaming allows quantitative tracking of performance, allowing therapists to monitor progress and adjust interventions accordingly. By making rehabilitation more enjoyable and less monotonous, exergaming helps to maintain long-term participation, which is crucial to achieving meaningful recovery in upper limb function, as is explored in 11% of the reviewed works [18, 24, 60]. However, some works have also noted variability in game design quality and a lack of standardized engagement metrics, showing the need for more rigorous development and evaluation frameworks [61].

Finally, evaluating the user experience of immersive technologies is essential to ensure effectiveness and patient comfort. Commonly used assessment tools include the System Usability Scale (SUS), as is evidenced in seven documents (16%) [11, 15, 22, 24, 37, 49, 50], which provides a quick measure of perceived usability; the NASA Task Load Index (NASA-TLX) (5%) [24, 29], which assesses perceived workload across dimensions such as mental demand and effort; and the Simulator Sickness Questionnaire (SSQ) (9%) [11, 19, 22, 50], which evaluates symptoms such as nausea, oculomotor strain, and disorientation that may arise from virtual environments. These tools help researchers and clinicians understand how stroke patients interact with VR-based rehabilitation systems, ensuring that the technology supports recovery without causing undue strain or discomfort.

Finally, Appendix A, **Table 3**, summarizes the main characteristics of the included works.

3.4 MR integration with an exoskeleton glove for poststroke rehab

This section describes our progress in developing an integration of a mixed reality application, combined with an as-needed assisted exoskeleton previously developed [62, 63], aimed at enhancing patient recovery capabilities.

3.4.1 Architecture

The general architecture is presented in **Figure 3**. The system mainly consists of the user, the robotic exoskeleton, and the immersive headsets. The mixed reality application is composed of different modules that aim to enhance the user experience through two main tasks: implementing a game in mixed/virtual reality and integrating the existing robotic exoskeleton into an interactive mixed reality system.

The therapy process begins once the user puts on and turns on the immersive headsets. When the mixed reality application starts, the user is presented with the possible therapy activities: a mixed/virtual reality serious game or recovery routines with the exoskeleton. If the user selects the game, they are taken to the game's start interface, where they will need to rely on exercises used during recovery routines to complete the game's challenges and dynamics. However, if the user selects the recovery routine option, an information guide is displayed, indicating the components of the robotic exoskeleton system and how to interact with them correctly during therapy sessions.

Once the user sets up the system, the user interface is presented to execute routines with the exoskeleton. In this interface, the user can preview the exercise to be performed and visualize the movements executed using a digital twin of the real exoskeleton to provide feedback on the exercise performed. The routine execution begins when the user selects one of the options in the interface; with this, the HMD communicates with the robotic exoskeleton, and a bidirectional communication is maintained to carry out the mentioned actions. At any moment, the user can end the therapy and receive feedback on the work done during the session.

3.4.2 Exoskeleton digital twin

In **Figure 3**, we can observe the main elements interacting in specific ways to ensure proper functionality. First, we have the user selection, which serves as the

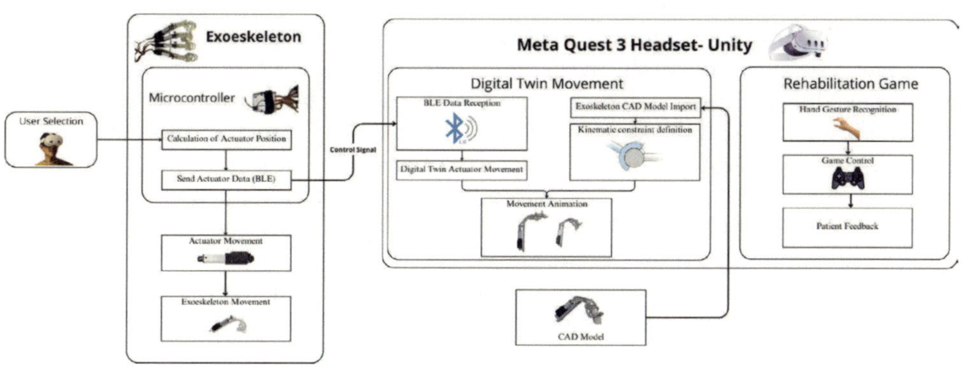

Figure 3.
System Architecture. A mixed reality system composed of two modalities: integration with a robotic exoskeleton and a standalone mixed reality game. This system aims to stimulate the bidigital pinch movement in the hand.

initial input to indicate the routine that the system must execute. After the user makes the selection, this signal is sent to the microcontroller, where, depending on the chosen routine, it calculates the actuator positions for each finger. Once the system determines these positions, the data is transmitted *via* the Bluetooth Low Energy (BLE) module to enable wireless communication. This signal is directed to two different components. First, it is sent to the exoskeleton to initiate the movement of the actuators, aligning with the selected routine. Simultaneously, the actuator data is transmitted to the Meta Quest 3 headset, where a specific module receives the signal and forwards it to the digital twin actuators.

To ensure accurate movement animation, additional considerations are necessary. The digital twin must replicate the behavior of the physical exoskeleton precisely. To achieve this, the computer-assisted design (CAD) model of the exoskeleton is imported into the Meta Quest 3 environment. Once all components are integrated, the kinematic constraints and relationships between the parts are defined. These constraints are designed based on the mechanical design principles established in Refs. [62, 63], ensuring that the digital twin mirrors the physical exoskeleton's movements accurately. With these elements in place, the system is capable of reflecting real-time motion.

3.4.3 Bluetooth LE connection

This sub-task is dedicated to creating a two-way communication link between the robotic exoskeleton and the Meta Quest 3S headset. Essentially, this component seeks to establish a communication framework that allows sending and receiving data between the two devices. The exoskeleton's control system utilizes the Bluetooth Low Energy (BLE) protocol for communication, and thus the application is designed accordingly to support this protocol. This module is involved in development subtasks such as the design of the therapy graphical interface and the visual feedback of recovery movements performed through the digital twin of the exoskeleton.

As illustrated in **Figure 3**, the architecture involves the user, the Meta Quest 3S headset, and the robotic exoskeleton. The flow begins with the user's interaction: the individual must wear the immersive headset and interact with the Unity-developed interface. During therapy, the user can execute recovery routines through buttons or signals in the interface; the user sends commands to transmit data from the headset to the exoskeleton while also enabling the reception of information from the physical model (e.g., actuator positions).

To support the development of modules such as the therapy interface and digital twin-based visual feedback, the implementation of four core communication functions is considered: connection request, transmission of exercise routine parameters, device disconnection, and reception of actuator state data. Much of this development lies in software implementation. Initially, it is necessary to define and establish the required permissions for BLE usage, based on the Android version used by the Meta Quest 3S headset; these permissions are essential, as they ensure the continuous operation of communication functions.

As a follow-up activity, an Android library is to be created using an Android Integrated Development Environment (IDE) (e.g., Android Studio), which integrates the necessary permissions and core functionalities, as shown in **Figure 4**. Since the main project is developed in a mixed reality-oriented engine, this library must be imported into the application so that these custom communication features can be efficiently integrated into the user interface. Once the library is imported, its

DOI: http://dx.doi.org/10.5772/intechopen.1011761

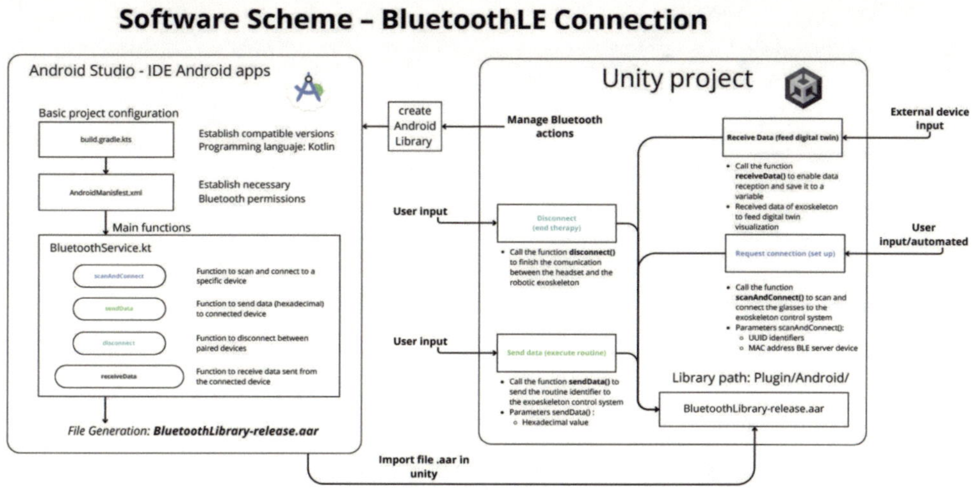

Figure 4.
Software Scheme – Bluetooth LE Connection. Development architecture of a custom Android library designed to manage Bluetooth Low Energy (BLE) functionalities on Meta Quest 3S immersive headsets. This task is part of the exoskeleton integration modality through communication among devices.

functions are linked to interactive elements in the system's main interface. As a result, when the user triggers a control signal from the therapy interface, the corresponding function in the Android library is invoked; this function will execute the predefined communication actions with the exoskeleton.

Again, this module operates as a subcomponent in other system sub-tasks; it facilitates the integration of multiple tools and resources that enhance the overall functionality of the proposed system.

3.4.4 Exoskeleton and gesture recognition

As illustrated in **Figure 5**, the software recognition architecture comprises four sequential phases to enable robust integration with the Meta Quest 3S. For this stage, the computer vision model for real-time object detection, YOLOv5 (You Only Look Once version 5) [64], is integrated.

- Phase 1: Data collection involves capturing images *via* mobile devices as raw input. These images are labeled using tools like Makesense.ai and structured into a dataset divided into training and validation subsets, governed by a data.yaml configuration file. A critical challenge at this stage is dataset inefficiency, which could compromise downstream model performance.

- Phase 2: YOLOv5 model training begins by cloning the YOLOv5 GitHub repository. The model undergoes training utilizing the prepared dataset, while key metrics like precision, recall, and mean average precision (mAP) are tracked. Insufficient dataset diversity or labeling errors may necessitate reverting to Phase 1 for adjustments.

- Phase 3: Model integration in Unity requires exporting the trained YOLOv5 model to open neural network exchange (ONNX) format *via* PyTorch. The ONNX file is imported into Unity using the Sentis engine, and a custom C#

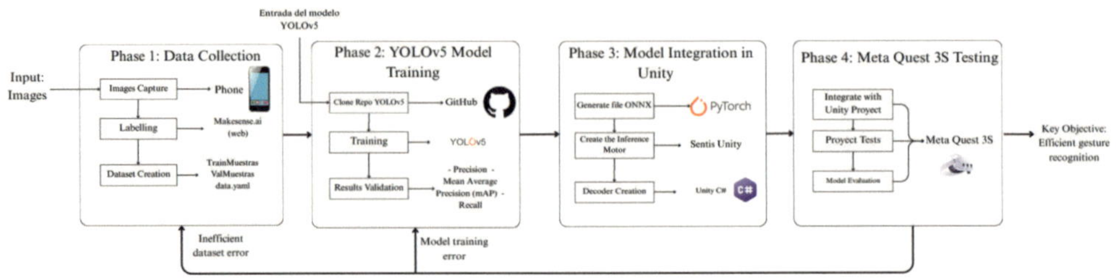

Figure 5.
Software recognition architecture composed of four sequential phases to enable the integration with the Meta Quest 3S. The block diagram of the interaction system using Meta Quest 3S headsets (software) illustrates the use of Unity for the user interface and computer vision algorithms for object recognition and classification.

decoder is developed to translate model outputs into actionable commands within Unity's scripting environment, enabling real-time gesture-to-action mapping.

- Phase 4: The final phase involves integrating the gesture/exoskeleton recognition module into a Unity project designed for Meta Quest 3S. Several rounds of project testing and model evaluation are conducted directly on the headset to validate recognition accuracy and system responsiveness.

Figure 6 shows how the Meta Quest 3S's built-in camera is integrated into the Unity-based application to enable dynamic object recognition. The process begins when the user interacts with the headset, where a Unity project manages core functionalities beyond object detection (rehabilitation routines or a game). Moreover, the headset camera captures environmental data, which is processed in real time by the object recognition module. The module identifies and classifies objects within the camera's field of view using a pretrained machine learning model. Classification results are relayed back to Unity, triggering context-specific responses such as behavioral modifications, interactive enhancements, or user feedback. This closed-loop system—spanning camera input, real-time recognition, and Unity-driven output—enables continuous synchronization between physical and virtual elements, achieving cohesive mixed reality integration.

3.4.5 Exoskeleton therapy assisted with immersive MR digital twin

The system is composed of two main components: the exoskeleton and its corresponding digital twin, which is visualized through the Meta Quest 3 headset, as

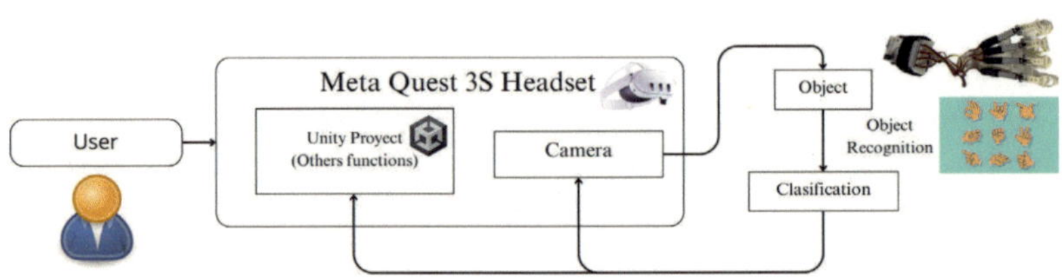

Figure 6.
Dynamic object recognition on HMD: Block diagram of the interaction system using Meta Quest 3S headsets (hardware), integrating Unity for the user interface and computer vision algorithms for object recognition and classification, including the exoskeleton and hand gestures.

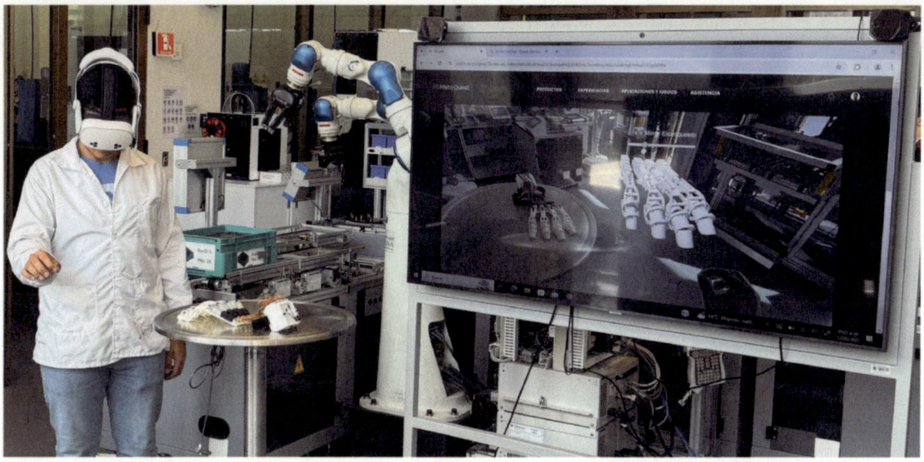

Figure 7.
Exoskeleton and digital twin visualization on the HMD. Implementation of a digital twin of the robotic exoskeleton in Unity to provide visual feedback and real-time tracking of the physical model on the head-mounted display (HMD).

shown in **Figure 7**. The exoskeleton is designed to assist the patient in performing rehabilitation exercises with precision and consistency. Simultaneously, the digital twin mirrors the exoskeleton's movements in real-time, providing the patient with visual feedback that enhances spatial awareness and motor learning. This synchronized representation allows for more efficient and engaging therapy sessions, as patients can observe their own movements in an augmented reality environment, facilitating better alignment and correction during rehabilitation.

The interaction between the exoskeleton and its digital model is facilitated by Bluetooth technology, which allows for instant data transfer regarding the actuator's positions. This smooth linkage guarantees that the digital twin precisely mirrors every motion of the exoskeleton, enabling the therapist and patient to track progress and adjust as necessary. This synergy not only enhances the rehabilitation process but also closes the divide between physical and digital therapy, crafting an engaging and interactive environment that supports better recovery results.

The system is designed to execute AR interventions utilizing an active support approach, facilitated by a robotic-assisted exoskeleton [62, 63]. This robotic setup modulates the exoskeleton's velocity during rehabilitation therapy by incorporating the patient's EMG muscle activity. Additionally, thanks to the bidirectional interaction between the exoskeleton and the AR system, it can incorporate EMG signals in both the design and evaluation of AR interventions.

To assess the effectiveness of our proposed system, multiple studies emphasize the significance of using standardized questionnaires for evaluating usability. The System Usability Scale (SUS), the Virtual Reality Sickness Questionnaire (VRSQ), and customized user feedback forms, designed specifically for the system in question, are frequently employed. These tools are integral for gauging user satisfaction with virtual environments and for detecting VR-related symptoms, such as dizziness, fatigue, or discomfort. Such methodology has been regularly utilized in research, including Refs. [11, 25, 48], where usability assessments were crucial for validating immersive systems aimed at upper limb rehabilitation.

Besides usability evaluation, clinical outcomes are taken into account for functional validation. Employing a methodology similar to that suggested in Ref. [13], participants will be split into a control group undergoing standard rehabilitation and an intervention group receiving the same treatment enhanced by immersive VR sessions. The results will then be evaluated through clinical scales like the Fugl-Meyer Assessment for Upper Extremity (FMA-UE), which assesses motor control, reflex function, and coordination.

4. Discussion

Utilizing a structured approach grounded in PRIMSA-ScR, a total of 43 published papers were examined, each concentrating on poststroke upper limb rehabilitation using immersive technologies. These studies specifically addressed various interventions, assessment techniques, and engagement evaluations.

Utilizing VOSviewer for co-authorship analysis, both at the author and country levels, derived from the 43 chosen documents, 10 are published from China (with a total of 195 citations), 9 from the USA (298 citations), 6 from Germany (86 citations), 4 from Italy (72 citations), and 4 from Japan (13 citations), among others. By examining the authors, it is observed that just 9 of them feature in more than two publications. In general, this indicates that research in this area is spread across numerous authors and institutions worldwide, as **Figure 8** shows.

Analyzing the technology, VR creates computer-generated environments that simulate real-life scenarios, allowing patients to perform task-specific training and receive immediate feedback. This approach has been shown to improve motor function, cognitive skills, and overall quality of life [51, 60]. Alternatively, AR superimposes virtual entities onto the physical world, creating a hybrid setting that allows patients to engage with both tangible and virtual components. This method has been used to improve upper limb motor function by replacing the paralyzed arm with a virtual one

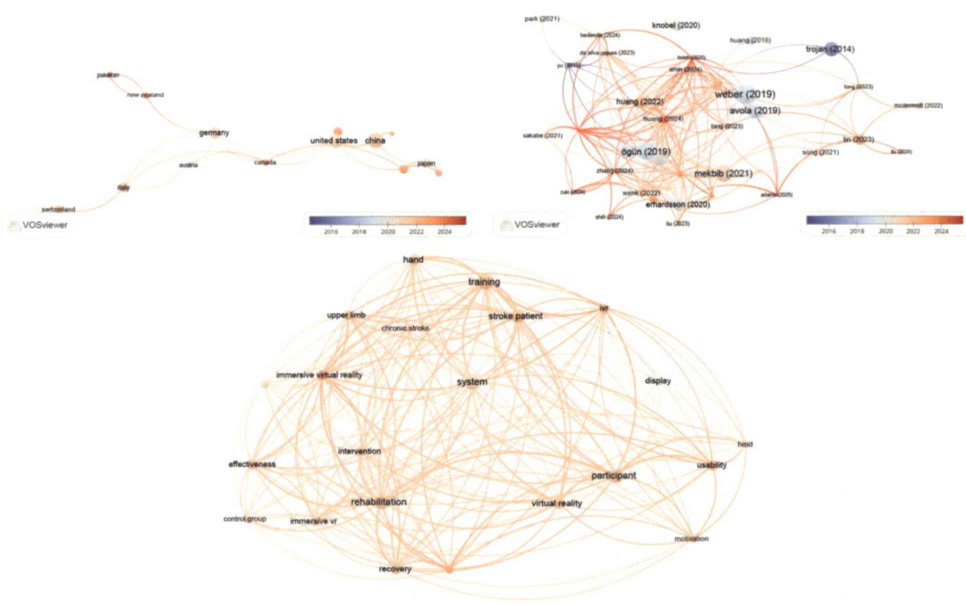

Figure 8.
Relations maps from reviewed papers. Top Left. Country relation map; Top Right: Bibliographic coupling; Bottom: Keywords concept map.

in real-time images [37, 41, 56]. MR combines elements of both VR and AR, allowing patients to interact with tangible objects within a virtual environment. The MR-board, for example, includes gamified programs that train upper extremity movements using real objects, leading to significant improvements in hand function and patient satisfaction. Therefore, MR systems have been shown to be effective self-training tools, enabling patients to perform rehabilitation exercises independently [28, 54].

It is important to recognize that although VR/AR-based rehabilitation for upper extremity management is considered a standalone approach in the literature [3], it is frequently used in conjunction with conventional methods such as MR (19% of the studies), BAT (12%), CIMT (7%), and MI (2%). Notably, its combination with robotics and exoskeletons (14%) for dynamic assistance as needed has been shown to expedite the recovery process [17, 27, 28, 55].

Virtual reality (VR), augmented reality (AR), and mixed reality (MR) have shown significant positive effects on improving upper limb (UL) recovery and activities of daily living (ADL) in stroke rehabilitation [46]. These technologies have been found to be superior to conventional treatment in UL impairment and daily function outcomes. VR, AR, and MR have demonstrated promising clinical outcomes in stroke rehabilitation, particularly in improving upper extremity motor function, upper extremity activity, participation, functional independence, balance, functional mobility, and cognitive function [46, 51, 60].

VR, AR, and MR have demonstrated a variety of advantages concerning functional capacity, encompassing enhancements in functional capacity assessed by the Functional Independence Measure (FIM) (2% of reviewed works), the Action Research Arm Test (ARAT) (16%), the Box and Block Test (BBT) (12%), and the Fugl-Meyer Assessment (FMA) (37%) of physical performance, strength, and balance outcomes.

These technologies have the potential to maximize recovery through increased motivation and adherence, particularly in the rehabilitation of stroke patients' hand motor skills. However, the evidence demonstrating considerably distinct effects of VR as opposed to traditional rehabilitation on cognitive function and participation was insufficient, indicating the need for further and advanced studies [22, 43, 51].

The literature often misuses the terms VR, AR, and MR to describe tools that do not fully meet the definitions, such as PC video games, flat displays, and QR codes. It is crucial to clarify VR and AR terminology, distinguishing between immersive and non-immersive VR and AR. Immersive applications create a deep sense of presence using equipment like head-mounted displays (HMDs) or VR goggles, allowing extensive interaction through free navigation and specialized input devices. Non-immersive VR, on the other hand, offers less immersion and relies on regular screens and conventional input methods like keyboards and touchscreens. Evidence shows that immersive VR can induce a strong sense of presence, leading to realistic responses to virtual stimuli and physiological reactions similar to real-life experiences [51]. Immersion is also more effective for upper extremity motor recovery. The feeling of presence allows people to react authentically to virtual stimuli, eliciting physiological reactions similar to those experienced in an actual environment. Future research should focus on identifying the best VR, AR, or MR treatment protocols for promoting upper limb recovery.

Despite the growth of VR and AR usage in poststroke upper limb rehabilitation, published VR research to date often does not extend beyond pilot trials and case studies. As mentioned in Ref. [43], given the lack of large-scale RCTs examining the clinical effectiveness of immersive VR for poststroke, research on evaluating effectiveness and engagement is still valid.

Presently, robot-assisted systems are not fully harnessing the capabilities of VR. Many systems that integrate virtual reality with exoskeletons and robotics operate within simulated environments displayed on flat screens, despite having been designed for three-dimensional scenarios [58].

Virtual reality (VR), augmented reality (AR), and mixed reality (MR) technologies present various hardware-related limitations, particularly when developing applications with high graphical demands. In such cases, latency issues and significant increases in device temperature are common, affecting sustained performance. One critical factor in these environments is battery life, as headsets—being portable and continuously rendering complex graphics—exhibit limited autonomy. Additionally, tracking of hands, eyes, or the environment can be impaired by unfavorable lighting conditions, such as dim, excessive, or reflective environments. In the case of AR, the limited field of view for holograms remains a challenge, reducing immersion in prolonged experiences. In VR, physical movement becomes a constraint, as the user, fully immersed in a virtual space, may accidentally collide with real-world objects. Furthermore, the weight of the devices can cause discomfort or physical fatigue during extended use.

In this specific project, Meta Quest 3 headsets were used, which exhibit some of the aforementioned limitations. One of the most relevant issues is the sensitivity of the hand-tracking system to lighting conditions. Environments with poor or excessive lighting, or with reflective surfaces, significantly affect tracking accuracy. Additionally, if the hands are too close to the headset or if controllers are used simultaneously, gesture recognition may suffer from interference or inconsistency. For this reason, it is advisable to configure the application to operate exclusively with hand tracking if that is the intended input method. It is also important to avoid hand overlap or crossing, as this can cause temporary loss of tracking. High graphical loads within the application directly impact the headset's performance, making it essential to optimize resource usage and set the refresh rate to the highest possible level. Finally, frequent updates to the Meta Guardian system and software development kit (SDK) may alter the behavior of the virtual environment, so regular compatibility checks are necessary.

In order to demonstrate what these technologies are capable of, we developed a hardware-software framework that integrates a mixed reality (MR) system with an exoskeleton, offering support based on patients' EMG signals. The architecture of this platform allows for the assessment of various intervention combinations using VR, AR, and MR, exoskeleton feedback, and EMG signals.

4.1 Challenges and limitations

The use of VR, AR, and MR in stroke rehabilitation presents challenges such as the need for further high-quality trials that examine their effects on measures of UL function, with an emphasis on subgroup meta-analysis by stroke type and recovery stage.

Despite promising outcomes, high-quality evidence for the routine use of VR in stroke treatment is lacking, and further research is needed to determine the treatment modality, duration, and long-term effects of these technologies on stroke populations.

5. Conclusions

Immersive technologies such as VR, AR, and MR have shown a strong potential to improve upper limb function and daily activities in poststroke rehabilitation. These technologies offer interactive, task-specific environments that improve motor function, cognitive engagement, and daily living activities. Notably, immersive systems, those utilizing head-mounted displays and motion tracking, have shown superior outcomes compared to non-immersive setups, largely due to their ability to evoke realistic physiological responses and a heightened sense of presence. However, more large-scale clinical trials are needed to confirm their long-term effectiveness.

Given this consideration, a novel hardware-software platform integrating a mixed reality (MR) system with an exoskeleton capable of offering assistance based on patients' EMG signals is introduced. This architectural framework is designed for assessing various intervention combinations utilizing virtual reality (VR), augmented reality (AR), MR, exoskeleton feedback, and EMG signals.

Acknowledgements

This work was funded by the project "iREHAB: Sistema inteligente de Rehabilitación usando un Exoesqueleto para recuperar Habilidad motora en discapacidades post-ACV, usando señales Biológicas del paciente" sponsored by the Ministry of Science, Technology and Innovation (MinCiencias), program 918-2022 under GRANT CTO: 622-2022, Award ID: 91805.

Abbreviations

VR	virtual reality
AR	augmented reality
MR	mixed reality
DALYs	disability-adjusted life years
CIMT	constraint-induced movement therapy
MI	motor imagery
AO	action observation
TOT	task-oriented therapy
BAT	bilateral arm training (BAT)
ST	strength training (ST)
ROM	range of motion (ROM)
MP	mental practice
FES	functional electrical stimulation
HMD	head-mounted displays
CAVE	cave automatic virtual environment
PRISMA-ScR	preferred reporting items for systematic review and meta-analyses extension for scoping reviews
FMA	Fugl-Meyer Assessment
FMA-UE	Fugl-Meyer Assessment Upper Extremity
BBT	box and block test
NHPT	nine-hole peg test
WMFT	wolf motor function test
BI	Barthel Index (BI)
MBI	Modified Barthel Index (MBI)
SSQOL	stroke-specific quality of life
ARAT	action research arm test

FIM	functional independence measure
PAS	performance assessment of self-care skills
SUS	system usability scale
SSQ	simulator sickness questionnaire
ADL	activities of daily living
EMG	electromyography
EEG	electroencephalography
BLE	bluetooth low energy
YOLOv5	you only look once version 5 (computer vision model for real-time object detection)

A. Appendix

Technology	Intervention method	Assessment	Engagement	Main results	Ref.
HTC VIVE Pro, Leap Motion controller				No significant difference between immersive vs. non-immersive in fNIRS.	[25]
HTC VIVE, Leap Motion Controller tracking technology	Bilateral training	BI/MBI		The VR group has significant improvements in FM-UE scores compared to the control group.	[39]
HMD HTC and Oculus Rift + HTC VIVE motion trackers + SteamVR drivers + EEG + BCI emotion detection	CIMT	EEG/EMG		Home-based system effective with emotion/adherence feedback.	[14]
HMD VR + 7° DOF exoskeleton	Robotic-assisted exoskeleton	FMA + WMFT		Patients increased the score in both the FMA and WMFT assessments. Subjects did not experience any problems when handling the device during the intervention.	[44]
Meta Quest 2 HMD + Iterative VR serious game with usability ratings			SUS (or equivalent)	Ease of use and feasibility for patients with limited hand function.	[15]
HTC VIVE PRO EYE, Unity3D Game Engine + VR basketball task with MI + AO + EMG/EEG	Motor imagery + Bilateral training	BI/MBI + EEG/EMG		Motor imagery + Action observation showed the strongest neural/muscular response. Generate more pronounced Event-related Desynchronization (ERD) in the alpha band.	[26]
Z800 3DVisor + eMagin + Imaging Development Systems cameras				Users improved across tasks; suitable for long-term use. High motivation, significant performance increase.	[56]
Time-of-Flight (ToF) camera, IR stereo camera, head-mounted display (HMD)		BI/MBI	Cognition	Significant gradual recovery of the patients' skills.	[45]
HMD VIVE-P130, HTC + upper limb exoskeleton robotic arm with CNN + SE BCI interface	Robotic-assisted exoskeleton	BI/MBI + EEG/EMG	Neuroplasticity + Cognition	VR + Upper limb exoskeleton enhanced motor imagery (MI) model improved task success (up to 88.48%), especially in exoskeleton control.	[27]
HTC VIVE virtual reality headset + EEG-based brain-computer interfaces (BCIs) + Valve Index Knuckle Controllers		EEG/EMG		Informative artifacts are a helpful friend in BCI-based communication applications.	[34]

Technology	Intervention method	Assessment	Engagement	Main results	Ref.
Meta Quest 2 head-mounted display (HMD) + Oculus App Version			SUS (or equivalent)	Virtual environments add value to motivation and engagement in VR stroke rehabilitation.	[16]
HTC VIVE headset + Leap Motion controller + Intelligent glove	Robotic-assisted exoskeleton + Bilateral training	EEG/EMG		Multimodal feedback improved EEG alpha power and EMG in traumatic brain injury (TBI) patients. Neurotypicals' performance worsened with additional visual cues.	[28]
Soft robotic glove + Virtual reality glasses holder + NirSmart fNIRS system	Robotic-assisted exoskeleton + Bilateral training			Robotic glove joint with VR tasks induced activation of larger cortical areas, with the stroke group showing higher average cortical activation measured with a functional near-infrared spectroscopy (fNIRS) device.	[17]
VR HMD motor rehabilitation serious game			Exergaming	VR rehabilitation serious game design framework improves long-term patient engagement.	[18]
Cell phone-based immersive VR goggles	Mirror therapy	FMA	SUS (or equivalent) + NASA-TLX	Both mirror therapy (MT) and VR had similar levels of perceived usability based on the SUS test, with MT being more adaptable and causing less overall discomfort.	[29]
HTC VIVE Focus 3 + Custom-built system with Unity/Blender	Mirror therapy		SUS (or equivalent) + SSQ	The VR mirrored-hand system shows promise for clinical application in poststroke upper limb rehabilitation.	[11]
DK2 Oculus Rift + Oculus Rift controller	Bilateral training	EEG/EMG		Both VR-based bilateral arm training (VRBAT) and normal-based bilateral arm training (NBAT) improve UL function (motor test) and electroencephalographic EEG activity in patients with chronic stroke.	[40]
Leap Motion device mounted on HMD (not defined)		FMA + FIM		All scores improved more in the VR group; FMA-UE and ARAT exceeded clinical significance thresholds. Immersive VR rehabilitation is effective in improving upper extremity function and self-care skills, but not for functional independence.	[47]
Oculus Quest 2 virtual reality device. Four VR games with full immersion (specific hand motion design)		FMA + BBT + BI/MBI	SSQ	Using immersive VR for poststroke motor rehabilitation is potentially effective, safe, and acceptable in poststroke patients. The VR group showed significantly better outcomes in FMA, MBI, BBT, and stroke-specific quality of life (SSQOL).	[19]

Technology	Intervention method	Assessment	Engagement	Main results	Ref.
HMD HTC VIVE Pro + wireless handheld controller for interaction with exercise system		FMA + WMFT		Patients show clinical benefits after 2 weeks, demonstrated in the outcome of active range of motion (AROM), perceived upper limb motor function, and quality of life (QoL). In addition, statistically significant improvements in coordination/speed (Fugl-Meyer Assessment for Upper Extremity).	[30]
HMD VR with action observation + focal vibration	Mirror therapy	BBT + NHPT		An improvement in the NHPT score was found for the paretic upper limb during the B-phase. No differences were found in the Box and Block Test.	[12]
"HTC VIVE HMD + IR emitters + five VR tasks		FMA + BI/MBI	Neuroplasticity	Significant biomarker and motor improvement in the VR group. Results found significant the AROM-Elbow Extension, AROM-Forearm Pronation, and FMA-UE-Shoulder/Elbow/Forearm.	[35]
""Vive (HTC) HMD + fish-catching task game				VR outperformed conventional and AR settings for grasp tasks. Results in rehabilitation therapy by improving patients' motivation and willingness to participate in, by demonstrating changes in the Test of Upper Limb Apraxia (TULIA).	[41]
"HMD (Oculus Rift DK2) + Leap Motion sensor	CIMT			Immersive virtual reality (IVR) with visual enhancement can positively influence hand-use decision-making, even after the visual feedback is removed. This suggests a lasting neurocognitive effect that could support the use of the impaired limb in stroke rehabilitation.	[42]
HMD HTC VIVE-VR + 2 wireless controllers		FMA		Immersive VR-based rehabilitation improves upper limb motor recovery and quality of life in stroke patients more effectively than traditional therapy.	[48]
Large screen 3D + Microsoft Kinect + Gamified VR-based upper limb training (custom)		FMA + WMFT		Individuals with stroke demonstrated reduced paretic arm motor impairment and increased function after the intervention with gamified practice.	[20]

Technology	Intervention method	Assessment	Engagement	Main results	Ref.
HMD (HTC VIVE)				System usability and acceptance were rated as high both in stroke patients and healthy controls, showing high usability and minimal adverse effects when using VR therapy.	[49]
HMD (Oculus Rift) + Leap Motion sensor + real-time feedback	CIMT	FMA	Neuroplasticity	The VR group showed improved upper limb function vs. control. The IVR group exhibited significant improvements in FMA scores, suggesting motor learning and recovery. The patients were highly engaged and motivated during the sessions because they felt like they were in charge of controlling the virtual image of their upper body.	[13]
HMD -Oculus Rift + tabletop infrared LED sensors + hand controllers	Mirror therapy	FMA	SUS (or equivalent) + SSQ	Immersive virtual reality (IVR) mirror therapy for patients with chronic stroke was safe, well-tolerated, and without adverse events, such as simulator sickness. Motor outcomes revealed improvement for the Fugl-Meyer Upper Extremity.	[50]
HMD Oculus Quest + VR apps for pain distraction and upper limb rehab		FMA		VR can be implemented in both clinical settings and people's own homes, where engagement in ongoing self-management approaches is often most challenging.	[43]
HMD (HTC VIVE-VR) + wireless controllers		FMA + BI/MBI		Trials on 40 patients divided into intention-to-treat (ITT) and per-protocol (PP) demonstrated the effectiveness of imVR-based rehabilitation. Significant gains in FM-UE and BI correlated with brain connectivity shifts.	[21]
KINVIS therapy with therapeutic exercise. Kinesthetic illusion using visual stimulation (KINVIS) with VR	Mirror Therapy	FMA + MAS		Kinesthetic illusion induced by visual stimulation, KINVIS therapy with VR, resulted in significant improvements in upper limb motor function, and the effect size was moderate.	[36]
HTC VIVE Pro + HTC VIVE tracker + Myo Armband EMG sensors + IMU	Mirror therapy	BBT + EEG/EMG	Neuroplasticity + SUS (or equivalent) + SSQ	VR shows positive outcomes from SUS and PQ, negligible adverse symptoms, and no significant distinctions between visual feedback configurations. Bimanual feedback improved task illusion and was highly usable.	[22]

Technology	Intervention method	Assessment	Engagement	Main results	Ref.
HTC VIVE Pro + HTC VIVE trackers; Meta 2 AR-HMD. 2D screen				IVR and AR show better performance compared with the 2D screen VR system. Comparison shows improved movement quality, high usability, preliminary clinical results, and suggests benefits for brain-injured patients. IVR using HMD yielded better movements; usability was rated high in the elderly and patients.	[37]
CUREO® immersive (HMD (Oculus Quest) vs. ARMEOSpring® device)				IVR-based training was not inferior to electromechanically assisted training, with 84% of patients showing improvement. IVR led to more patients achieving clinically relevant gains than EM-assisted training.	[31]
HTC VIVE HMD bimanual action (game-like system)	Robotic-assisted exoskeleton	EEG/EMG		Using VR with visual feedback is adequate for transferring coordination skills to the paretic hand, improving cortical network efficiency measured using EEG.	[32]
HTC VIVE HMD, 5 VR tasks		BBT + BI/MBI		Rehabilitation therapy using virtual reality (VR) shows significant functional improvement in all outcome measures (MBI, BBT, ARAT) after training. Also shows high overall satisfaction assessed using a self-reported questionnaire.	[53]
HMD Pico 3 VR		BI/MBI	SUS (or equivalent)	IVR based on five scenarios for rehabilitation. The result of the User Satisfaction Evaluation Questionnaire and the modified Intrinsic Motivation Inventory shows varied levels of enjoyment and engagement and recommendations for tailoring scenarios to match varied upper limb capacities.	[23]
Oculus Quest 2 VR, App Virtual Mirror Hand 1.0	Mirror therapy	FMA	SUS (or equivalent)	VR mirror therapy results in a positive upper limb functionality score by FMA-UE, and SF-36 improvements occurred in both the study and the control group.	[33]
HTC VIVE		BBT + BI/MBI		Head-mounted-display VR has potential for upper extremity rehabilitation in individuals with chronic stroke.	[54]

Technology	Intervention method	Assessment	Engagement	Main results	Ref.
HMD Oculus Rift DK2	Task-specific training + Robotic-assisted exoskeleton	FMA + BI/MBI	Neuroplasticity	System combining adaptive assist-as-needed control (hand rehab robot) and immersive virtual environment (VE) enhances the efficiency of fine hand motion rehabilitation training by 35% on average on FMA, MAS, and kinematic ROM.	[55]
Meta Quest 2 device SDKs + computer vision algorithms for hand and finger tracking			SUS (or equivalent) + NASA-TLX + Exergaming	VR in a home-based environment has demonstrated that users and experts have received the application positively when it is tested considering standard measures related to usability, immersion, workload, and simulator sickness (SUS, NASA-TLX, and Simulator Sickness Questionnaire (SSQ)).	[24]
HMD Oculus CV1 + Leap Motion sensor	Mirror therapy	FMA + BI/MBI	SUS (or equivalent)	Immersive VR systems and mirror therapy protocols are feasible for clinical use. A large part of the participants showed some improvement in their affected hand after the intervention. Someone reported experiencing some psycho-physical effects, such as tingling or paresthesia on the affected limb.	[38]

Table 3.
Characteristics included works.

Author details

Iván F. Mondragón B.[1*†], Wilson A. Henández M.[1†], Catalina Alvarado-Rojas[1†], Diego Mendez[1†], Jeronimo Rueda[1†], David E. González[1†], Guillermo A. Aguilera[1†] and Julian D. Colorado[1,2†]

1 Pontificia Universidad Javeriana, School of Engineering, Carrera, Bogotá, DC, Colombia

2 The Omics Science Research Institute, iOMICAS, Pontificia Universidad Javeriana, Cali, Colombia

*Address all correspondence to: imondragon@javeriana.edu.co

† These authors contributed equally.

References

[1] Organization WH. World Health Statistics 2023: Monitoring Health for the Sdgs, Sustainable Development Goals. Vol. 27. Geneva: World Health Organization; 2023

[2] Pu L, Wang L, Zhang R, Zhao T, Jiang Y, Han L. Projected global trends in ischemic stroke incidence, deaths and disability-adjusted life years from 2020 to 2030. Stroke. 2023;**54**(5):1330-1339

[3] Teasell R, Hussein N, Mirkowski M, Vanderlaan D, Saikaley M, Longval M, et al. Stroke rehabilitation clinician handbook. Heart and Stroke Foundation. 2020;**1**(4):1-60

[4] Wang H, Arceo R, Chen S, Ding L, Jia J, Yao J. Effectiveness of interventions to improve hand motor function in individuals with moderate to severe stroke: A systematic review protocol. BMJ Open. 2019;**9**(9):e032413

[5] Everard G, Declerck L, Detrembleur C, Leonard S, Bower G, Dehem S, et al. New technologies promoting active upper limb rehabilitation after stroke: An overview and network meta-analysis. European Journal of Physical and Rehabilitation Medicine. Aug 2022;**58**(4):530-548. Minerva Medica. DOI: 10.23736/S1973-9087.22.07404-4

[6] Doerner R, Broll W, Jung B, Grimm P, Göbel M, Kruse R. Introduction to Virtual and Augmented Reality. Cham, Switzerland: Springer International Publishing; 2022. pp. 1-37

[7] Muhanna MA. Virtual reality and the CAVE: Taxonomy, interaction challenges and research directions. Journal of King Saud University - Computer and Information Sciences. 2015;**27**(3):344-361. ISSN 1319-1578

[8] Tricco AC, Lillie E, Zarin W, O'Brien KK, Colquhoun H, Levac D, et al. PRISMA extension for scoping reviews (PRISMA-ScR): Checklist and explanation. Annals of Internal Medicine. 2018;**169**(169):467-473

[9] van Eck NJ, Waltman L. Software survey: VOSviewer, a computer program for bibliometric mapping. Scientometrics. 2010;**84**:523-538

[10] Peters MDJ, Marnie C, Tricco AC, Pollock D, Munn Z, Alexander L, et al. Updated methodological guidance for the conduct of scoping reviews. JBI Evidence Synthesis. 2020;**18**(10):2119-2126

[11] Hsieh YW, Howe TH, Lee MT, Tai RY, Chen CC. Design and usability evaluation of an immersive virtual reality mirrored hand system for upper limb stroke rehabilitation. Scientific Reports. 2025;**15**:5781

[12] Adamo P, Leo DD, Fava T, Binda S, Avanzini P, Fabbri-Destro M, et al. Effects of immersive virtual reality-based action observation training integrated with focal muscle vibration on upper extremity in a patient with chronic disability following stroke: A single-subject study. Physiotherapy Theory and Practice. 2025;**3**:1-9

[13] Altukhaim S, Sakabe N, Nagaratnam K, Mannava N, Kondo T, Hayashi Y. Immersive virtual reality enhanced reinforcement induced physical therapy (EVEREST). Displays. 2025;**87**:102962

[14] Shih CH, Lin PJ, Chen YL, Chen SL. A post-stroke rehabilitation system with compensatory movement detection using virtual reality and electroencephalogram technologies. IEEE Access. 2024;**12**:61418-61432

[15] Bressler M, Merk J, Gohlke T, Kayali F, Daigeler A, Kolbenschlag J, et al. A virtual reality serious game for the rehabilitation of hand and finger function: Iterative development and suitability study. JMIR Serious Games. 2024;**12**:e54193

[16] Zuki FSM, Sulaiman S, Mérienne F, Ricca A, Guillet C, Saad MNM. Assessing the impact of enriched virtual reality on motivation and engagement in stroke rehabilitation. IEEE Access. 2024;**12**:143585-143598

[17] Liu P, Yang X, Han F, Peng G, Li Q, Huang L, et al. Brain activation pattern caused by soft rehabilitation glove and virtual reality scenes: A pilot fNIRS study. IEEE Transactions on Neural Systems and Rehabilitation Engineering. 2024;**32**:3848-3857

[18] Zhang C, Yu S, Ji J. CFI: A VR motor rehabilitation serious game design framework integrating rehabilitation function and game design principles with an upper limb case. Journal of NeuroEngineering and Rehabilitation. 2024;**21**:113

[19] Amin F, Waris A, Syed S, Amjad I, Umar M, Iqbal J, et al. Effectiveness of immersive virtual reality-based hand rehabilitation games for improving hand motor functions in subacute stroke patients. IEEE Transactions on Neural Systems and Rehabilitation Engineering. 2024;**32**:2060-2069

[20] Rubino C, Lakhani B, Larssen BC, Kraeutner SN, Andrushko JW, Borich MR, et al. Gamified practice improves paretic arm motor behavior in individuals with stroke. Neurorehabilitation and Neural Repair. 2024;**38**:832-844

[21] Huang Q, Jiang X, Jin Y, Wu B, Vigotsky AD, Fan L, et al. Immersive virtual reality-based rehabilitation for subacute stroke: A randomized controlled trial. Journal of Neurology. 2024;**271**(3):1256-1266

[22] Capsi-Morales P, Geier T, Hermsdörfer J, Piazza C. Impact of visual feedback configurations in a task-oriented immersive virtual reality Mirror therapy. IEEE Transactions on Neural Systems and Rehabilitation Engineering. 2024;**32**:3923-3932

[23] Isbel S, Holloway H, Greber C, Nguyen K, Frost J, Pearce C, et al. Virtual reality after stroke: Identifying important characteristics when designing experiences to improve engagement in upper limb rehabilitation. Digital Health. 2024;**1**:10

[24] Bedendo V, Aruanno B, Dozio N, Covarrubias M, Ferrise F, Bordegoni M. Exploiting virtual reality to design exercises for the recovery of stroke patients at home. Computer-Aided Design and Applications. 2023;**9**:463-473

[25] Dordevic M, Maile O, Das A, Kundu S, Haun C, Baier B, et al. A comparison of immersive vs. non-immersive virtual reality exercises for the upper limb: A functional near-infrared spectroscopy pilot study with healthy participants. Journal of Clinical Medicine. 2023;**12**:5781

[26] Lin M, Huang J, Fu J, Sun Y, Fang Q. A VR-based motor imagery training system with EMG-based real-time feedback for post-stroke rehabilitation. IEEE Transactions on Neural Systems and Rehabilitation Engineering. 2023;**31**:1-10

[27] Tang Z, Wang H, Cui Z, Jin X, Zhang L, Peng Y, et al. An upper-limb rehabilitation exoskeleton system controlled by MI recognition model with deep emphasized informative features in a VR scene. IEEE Transactions on Neural

Systems and Rehabilitation Engineering. 2023;**31**:4390-4401

[28] Liu M, Wilder S, Sanford S, Glassen M, Dewil S, Saleh S, et al. Augmented feedback modes during functional grasp training with an intelligent glove and virtual reality for persons with traumatic brain injury. Frontiers in Robotics and AI. 2023;**11**:10

[29] da Silva JE, Figueiredo AI, Schiavo A, Loss BP, da Silveira GH, Sangalli VA, et al. Conventional Mirror therapy versus immersive virtual reality Mirror therapy: The perceived usability after stroke. Stroke Research and Treatment. 2023;**2023**:1-8

[30] Chen J, Or CK, Li Z, Yeung EHK, Zhou Y, Hao T. Effectiveness, safety and patients' perceptions of an immersive virtual reality–based exercise system for poststroke upper limb motor rehabilitation: A proof-of-concept and feasibility randomized controlled trial. Digital Health. 2023;**1**:9

[31] Lülsdorff K, Junker FB, Studer B, Wittenberg H, Pickenbrock H, Schmidt-Wilcke T. Neurorehabilitation of the upper extremity – Immersive virtual reality vs. electromechanically assisted training. A comparative study. Frontiers in Neurology. 2023;**14**:1290637, 01-09. Frontiers Media. DOI: 10.3389/fneur.2023.1290637

[32] Long J, Shen L, Cai Q, Xiao S, Chen Z. Novel approach to transfer of coordination skills to the paretic hand by improving the efficiency of cortical network. IEEE Transactions on Neural Systems and Rehabilitation Engineering. 2023;**31**:326-334

[33] Sip P, Kozłowska M, Czysz D, Daroszewski P, Lisiński P. Perspectives of motor functional upper extremity recovery with the use of immersive virtual reality in stroke patients. Sensors. 2023;**23**:712

[34] McDermott EJ, Raggam P, Kirsch S, Belardinelli P, Ziemann U, Zrenner C. Artifacts in EEG-based BCI therapies: Friend or foe? Sensors. 2021;**22**:96

[35] Huang CY, Chiang WC, Yeh YC, Fan SC, Yang WH, Kuo HC, et al. Effects of virtual reality-based motor control training on inflammation, oxidative stress, neuroplasticity and upper limb motor function in patients with chronic stroke: A randomized controlled trial. BMC Neurology. 2022;**22**(1):21

[36] Kuwahara W, Miyawaki Y, Kaneko F. Impact of the upper limb physiotherapy on Behavioral and brain adaptations in post-stroke patients. Journal of Robotics and Mechatronics. 2022;**34**:718-725

[37] Wenk N, Buetler KA, Penalver-Andres J, Müri RM, Marchal-Crespo L. Naturalistic visualization of reaching movements using head-mounted displays improves movement quality compared to conventional computer screens and proves high usability. Journal of NeuroEngineering and Rehabilitation. 2022;**12**(19):137

[38] Heinrich C, Morkisch N, Langlotz T, Regenbrecht H, Dohle C. Feasibility and psychophysical effects of immersive virtual reality-based mirror therapy. Journal of NeuroEngineering and Rehabilitation. 2022;**19**:107

[39] Mekbib DB, Debeli DK, Zhang L, Fang S, Shao Y, Yang W, et al. A novel fully immersive virtual reality environment for upper extremity rehabilitation in patients with stroke. Annals of the New York Academy of Sciences. 2021;**1493**:75-89

[40] Song YH, Lee HM. Effect of immersive virtual reality-based

bilateral arm training in patients with chronic stroke. Brain Sciences. 2021;**11**(8):1032

[41] Park W, Kim J, Kim M. Efficacy of virtual reality therapy in ideomotor apraxia rehabilitation. Medicine. 2021;**100**:e26657

[42] Sakabe N, Altukhaim S, Hayashi Y, Sakurada T, Yano S, Kondo T. Enhanced visual feedback using immersive VR affects decision making regarding hand use with a simulated impaired limb. Frontiers in Human Neuroscience. 2021;**6**:15

[43] Tran JE, Fowler CA, Delikat J, Kaplan H, Merzier MM, Schlesinger MR, et al. Immersive virtual reality to improve outcomes in veterans with stroke: Protocol for a single-arm pilot study. JMIR Research Protocols. 2021;**10**(5):e26133

[44] Yu H, Xie L, Lv C, Shao W, Wang Y, Wang J, et al. A system for upper limb rehabilitation and motor function evaluation. Journal of Mechanics in Medicine and Biology. 2015;**15**:1550010

[45] Avola D, Cinque L, Foresti GL, Marini MR. An interactive and low-cost full body rehabilitation framework based on 3D immersive serious games. Journal of Biomedical Informatics. 2019;**89**:81-100

[46] Kim WS, Cho S, Ku J, Kim Y, Lee K, Hwang HJ, et al. Clinical application of virtual reality for upper limb motor rehabilitation in stroke: Review of technologies and clinical evidence. Journal of Clinical Medicine. 2020;**9**(10):3369

[47] Ögün MN, Kurul R, Yaşar MF, Turkoglu SA, Avci Ş, Yildiz N. Effect of leap motion-based 3D immersive virtual reality usage on upper extremity function in ischemic stroke patients. Arquivos de Neuro-Psiquiatria. 2019;**77**(10):681-688

[48] Huang Q, Wu W, Chen X, Wu B, Wu L, Huang X, et al. Evaluating the effect and mechanism of upper limb motor function recovery induced by immersive virtual-reality-based rehabilitation for subacute stroke subjects: Study protocol for a randomized controlled trial. Trials. 2019;**20**:104

[49] Knobel SEJ, Kaufmann BC, Gerber SM, Cazzoli D, Müri RM, Nyffeler T, et al. Immersive 3D virtual reality cancellation task for visual neglect assessment: A pilot study. Frontiers in Human Neuroscience. 2020;**5**:14

[50] Weber LM, Nilsen DM, Gillen G, Yoon J, Stein J. Immersive virtual reality Mirror therapy for upper limb recovery after stroke. American Journal of Physical Medicine & Rehabilitation. 2019;**98**(9):783-788

[51] Ceradini M, Losanno E, Micera S, Bandini A, Orlandi S. Immersive VR for upper-extremity rehabilitation in patients with neurological disorders: A scoping review. Journal of NeuroEngineering and Rehabilitation. 2024;**21**:75

[52] Matamala-Gomez M, Slater M, Sanchez-Vives MV. Impact of virtual embodiment and exercises on functional ability and range of motion in orthopedic rehabilitation. Scientific Reports. 2022;**12**:5046

[53] Lee SH, Jung H, Yun SJ, Oh B, Seo HG. Upper extremity rehabilitation using fully immersive virtual reality games with a head mount display: A feasibility study. PM&R. 2020;**12**(3):257-262

[54] Erhardsson M, Murphy MA, Sunnerhagen KS. Commercial

head-mounted display virtual reality for upper extremity rehabilitation in chronic stroke: A single-case design study. Journal of NeuroEngineering and Rehabilitation. 2020;**12**(17):154

[55] Huang X, Naghdy F, Du H, Naghdy G, Murray G. Design of adaptive control and virtual reality-based fine hand motion rehabilitation system and its effects in subacute stroke patients. Computer Methods in Biomechanics and Biomedical Engineering: Imaging & Visualization. 2017;7:1-9

[56] Trojan J, Diers M, Fuchs X, Bach F, Bekrater-Bodmann R, Foell J, et al. An augmented reality home-training system based on the mirror training and imagery approach. Behavior Research Methods. 2014;**9**(46):634-640

[57] Tuominen PPA, Saarni LA. The use of virtual technologies with music in rehabilitation: A scoping systematic review. Frontiers in Virtual Reality. 2024;**5**:5

[58] Oña ED, Garcia-Haro JM, Jardón A, Balaguer C. Robotics in health care: Perspectives of robot-aided interventions in clinical practice for rehabilitation of upper limbs. Applied Sciences. 2019;**9**:2586

[59] Khan A, Imam YZ, Muneer M, Jerdi SA, Gill SK. Virtual reality in stroke recovery: A meta-review of systematic reviews. Bioelectronic Medicine. 2024;**10**:23

[60] Khizhnikova AE, Klochkov AS, Kotov-Smolenskiy AM, Suponeva NA, Chernikova LA. Virtual reality as an upper limb rehabilitation approach. Human Physiology. 2017;**43**:855-862

[61] Rodrigues P, Quaresma C, Costa M, Luz F, Fonseca MM. Virtual Reality-Based Telerehabilitation for Upper Limb Recovery Post-Stroke: A Systematic Review of Design Principles, Monitoring, Safety, and Engagement Strategies. arXiv:2501.06899. 2025. DOI: 10.48550/arXiv.2501.06899

[62] Castiblanco JC, Mondragon IF, Alvarado-Rojas C, Colorado JD. Assist-as-needed exoskeleton for hand joint rehabilitation based on muscle effort detection. Sensors (Basel). 2021;**21**(13):4372, 01-16. MDPI. DOI: 10.3390/s21134372

[63] Bonilla D, Bravo M, Bonilla SP, Iragorri AM, Mendez D, Mondragon IF, et al. Progressive rehabilitation based on EMG gesture classification and an MPC-driven exoskeleton. Bioengineering. 2023;**6**(10):770

[64] Jocher G. ultralytics/yolov5: v7.0 - YOLOv5 SOTA realtime instance segmentation (v7.0). 2022. Available from: https://GithubCom/Ultralytics/Yolov5/Tree/V70

Section 2

Aging, Frailty, and Postural Control

Chapter 4

Age-Related Changes in Upper Limb Motor Function, Focusing on Bimanual Coordination

Yusuke Shizuka, Shun Sawai, Takato Nishida, Shoya Fujikawa, Ryosuke Yamamoto, Naoki Shimizu and Hideki Nakano

Abstract

In an international society where the elderly population is increasing annually, developing preventive measures to extend healthy life expectancy and support independence in activities of daily living is considered one of the most critical issues. It has been pointed out that upper limb function in older adults declines with age, especially in bimanual coordination, and that this decline significantly impacts daily life. Therefore, it is essential to properly evaluate, maintain, and improve bimanual coordination in older adults so that they can lead healthy lives. In this chapter, we review the latest findings on bimanual coordination performance in older adults and outline aging-related changes. The motor control mechanisms of bimanual coordination and specific measurement methods are also introduced.

Keywords: older adults, age-related changes, upper limb motor function, bimanual coordination, motor control mechanisms

1. Introduction

1.1 Relationship between the current aging society and the activities of daily living of the older adult

The proportion of older adults worldwide has increased in recent years. According to the United Nations World Population Prospects 2022, the global proportion of older adults—defined as individuals aged 65 years and older—is projected to increase from less than 10% in 2021 to approximately 17% by 2050. The global population of older adults is projected to triple from approximately 260 million in 1980 to 761 million in 2021, quadruple to over one billion by 2030, and rise to more than 1.6 billion by 2050. The global population of older adults is expected to reach nearly 2.5 billion by the end of the twenty-first century [1]. According to the United Nations World Social Report 2023, one in ten people worldwide was aged 65 or older in 2021, and by 2050, one in six people will be in this age group [2]. These facts indicate that life expectancy is increasing worldwide, and the rate of population aging is much faster than in the past.

It is becoming increasingly difficult for older adults to lead independent lives. Age-related changes may affect independent living in older adults [3]. A decline in physical function, including muscle strength, endurance, and walking speed, is associated with the loss of the ability to live independently and poses a challenge to public health [4]. Cognitive decline makes it difficult for patients to perform activities of daily living, including bathing, toileting, and instrumental activities of daily living, such as using the telephone, taking medications, and managing money [5]. In addition, physical and cognitive decline contribute to reduced motivation in daily life as social networks decrease [6], and psychological functions—including self-efficacy, anxiety, and depression—can become problematic [7]. In light of the above, it is essential to maintain and improve the physical, cognitive, social, and psychological functions of older adults so they can lead independent lives in familiar settings.

In recent years, the relationship between independence in activities of daily living and upper limb dysfunction in older adults has become clear [8]. Therefore, there is a close relationship between upper limb function and activities of daily living in older adults. Older adults frequently use their upper limbs because they often move and manipulate objects during daily lives [9]. The age-related decline in upper limb function decreases the ability to perform activities of daily living, such as eating and changing clothes [10]. It has been suggested that the decline in upper limb function in older adults may also be a factor limiting their activities, affecting their quality of life and independence in daily living [11].

Therefore, we believe that it is necessary to focus on upper limb function to improve the independence of older adults in their daily lives.

1.2 Upper limb function and age-related changes in older adults

We previously described the potential impact of decreased upper limb function on activities of daily living in older adults. Upper limb function includes joint range of motion, muscle strength, and sensation. Bland et al. administered the Jebsen–Taylor hand function test to 18 young adults (mean age 27 ± 4 years) and 15 older adults (mean age 67 ± 6 years) under restricted upper extremity joint range of motion. Previous studies have reported that the completion time for the Jebsen–Taylor hand function test is longer in older adults than in young adults when movements of the elbow, forearm, wrist, and fingers are deliberately restricted [12]. Delbaere et al. evaluated isometric and isokinetic maximal muscle strength in the upper extremities of 111 men and women aged 20–89 years. It has been reported that maximal muscle strength decreases with age, ranging from 34 to 45% in men and 11–32% in women [13]. Grip strength, a measure of upper limb muscle strength, declines with age. Therefore, longitudinal changes in grip strength are associated with lifestyle and health status in older adults, suggesting its potential as an indicator of healthy aging [14]. Additionally, grip strength is a component of the Kihon Checklist (KCL), an internationally recognized tool for assessing frailty; values below 28 kg in men and 18 kg in women are considered indicative of muscle weakness [15, 16]. Therefore, upper limb function progressively declines with age in frail older adults.

Cui et al. conducted a systematic review of grip strength and the risk of cognitive decline and dementia in older adults. The review found that reduced upper limb muscle strength was significantly associated with increased risk of cognitive decline and higher prevalence of dementia [17]. Thus, upper extremity function declines with age among older adults with dementia. In another study, Stevens et al. compared tactile acuity in 19 young adults (aged 18–28 years) and 60 older adults (aged ≥65 years) using two-point discrimination thresholds on the dorsal and palmar surfaces of the index finger, foot, and forearm. Reports indicate that tactile thresholds of the forearm are approximately 22% higher in older adults than in younger adults, while those in the foot and fingers are about 80% higher, suggesting age-related decline in upper extremity sensory perception [18].

These findings indicate that upper limb function declines with age in older adults. In particular, reports on age-related decline in upper limb function among older adults more commonly focus on motor function than sensory function. Motor function is often used as a disease-specific evaluation index, suggesting the importance of prioritizing motor function in assessments of upper limb functions.

2. Upper limb motor function in older adults compared to young adults

Understanding the characteristics of the upper limb motor function in older adults is critical for their independence in daily living. In daily life, older adults frequently use their upper limbs and often engage in tasks that require the use of both hands. In recent years, research has shown that certain aspects of bimanual movement in older adults are notably reduced, with this reduction varying depending on task characteristics and sex. In this section, we first review age-related changes in upper limb motor function in older adults, as well as related factors. Next, we review findings on the age-related decline in upper limb motor function and associated sex differences, with a focus on activities of daily living. We compare the bimanual motor function of older adults and young adults based on data from the previous studies. These comparisons enabled a better understanding of the characteristics of bimanual motor function in older adults from various perspectives. Furthermore, clarifying the differences in bimanual motor function between young and older adults contributes to a comprehensive understanding of age-related changes.

2.1 Characteristics of upper extremity motor function in the elderly

The upper extremities are frequently used in daily life, with the hands playing the most active and important role. The hand is significantly affected by various physiological and anatomical changes associated with aging. Therefore, it has been shown that hand function declines with age in both men and women, but the decline is particularly pronounced after the age of 65 [19]. It has been suggested that the decline in hand function may result from age-related deterioration in sensorimotor function—such as muscle weakness and sensory-perceptual blunting [14, 18]—changes in the central nervous system (e.g., the motor cortex and corpus callosum) [20], and the peripheral nervous system, such as reduced nerve conduction velocity and impaired excitation-contraction linkage in motor units [21]. It has also been suggested that this may affect older adults' abilities to perform daily activities [11]. Therefore, special attention should be given to hand motor function as a key component of upper limb functions in the daily lives of older adults.

In real life, upper limb movements in older adults primarily consist of two types: one-handed and two-handed movements. Older adults perform more bimanual than one-handed activities [9]. In general, studies have reported that with aging, the frequency of one-handed movements increases more in the dominant hand than in the non-dominant hand [22], and that decreased dominant hand use due to an inactive lifestyle may lead to a shift toward ambidexterity [23]. This shift is based on the concept of use-dependent plasticity. Use-dependent plasticity refers to the phenomenon in which repetitive movements induce plastic reorganization in the motor cortex [24]. Aging and a sedentary lifestyle may reduce the frequency and dominance of dominant hand use, resulting in older adults performing bimanual movements more frequently than one-handed movements. Examples of time-consuming daily bimanual tasks performed by older adults include pouring milk and taking money out of their wallets. The ability to perform these functional movements gradually declines after the age of 65 [10]. Therefore, greater attention should be given to two-handed movements rather than one-handed movements in the daily activities of older adults.

In recent years, the characteristics of bimanual motor performance in older adults have become increasingly well understood, with several age- and task-related aspects identified. Krehbiel et al. conducted a systematic review and meta-analysis of age-related changes in bimanual movements. Bimanual movements in older adults have been shown to result in reduced accuracy, greater variability, and longer execution time, all of which impair motor performance [25]. Kang et al. also conducted a systematic review and meta-analysis of task-specific bimanual motor impairments in this population. Bimanual motor performance in older adults is more impaired in asymmetric bimanual movements than in symmetric bimanual movements [26].

It has also been reported that bimanual motor performance in older adults differs between men and women. Buchman et al. measured grip and pinch strength, finger-tapping speed, and performance on the Purdue Pegboard in 764 older adults (530 women) aged 65 years and older with no clinical evidence of dementia. The results showed that muscle strength was higher in men than in women. Muscle strength and finger-tapping speed were greater in men than in women, whereas Purdue Pegboard scores were higher in women [27]. These studies suggest that men tend to perform better in tasks requiring motor speed, such as finger-tapping, whereas women may perform better in tasks requiring fine motor skills, such as the Purdue Pegboard task. These results further indicate that men emphasize movement speed, whereas women outperform men in tasks requiring fine motor control, such as the Purdue Pegboard task. These differences reflect distinct motor strategies between men and women, with men emphasizing movement speed and women prioritizing movement accuracy [28].

Furthermore, it has been reported that bimanual motor performance in older adults differs between men and women. Vasylenko et al. compared movement times and kinematics of one- and two-handed Purdue Pegboard tasks in 45 young adults aged 19–31 years and 55 older adults aged 60–88 years. They reported that older men had greater movement latencies than older women [29]. In contrast, Sebastjan et al. reported that older women showed significantly lower movement dexterity than older men in finger-tapping and peg insertion tasks [30]. Although sex differences in bimanual motor performance have been reported in older adults, studies on motor dysfunction remain limited and inconsistent. However, some factors have been suggested to contribute to the decline in motor function.

These findings suggest that bimanual motor performance in older adults is influenced by three factors—accuracy, variability, and execution time—and may vary depending on task and sex. Given that bimanual movements are commonly used than one-handed movements in the daily lives of older adults, it is necessary to examine how factors such as aging, task type, and sex influence bimanual motor performance.

2.2 Comparison of bimanual motor function between young and elderly

The bimanual motor performance of older adults declines with age compared with that of the young. In particular, older adults' bimanual motor performance has reduced accuracy, greater variability, and longer execution times than that of younger adults [25]. In addition, studies have shown that motor performance in asymmetric tasks is lower than in symmetric tasks [26]. Serbruyns et al. compared the motor performance of 33 young adults (17 females, average age 25.40 ± 4.66 years) and 33 older adults (17 females, average age 69.33 ± 5.56 years) on finger-tapping and Purdue Pegboard tasks. The results showed that younger adults (96.03 taps ±2.29) performed more tapping than older adults (70.65 taps ±2.33) in the finger-tapping task and manipulated more pegs (12.35 ± 0.25) than the older adults (9.59 ± 0.25) in the Purdue Pegboard task. It has been reported that older adults have reduced accuracy in bimanual movements and longer execution times than younger adults [31]. Fling et al. also compared the motor performance of 14 young adults (five females, 23.1 ± 3.2 years) and 16 older adults (seven females, 71.9 ± 5.2 years) in symmetric and asymmetric finger-tapping tasks. The results showed that older adults had greater variability in bimanual movements in the asymmetric task than younger adults [32]. These findings indicate that bimanual movement performance in older adults is significantly lower than in younger adults in terms of accuracy, variability, and execution time.

People aged 65 years or older are referred to as older adults. This age classification is defined by the World Health Organization [1]. However, individuals aged 65–75 and those aged 90 or older are classified under the same category of older adults. As bimanual motor performance declines with age, there may be significant differences in motor performance among older adults of all ages. Therefore, a more detailed classification of older adults is necessary. Hoogendam et al. investigated the relationship between age and hand fine motor performance using the Archimedes' spiral drawing test in 1912 community-dwelling subjects aged 45 years and older (average age: 77.4 years). They reported that adults over 75 years of age showed increased deviation from the template when drawing spirals and decreased accuracy in that movement [33]. In addition, Shiffman compared daily bimanual fine motor tasks such as pouring milk and retrieving money from a walkway in 10 adults aged 24–87. Consequently, it was reported that the fine motor performance of both hands began to gradually decline from the age of 65 years, with a marked decrease in motor performance after the age of 75 years [10]. Furthermore, most adults over the age of 75 have, on average, three or more chronic diseases and at least one-quarter experience severe functional disabilities. This trend reportedly increases exponentially with age [34]. These findings suggest that it may be important to subdivide older adults according to age.

The most widely recognized international classification system for the older adults categorizes them as "early-stage elderly" and "late-stage elderly." In this system, young-old adults are defined as those aged 65–74 years, while old-old adults are those aged 75 years and older [35]. Recently, bimanual motor performance in early- and late-aged adults has been reported. Lee et al. conducted symmetric and asymmetric tasks in 12 young adults aged 20–22 years (nine females, average age 21.7 years) and 12 older adults aged 65–74 years (nine females, average age 68.8 years). They compared the performance of both hands in slicing handle movements in symmetric and asymmetric tasks. In this context, coordination refers to both accuracy and variability in bimanual coordination performance. It has been reported that young adults exhibit lower performance in asymmetric bimanual motor tasks compared to older adults [36]. Rudisch et al. compared bimanual force control performance in symmetric, asymmetric, and complexity tasks in 19 young adults aged 21–30 years (nine females, average age 21.0 ± 2.6 years) and 52 old-old adults aged 80–91 years (32 females, average age 82.3 ± 2.4 years). The results showed that old-old adults had lower coordination in both symmetric and asymmetric bimanual force control tasks than young adults [37].

We compared bimanual coordination and motor performance in symmetric and asymmetric tasks among 97 young adults (72 females, mean age 20.73 ± 1.43 years), 102 young-old adults (85 females, average age 70.77 ± 2.70 years), and 222 old-old adults (170 females, average age 80.71 ± 4.38 years). The results showed that bimanual coordination performance was significantly lower in the more difficult asymmetric task than in the less difficult symmetric task and was also significantly lower in the non-dominant left hand than in the dominant right hand. The number and frequency of taps, indicating performance speed in the bimanual coordination task, decreased significantly across groups in the order of young adults, young-old adults, and old-old adults, while the average tapping intervals, representing rhythm variability, increased significantly. These parameters may serve as useful indicators for evaluating age-related changes in bimanual coordination (**Figure 1**) [38].

These findings suggest age-related differences in bimanual motor performance, particularly between young-old and old-old adults compared to young adults, with more pronounced impairments observed in bimanual coordination. Therefore, it is necessary to focus on bimanual coordination.

3. Bimanual coordination and its motor control mechanism

Understanding the characteristics of bimanual motor function in older adults requires clarifying the performance features of both simple and bimanual coordination movements. Additionally, the bimanual coordination performance in older adults is task-dependent. Recent findings indicate that neurological and functional factors are involved in the motor control mechanisms underlying bimanual coordination. In this section, we first review the definition of bimanual coordination and its relationship to daily activities. The following section describes various bimanual coordination tasks. Next, the classification and characteristics of bimanual coordination tasks are reviewed based on specific examples. Furthermore, the motor control mechanisms of bimanual coordination have been clarified from both neurological and functional perspectives. This study aimed to reaffirm age-related changes in bimanual coordination and examine their impact on the daily lives of older adults.

3.1 What is bimanual coordination?

We perform voluntary movements daily to fulfill specific purposes. These voluntary movements require not only individual manipulation of the dominant and non-dominant hands, but also frequent coordination of both hands simultaneously or synchronously. Therefore, bimanual coordination is essential for performing daily activities. Bimanual coordination refers to cooperative movement involving interactions between both hands. Bimanual coordination is essential for the efficient performance of a wide variety of daily activities, such as grasping and moving objects, writing, and playing musical instruments [39]. Kang et al. recently conducted a systematic review and meta-analysis of task-specific bimanual coordination in older adults. The review identified 48 bimanual coordination tasks across 47 reported

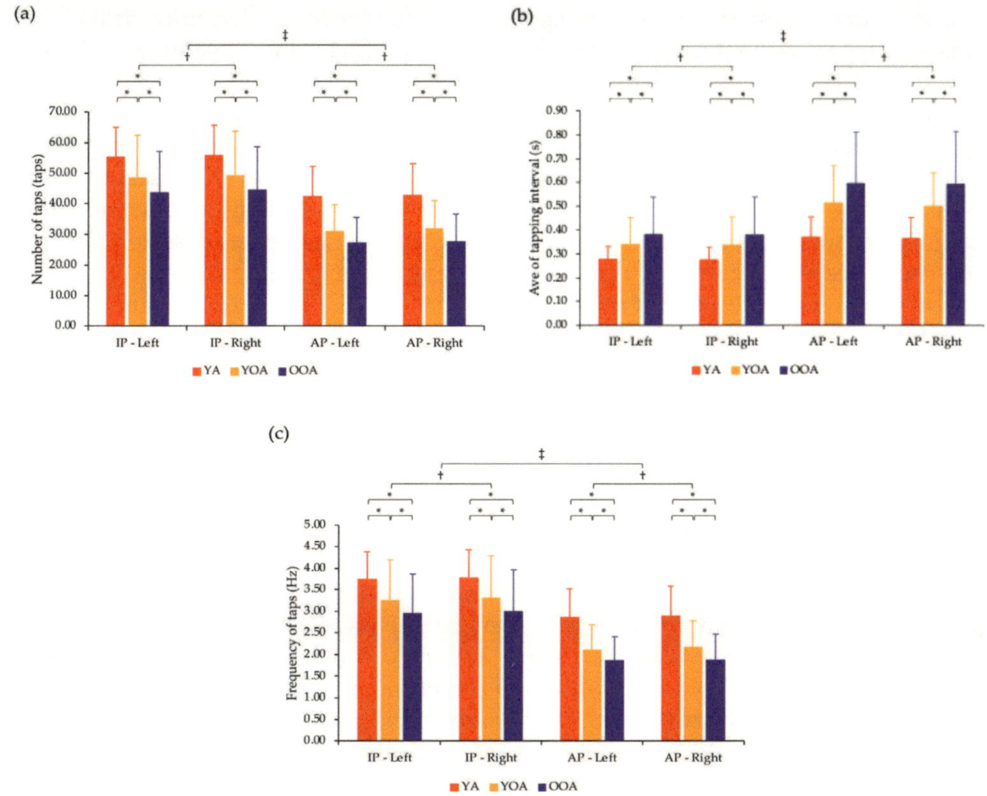

Figure 1.
Comparison of in-phase and anti-phase tasks and dominant versus non-dominant hand performance based on the number of taps, average tapping interval, and frequency of taps. (a) The number of taps showed a significant interaction effect between task and group factors ($p < 0.05$), as well as significant main effects for hand, task, and group factors ($p < 0.05$). Post-hoc tests indicated that the number of taps in both in-phase and anti-phase tasks decreased significantly in the following order: young adults, young-old adults, and old-old adults ($p < 0.05$). Additionally, the number of taps was significantly lower for the left hand than for the right hand († $p < 0.05$). Moreover, across all groups, the number of taps was significantly lower during the anti-phase task than the in-phase task (‡ $p < 0.05$). (b) The average tapping interval showed a significant interaction effect between the task and group factors ($p < 0.05$). Additionally, the average tapping interval demonstrated significant main effects for hand, task, and group factors ($p < 0.05$). Post-hoc test results indicated that the average tapping interval in both in-phase and anti-phase tasks significantly increased in the order: young adults, young-old adults, and old-old adults (* $p < 0.05$). Furthermore, the average tapping interval was significantly longer for the left hand than for the right hand († $p < 0.05$). Finally, the average tapping interval in the young, young-old, and old-old adult groups was significantly longer during the anti-phase task than in the in-phase task (‡ $p < 0.05$). (c) The tap frequency showed a significant interaction effect between task and group factors ($p < 0.05$). Additionally, tap frequency demonstrated significant main effects for hand, task, and group factors ($p < 0.05$). Post-hoc tests indicated that tap frequency in both in-phase and anti-phase tasks decreased significantly in the order: young adults, young-old adults, and old-old adults (* $p < 0.05$). Furthermore, tap frequency was significantly lower in the left hand than in the right hand († $p < 0.05$). Finally, tap frequency in the young, young-old, and old-old adult groups was significantly lower during the anti-phase task than in the in-phase task (‡ $p < 0.05$). Abbreviations: Ave: Average; S: Second; IP: In-phase task; AP: Anti-phase task; YA: Young adult; YOA: Young-old adult; OOA: Old-old adult [38].*

studies. The review classified nine types of bimanual coordination tasks based on the included studies. (1) Tracking task: 11 studies; (2) force control task: five studies; (3) tapping task: 10 studies; (4) cyclical movement task: 11 studies; (5) reaching task: four studies; (6) grip or grasp task: two studies; (7) activity of daily living task: two studies; (8) reaction task: two studies; and (9) matching task: one study [38].

Bimanual coordination tasks are classified into four types. (1) Symmetrical bimanual coordination tasks, in which both hands perform simultaneous left-right movements, (2) asymmetrical bimanual coordination tasks, in which both hands perform alternating movements, (3) complex bimanual coordination tasks, involving integration of identical symmetrical and asymmetrical tasks, and (4) complex bimanual coordination tasks, in which different symmetrical and asymmetrical tasks are integrated [26]. Specific examples of bimanual coordination tasks include the finger-tapping task, Purdue Pegboard task, tracking task, circle description task, and force regulation task. For example, in the finger-tapping task, the in-phase task, in which the left and right fingers of both hands were tapped simultaneously, represented a symmetry task, while the anti-phase task, in which tapping occurred alternately, represented an asymmetry task (**Figure 2**) [38].

In conclusion, bimanual coordination is essential for the efficient execution of daily activities. Motor control mechanisms, particularly those involving neurological processes, are believed to play a critical role in executing such complex movements.

3.2 Motor control mechanisms in bimanual coordination

Bimanual coordination requires complex motor control mechanisms to perform various movements smoothly in daily life. Interhemispheric interactions via the corpus callosum (CC) play a key role in motor control during bimanual coordination. In particular, interhemispheric inhibition plays a fundamental role in motor control during bimanual coordination [40]. Interhemispheric inhibition refers to a motor control mechanism in which one cerebral hemisphere inhibits the other. Structural and functional connectivity of the corpus callosum undergo age-related changes that impair bimanual coordination performance [41, 42]. Tazoe et al. applied transcranial magnetic stimulation (TMS) to the left primary motor cortex during a visually guided bimanual force-tracking task in 11 healthy young males aged 22–35 years. Motor evoked potential (MEP) was recorded from the right short thumb abductor muscle

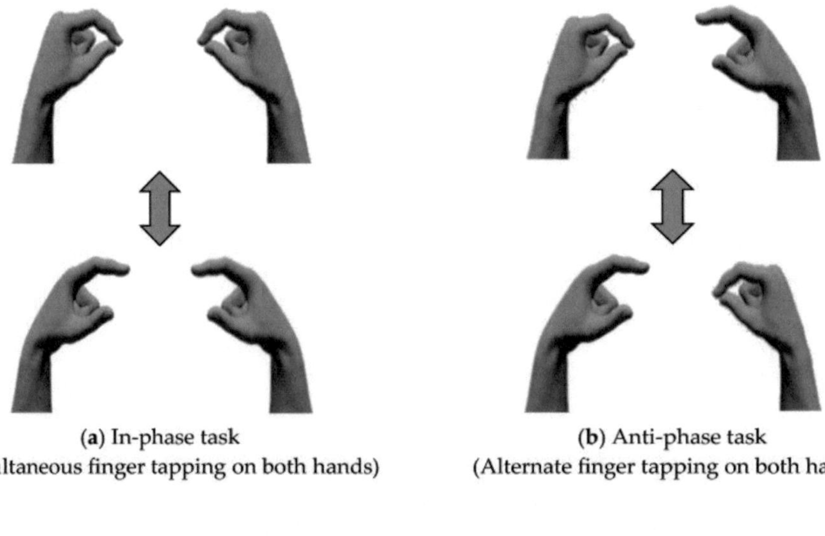

Figure 2.
Bimanual coordination task. (a) In-phase task: Participants performed tapping movements of the thumb and index finger simultaneously on both sides. (b) Anti-phase task: Participants performed tapping movements of the thumb and index finger alternately on both sides [38].

during in-phase and anti-phase tasks. The results showed that tracking accuracy was equivalent between the two motion conditions; however, synchronization of the left and right tracking trajectories was higher in the in-phase condition than in the anti-phase condition. These findings suggest that interhemispheric inhibition between the motor cortices—critical for bimanual coordination—is mediated via the corpus callosum [43].

Inter- and intra-hemispheric neural dynamics associated with bimanual coordination are involved in the planning, execution, and motor learning of such movements [44]. Meister et al. used functional magnetic resonance imaging (fMRI) to examine symmetric and asymmetric bimanual coordination movements in 13 young adults (five females; mean age 29.4 ± 6.1 years). The results further indicated that the degree of functional coupling between the primary motor cortices is associated with temporal coupling in bimanual coordination and that activity in the inferior parietal lobule and premotor cortex is related to temporal coupling [45]. Karabanov et al. used fMRI to examine brain activity during a bimanual pinch force control task in 25 young adults (10 females; mean age 26.1 ± 6.1 years). The results showed that increased activity in the dorsal premotor cortex was accompanied by enhanced connectivity to the supplementary motor cortex, which provided feedback to the sensory system regarding bimanual coordination [46]. Additionally, Debaere et al. reported an interaction between the dorsal premotor cortex and the cerebellum [47]. These findings suggest that interactions among the dorsal premotor cortex, supplementary motor area, and cerebellum play a critical role in controlling bimanual coordination.

Non-neurological factors influencing motor control in bimanual coordination have also been investigated. Lin et al. used a dynamometer to measure grip strength in a bimanual coordination control task in 21 young adults (six females; mean age 23.05 ± 3.15 years) and 10 older adults (2 females; mean age 80.5 ± 4.53 years). Bimanual coordination performance has been reported to decline with age-related changes in maximal grip force, potentially leading to difficulties in performing daily activities requiring bimanual coordination [48].

These results indicate that interactions between cerebral hemispheres play a crucial role in bimanual coordination. Other findings suggest that bimanual coordination is influenced not only by neurological factors, such as connectivity between motor-related brain regions, but also by functional factors, including grip and muscle strength.

4. Methods for measuring bimanual coordination

As previously mentioned, force regulation, the Purdue Pegboard test, tracking, and circle description tasks are specific bimanual coordination tasks. Numerous studies have reported on the relationship between bimanual coordination performance and brain function, using TMS and fMRI during these tasks. Recently, a magnetic sensor finger-tapping device (UB-2; Maxell, Japan) has attracted attention as a new method of measuring bimanual coordination (**Figure 3**) [49]. This device is equipped with a magnetic sensing system consisting of a magnetic induction coil, a sensing coil, and a circuit unit [50]. The coil voltage induced by the electromagnetic induction law varied with the distance between the two coils. As the coil voltage has a nonlinear relationship with the distance between the coils, the distance to the fingertip where the coils are attached can be estimated based on the measured voltage [51]. This

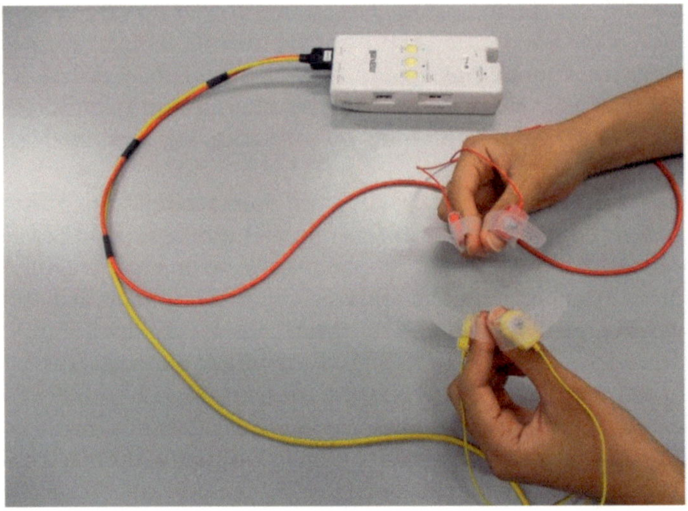

Figure 3.
Magnetic sensor finger-tapping device (UB-2, Maxell Ltd. Tokyo, Japan) [49].

device was confirmed to be highly reproducible and reliable across periods, devices, and measurements [52].

Two types of bimanual coordination tasks use a magnetic sensor finger-tapping device: an in-phase task in which the left and right fingers of both hands are tapped simultaneously, and an anti-phase task in which the left and right fingers of both hands are tapped alternately [38]. The magnetic sensor finger-tapping device can objectively evaluate the bimanual coordination performance from the following three perspectives using these finger-tapping tasks. (1) Distance: evaluates the range and magnitude of hand movement; (2) tap interval: evaluates the average speed of hand movement and the variation in tapping timing; and (3) phase difference: measures the temporal gap between the left- and right-hand taps [53].

Recently, many studies on bimanual coordination using this magnetic sensor finger-tapping device have been reported. The report by Fujikawa et al. on the characteristics of bimanual coordination in physical frailty has been highly evaluated internationally and has attracted considerable attention in the field of bimanual coordination research. Fujikawa et al. included 47 older adults with frailty (39 females, mean age 78.38 ± 5.73 years), 136 older adults with pre-frailty (109 females, mean age 77.94 ± 6.25 years), and 129 older adults with robust health (96 females, mean age 76.85 ± 6.04 years). Bimanual coordination during the in-phase and anti-phase tasks was evaluated by measuring thumb and index finger-tapping movements of both hands using a magnetic sensor finger-tapping device. Participants were verbally instructed to tap the thumb and index finger as quickly and rhythmically as possible. The participants were instructed to open their fingers 40 mm apart during a 15-second pre-practice and measurement period to minimize intersubject variability in amplitude. The results showed that the total traveling distance—interpreted as "momentum" in the bimanual coordination task—was significantly shorter in the frailty group than in the robust group. Regardless of frailty severity, participants showed lower bimanual coordination in the anti-phase task than in the in-phase task, and finger dexterity was lower in the left hand than in the right hand during the task [53].

Although older adults with frailty exhibited bimanual coordination performance similar to those with robust health, the overall coordination was lower than in healthy older adults [53]. The results of this international study not only deepen our understanding of bimanual coordination but also suggest its global importance as a novel approach to frailty prevention and rehabilitation. Furthermore, quantitative evaluation of bimanual coordination using a magnetic sensor finger-tapping device may contribute to addressing international health challenges for older adults by applying it to the early detection and prevention of frailty and other diseases. Furthermore, clarification of disease-specific indices in bimanual coordination may contribute to the design and application of individualized rehabilitation programs.

5. Conclusions

This study examines age-related changes in upper limb motor function, focusing on bimanual coordination and its underlying motor control mechanisms in older adults. In a super-aging society with a rapidly growing elderly population globally, a key academic challenge is to support daily independence and improve the well-being of older adults. Older adults rely more on their upper limbs and perform bimanual movements more frequently than one-handed movements in daily life. Bimanual coordination in older adults is evaluated in terms of accuracy, variability, and execution time and has been shown to be impaired with age. Therefore, it is essential to elucidate the motor control mechanisms involved in bimanual coordination in older adults and establish a simple and effective evaluation system. In this study, we review the latest findings on bimanual coordination performance in older adults and discuss evaluation methods in addition to motor control mechanisms. In particular, the magnetic sensor finger-tapping device allows objective and quantitative assessment of distance, velocity, and deviations in tapping timing and coordination. This measurement method may help address international health challenges in older adults by enabling early detection and prevention of frailty.

Acknowledgements

This work was supported by JSPS KAKENHI Grant Numbers JP23K10417 and JP 25KJ2198, as well as by the Yuumi Memorial Foundation for Home Health Care.

Conflict of interest

The authors declare no conflict of interest.

Appendices and nomenclature

KCL	Kihon Checklist
TMS	Transcutaneous Magnetic Stimulation
MEP	Motor Evoked Potential
fMRI	functional Magnetic Resonance Imaging

Author details

Yusuke Shizuka[1,2], Shun Sawai[1,3], Takato Nishida[1,4], Shoya Fujikawa[1,2], Ryosuke Yamamoto[1,5], Naoki Shimizu[1,2] and Hideki Nakano[1*]

1 Graduate School of Health Sciences, Kyoto Tachibana University, Kyoto, Japan

2 Department of Rehabilitation, Kyoto Kuno Hospital, Kyoto, Japan

3 Society for the Promotion of Science (JSPS), Research Fellow (DC), Japan

4 Faculty of Rehabilitation and Care, Seijoh University, Aichi, Japan

5 Department of Rehabilitation, Tesseikai Neurosurgical Hospital, Osaka, Japan

*Address all correspondence to: nakano-h@tachibana-u.ac.jp

References

[1] United Nations. World Population Prospects 2022. Online ed. Chapter One. New York: United Nations; 2022

[2] United Nations Department of Economic and Social Affairs. World Social Report 2023: Leaving No One Behind in an Ageing World. 2023. Available from: https://social.desa.un.org/publications/undesa-world-social-report-2023.

[3] Talarska D, Kropińska S, Strugała M, Szewczyczak M, Tobis S, Wieczorowska-Tobis K. The most common factors hindering the independent functioning of the elderly at home by age and sex. European Review for Medical and Pharmacological Sciences. 2017;**21**:775-785

[4] Brach JS, VanSwearingen JM. Physical impairment and disability: Relationship to performance of activities of daily living in community-dwelling older men. Physical Therapy. 2002;**82**:752-761

[5] Millán-Calenti JC, Tubío J, Pita-Fernández S, Rochette S, Lorenzo T, Maseda A. Cognitive impairment as predictor of functional dependence in an elderly sample. Archives of Gerontology and Geriatrics. 2012;**54**:197-201. DOI: 10.1016/j.archger.2011.02.010. Epub 2011 Mar 11

[6] Asakawa T, Koyano W, Ando T, Shibata H. Effects of functional decline on quality of life among the Japanese elderly. International Journal of Aging & Human Development. 2000;**50**:319-328. DOI: 10.2190/3TR1-4V6R-MA5M-U1BV

[7] Mendes de Leon CF, Seeman TE, Baker DI, Richardson ED, Tinetti ME. Self-efficacy, physical decline, and change in functioning in community-living elders: A prospective study. The Journals of Gerontology. Series B, Psychological Sciences and Social Sciences. 1996;**51**:S183-S190. DOI: 10.1093/geronb/51b.4.s183

[8] Mahdizadeh A, Farzad M, Bolghanabadi Z. The investigation of relationship between functional disorders of upper extremity with independence in activities of daily living and depression in elderly. Journal of Gerontology. 2019;**3**:59-69. DOI: 10.29252/joge.3.2.59

[9] Kilbreath SL, Heard RC. Frequency of hand use in healthy older persons. The Australian Journal of Physiotherapy. 2005;**51**:119-122. DOI: 10.1016/s0004-9514(05)70040-4

[10] Shiffman LM. Effects of aging on adult hand function. The American Journal of Occupational Therapy. 1992;**46**:785-792. DOI: 10.5014/ajot.46.9.785

[11] Incel NA, Sezgin M, As I, Cimen OB, Sahin G. The geriatric hand: Correlation of hand-muscle function and activity restriction in elderly. International Journal of Rehabilitation Research. 2009;**32**:213-218. DOI: 10.1097/MRR.0b013e3283298226

[12] Bland MD, Beebe JA, Hardwick DD, Lang CE. Restricted active range of motion at the elbow, forearm, wrist, or fingers decreases hand function. Journal of Hand Therapy. 2008;**21**:268-274. quiz 275. DOI: 10.1197/j.jht.2008.01.003

[13] Delbaere K, Bourgois J, Witvrouw EE, Willems TM, Cambier DC. Age-related changes in concentric and eccentric muscle strength in the lower and upper extremity: A

cross-sectional study. Isokinetics and Exercise Science. 2003;**11**:145-151. DOI: 10.3233/IES-2003-0141

[14] Kozakai R. Grip strength and healthy aging. The Journal of Physical Fitness and Sports Medicine. 2017;**6**:145-149. DOI: 10.7600/jpfsm.6.145

[15] Sentandreu-Mañó T, Cezón-Serrano N, Cebrià IMA I, Tortosa-Chuliá MA, Tomás JM, Salom Terrádez JR, et al. Kihon checklist to assess frailty in older adults: Some evidence on the internal consistency and validity of the Spanish version. Geriatrics & Gerontology International. 2021;**21**:262-267. DOI: 10.1111/ggi.14126. Epub 2021 Jan 3

[16] Satake S, Arai H. The revised Japanese version of the Cardiovascular Health Study criteria (revised J-CHS criteria). Geriatrics & Gerontology International. 2020;**20**:992-993. DOI: 10.1111/ggi.14005

[17] Cui M, Zhang S, Liu Y, Gang X, Wang G. Grip strength and the risk of cognitive decline and dementia: A systematic review and meta-analysis of longitudinal cohort studies. Frontiers in Aging Neuroscience. 2021;**13**:625551. DOI: 10.3389/fnagi.2021.625551

[18] Stevens JC, Alvarez-Reeves M, Dipietro L, Mack GW, Green BG. Decline of tactile acuity in aging: A study of body site, blood flow, and lifetime habits of smoking and physical activity. Somatosensory & Motor Research. 2003;**20**:271-279. DOI: 10.1080/08990220310001622997

[19] Carmeli E, Patish H, Coleman R. The aging hand. The Journals of Gerontology. Series A, Biological Sciences and Medical Sciences. 2003;**58**:146-152. DOI: 10.1093/gerona/58.2.m146

[20] Bernard JA, Seidler RD. Hand dominance and age have interactive effects on motor cortical representations. PLoS One. 2012;7:e45443. DOI: 10.1371/journal.pone.0045443. Epub 2012 Sep 25

[21] Laidlaw DH, Bilodeau M, Enoka RM. Steadiness is reduced and motor unit discharge is more variable in old adults. Muscle & Nerve. 2000;**23**:600-612. DOI: 10.1002/(sici)1097-4598(200004)23:4<600::aid-mus20>3.0.co;2-d

[22] Weller MP, Latimer-Sayer DT. Increasing right hand dominance with age on a motor skill task. Psychological Medicine. 1985;**15**:867-872. DOI: 10.1017/s0033291700005109

[23] Kalisch T, Wilimzig C, Kleibel N, Tegenthoff M, Dinse HR. Age-related attenuation of dominant hand superiority. PLoS One. 2006;**1**:e90. DOI: 10.1371/journal.pone.0000090

[24] Bütefisch CM, Khurana V, Kopylev L, Cohen LG. Enhancing encoding of a motor memory in the primary motor cortex by cortical stimulation. Journal of Neurophysiology. 2004;**91**:2110-2116. DOI: 10.1152/jn.01038.2003

[25] Krehbiel LM, Kang N, Cauraugh JH. Age-related differences in bimanual movements: A systematic review and meta-analysis. Experimental Gerontology. 2017;**98**:199-206. DOI: 10.1016/j.exger.2017.09.001. Epub 2017 Sep 7

[26] Kang N, Ko DK, Cauraugh JH. Bimanual motor impairments in older adults: An updated systematic review and meta-analysis. EXCLI Journal. 2022;**21**:1068-1083. DOI: 10.17179/excli2022-5236

[27] Buchman AS, Wilson RS, Bienias JL, Bennett DA. Gender differences in

upper extremity motor performance of older persons. Geriatrics & Gerontology International. 2005;**5**:59-65. DOI: 10.1111/j.1447-0594.2005.00266.x

[28] Rohr LE. Gender-specific movement strategies using a computer-pointing task. Journal of Motor Behavior. 2006;**38**:431-437. DOI: 10.3200/JMBR.38.6.431-137

[29] Vasylenko O, Gorecka MM, Rodríguez-Aranda C. Manual dexterity in young and healthy older adults. 1. Age- and gender-related differences in unimanual and bimanual performance. Developmental Psychobiology. 2018;**60**:407-427. DOI: 10.1002/dev.21619. Epub 2018 Mar 12

[30] Sebastjan A, Skrzek A, Ignasiak Z, Sławińska T. Age-related changes in hand dominance and functional asymmetry in older adults. PLoS One. 2017;**12**:e0177845. DOI: 10.1371/journal.pone.0177845

[31] Serbruyns L, Gooijers J, Caeyenberghs K, Meesen RL, Cuypers K, Sisti HM, et al. Bimanual motor deficits in older adults predicted by diffusion tensor imaging metrics of corpus callosum subregions. Brain Structure & Function. 2015;**220**:273-290. DOI: 10.1007/s00429-013-0654-z. Epub 2013 Oct 26

[32] Fling BW, Walsh CM, Bangert AS, Reuter-Lorenz PA, Welsh RC, Seidler RD. Differential callosal contributions to bimanual control in young and older adults. Journal of Cognitive Neuroscience. 2011;**23**:2171-2285. DOI: 10.1162/jocn.2010.21600. Epub 2010 Oct 18

[33] Hoogendam YY, van der Lijn F, Vernooij MW, Hofman A, Niessen WJ, van der Lugt A, et al. Older age relates to worsening of fine motor skills: A population-based study of middle-aged and elderly persons. Frontiers in Aging Neuroscience. 2014;**6**:259. DOI: 10.3389/fnagi.2014.00259

[34] Beales DL, Tulloch AJ. Community care of vulnerable older people: Cause for concern. The British Journal of General Practice. 2013;**63**:549-550. DOI: 10.3399/bjgp13X673892

[35] Tanaka M, Tsubouchi M, Kayashita J, Mizukami K. Factors associated with oral frailty among community-dwelling older people -A comparison between those <75 and ≥75 years old. Nihon Ronen Igakkai Zasshi. 2024;**61**:68-79. Japanese. DOI: 10.3143/geriatrics.61.68

[36] Lee TD, Wishart LR, Murdoch JE. Aging, attention, and bimanual coordination. Canadian Journal on Aging/La Revue canadienne du vieillissement. 2002;**21**:549-557. DOI: 10.1017/S0714980800002087

[37] Rudisch J, Müller K, Kutz DF, Brich L, Sleimen-Malkoun R, Voelcker-Rehage C. How age, cognitive function and gender affect bimanual force control. Frontiers in Physiology. 2020;**11**:245. DOI: 10.3389/fphys.2020.00245

[38] Shizuka Y, Murata S, Goda A, Sawai S, Fujikawa S, Yamamoto R, et al. Aging-related changes in bimanual coordination as a screening tool for healthy aging. Geriatrics (Basel). 2025;**10**:45. DOI: 10.3390/geriatrics10020045

[39] Rand D, Omer N, Levkoviz A, Assadi Khalil S. The bimanual observation of the hands (BOTH): Development, reliability, and validity for stroke rehabilitation. PLoS One. 2025;**20**:e0316356. DOI: 10.1371/journal.pone.0316356

[40] Gerloff C, Andres FG. Bimanual coordination and interhemispheric

interaction. Acta Psychologica. 2002;**110**:161-186. DOI: 10.1016/s0001-6918(02)00032-x

[41] Fling BW, Seidler RD. Fundamental differences in callosal structure, neurophysiologic function, and bimanual control in young and older adults. Cerebral Cortex. 2012;**22**:2643-2652. DOI: 10.1093/cercor/bhr349

[42] Fujiyama H, Soom JV, Rens G, Gooijers J, Leunissen J, Levin O, et al. Age-related changes in frontal network structural and functional connectivity in relation to bimanual movement control. The Journal of Neuroscience. 2016;**36**:1808-1822. DOI: 10.1523/JNEUROSCI.3355-15.2016

[43] Tazoe T, Sasada S, Sakamoto M, Komiyama T. Modulation of interhemispheric interactions across symmetric and asymmetric bimanual force regulations. The European Journal of Neuroscience. 2013;**37**:96-104. DOI: 10.1111/ejn.12026. Epub 2012 Nov 15

[44] Rueda-Delgado LM, Solesio-Jofre E, Serrien DJ, Mantini D, Daffertshofer A, Swinnen SP. Understanding bimanual coordination across small time scales from an electrophysiological perspective. Neuroscience and Biobehavioral Reviews. 2014;**47**:614-635. DOI: 10.1016/j.neubiorev.2014.10.003

[45] Meister IG, Foltys H, Gallea C, Hallett M. How the brain handles temporally uncoupled bimanual movements. Cerebral Cortex. 2010;**20**:2996-3004. DOI: 10.1093/cercor/bhq048. Epub 2010 Mar 31

[46] Karabanov AN, Chillemi G, Madsen KH, Siebner HR. Dynamic involvement of premotor and supplementary motor areas in bimanual pinch force control. NeuroImage. 2023;**276**:120203. DOI: 10.1016/j.neuroimage.2023.120203. Epub 2023 Jun 3

[47] Debaere F, Wenderoth N, Sunaert S, Van Hecke P, Swinnen SP. Cerebellar and premotor function in bimanual coordination: Parametric neural responses to spatiotemporal complexity and cycling frequency. NeuroImage. 2004;**21**:1416-1427. DOI: 10.1016/j.neuroimage.2003.12.011

[48] Lin CH, Chou LW, Wei SH, Lieu FK, Chiang SL, Sung WH. Influence of aging on bimanual coordination control. Experimental Gerontology. 2014;**53**:40-47. DOI: 10.1016/j.exger.2014.02.005. Epub 2014 Feb 15

[49] Takahashi S, Tomita Y, Tanaka S, Sakurai N, Kodama N. Prefrontal cerebral oxygenated hemoglobin concentration during the category fluency and finger-tapping tasks in adults with and without mild cognitive impairment: A near-infrared spectroscopy study. Brain Sciences. 2022;**12**:1636. DOI: 10.3390/brainsci12121636

[50] Kandori A, Yokoe M, Sakoda S, Abe K, Miyashita T, Oe H, et al. Quantitative magnetic detection of finger movements in patients with Parkinson's disease. Neuroscience Research. 2004;**49**:253-260. DOI: 10.1016/j.neures.2004.03.004

[51] Shima K, Tsuji T, Kan E, Kandori A, Yokoe M, Sakoda S. Measurement and evaluation of finger tapping movements using magnetic sensors. Annual International Conference of the IEEE Engineering in Medicine and Biology Society. 2008;**2008**:5628-5631. DOI: 10.1109/IEMBS.2008.4650490

[52] Sano Y, Kandori A, Shima K, Tamura Y, Takagi H, Tsuji T, et al.

Reliability of finger tapping test used in diagnosis of movement disorders. In: 2011 5th International Conference on Bioinformatics and Biomedical Engineering. 2011. pp. 1-4. DOI: 10.1109/icbbe.2011.5780409

[53] Fujikawa S, Murata S, Goda A, Sawai S, Yamamoto R, Shizuka Y, et al. Comparison of characteristics of bimanual coordinated movements in older adults with frailty, pre-frailty, and robust health. Frontiers in Aging. 2025;**6**:1519129. DOI: 10.3389/fragi.2025.1519129

Chapter 5

Transformation and Evaluation of Standing Postural Control in Older Adults: Mechanisms, Clinical Assessments, and Technological Advances

Takato Nishida, Shin Murata, Shun Sawai, Shoya Fujikawa, Ryosuke Yamamoto, Yusuke Shizuka, Naoki Shimizu and Hideki Nakano

Abstract

This chapter explores the mechanisms, age-related changes, and clinical assessments of standing balance control in older adults, with an emphasis on emerging technological approaches. It first outlines how multisensory integration of visual, vestibular, and somatosensory inputs contributes to maintaining postural stability and how aging impairs these processes through reduced sensory sensitivity, muscle strength, and neural processing speed. It then reviews conventional clinical assessments, ranging from simple screening tools such as the One-Leg Standing Test and Timed Up and Go test to comprehensive scales such as the Berg Balance Scale and Mini-BESTest, along with quantitative methods such as the Index of Postural Stability. Finally, the chapter highlights the technological innovations, including light-touch–based devices, virtual and augmented reality systems, and wearable sensors, that enable the detection of subtle balance deficits and monitoring in real-world contexts. By integrating these technologies into clinical practice, clinicians can achieve higher diagnostic precision, continuous monitoring, and personalized rehabilitation strategies that directly improve the functional outcomes. Collectively, these sections provide an integrated framework for understanding and evaluating postural control in aging populations.

Keywords: clinical evaluation measures, light-touch contact, older adults, postural control, rehabilitation

1. Introduction

Decreased postural control in older adults represents a global public health concern directly associated with increased requirement of long-term care and mortality

 IntechOpen

because of falls and fractures. International systematic reviews report an annual fall prevalence of approximately 26.5% among community-dwelling older adults, with the rate rising to 40–50% among those aged ≥80 years [1, 2]. According to the U.S. Centers for Disease Control and Prevention (CDC), approximately one in four adults aged ≥65 years experiences at least one fall annually, with 20% of these falls resulting in serious injuries, including fractures or head trauma [3]. Falls are also highly recurrent, and a single fall doubles the risk of subsequent falls, significantly impairing healthy life expectancy.

The decline in postural control among older adults is a common challenge across regions and countries, warranting urgent attention in aging societies worldwide. Accurately assessing the degree of decline in postural control among older adults is essential for understanding its underlying mechanisms and for extending healthy life expectancy. Furthermore, establishing objective evaluation methods to measure individual abilities and ensuring their applicability in clinical and community health settings is crucial.

Evidence cited in this chapter was mainly drawn from peer-reviewed journals and official guidelines published between 2000 and 2025, with selected seminal works before 2000 such as the Functional Reach Test. Studies demonstrating methodological rigor and standardized assessment protocols were prioritized.

This chapter first examines the fundamental mechanisms of standing postural control from neurological, sensory, and musculoskeletal perspectives and discusses age-related changes. Next, it outlines representative clinical assessment methods, categorizing them into screening and comprehensive evaluations. Finally, it reviews recent technological advances in standing postural control assessment and presents an integrated framework for evaluating standing postural control in older adults. This chapter aims to provide clinicians and researchers with a common foundation to strengthen efforts toward fall prevention and independent living support.

2. Mechanisms of standing postural control

In this chapter, we use center of mass (COM) to describe the body's mechanical reference point and center of pressure (COP) to refer to the ground reaction force-based measurement obtained from the stabilometric devices. To ensure terminological consistency, the term COG is not used.

Maintaining upright posture is a continuous regulatory process in which the central nervous system interprets sensory information and generates coordinated motor responses. The brain draws on visual cues, vestibular signals, and somatosensory input from the feet and joints to estimate body orientation and detect changes in movement. These multisensory cues are then integrated to produce both reflexive and voluntary adjustments of the musculoskeletal system, allowing fine-tuned control of balance during standing (**Figure 1**) [4, 5].

The primary goals of postural control can be broadly categorized into two aspects: "postural stability" and "postural orientation". Some literature refers to "postural stability" as "postural equilibrium," but these two terms are synonymous [6]. Postural stability refers to the unconscious function of maintaining and controlling the body's COM within its base of support. Meanwhile, postural orientation is the conscious ability to adjust the body's direction and spatial relationships according to the intended movement (**Figure 2**). In daily life, effective postural stability and orientation are necessary to enable safe and appropriate movement.

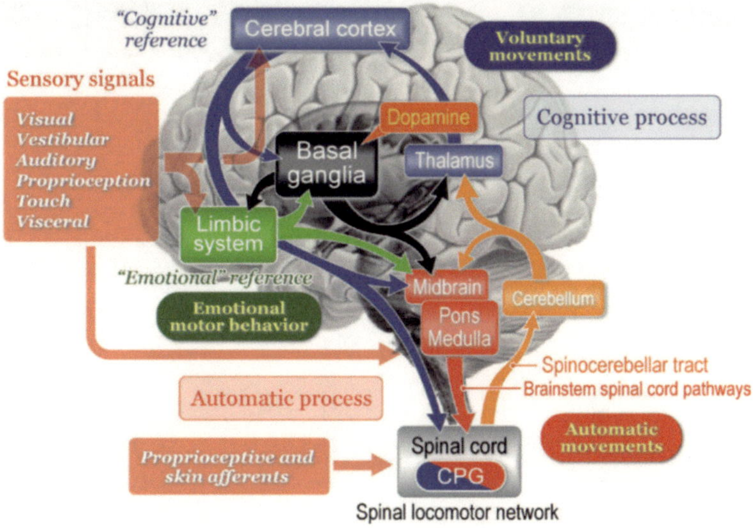

Figure 1.
Basic signal flow involved in postural control. This diagram depicts the neural mechanisms processing multisensory signals from visual, vestibular, auditory, and somatosensory inputs. Understanding the neural and sensory processes underlying postural control is essential for identifying and interpreting pathological changes in stability regulation in individual participants. Reproduced from Takakusaki [4]. Licensed under CC BY-NC 3.0.

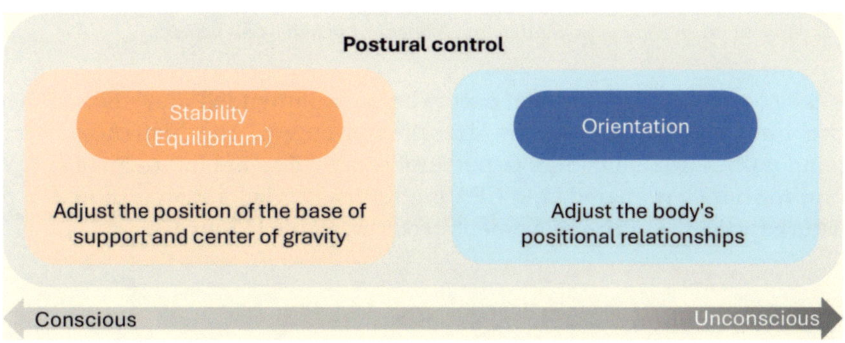

Figure 2.
Two aspects of the postural control. This schematic illustrates the dual roles of postural control: Orientation and stability. Differentiating these two aspects enables clinicians to select the appropriate balance assessments.

Anticipatory postural adjustments (APA) refer to the postural control mechanism that adjusts the COM before executing a targeted movement. This adjustment compensates for instability and facilitates smooth execution of the movement. Specifically, it involves pre-emptive activation of the trunk extensor muscles when rapidly raising the upper limbs or lifting a load, thereby maintaining a stable posture. In contrast, compensatory postural adjustments (CPA) occur as a post-action response to restore stability when posture is disrupted during an action [7]. CPA employ strategies to ensure postural stability within the base of support through ankle or hip joint movements, as well as stepping strategies, where a step is taken to change the base of support and regain stability when the body's COM is beyond the base of support [8, 9].

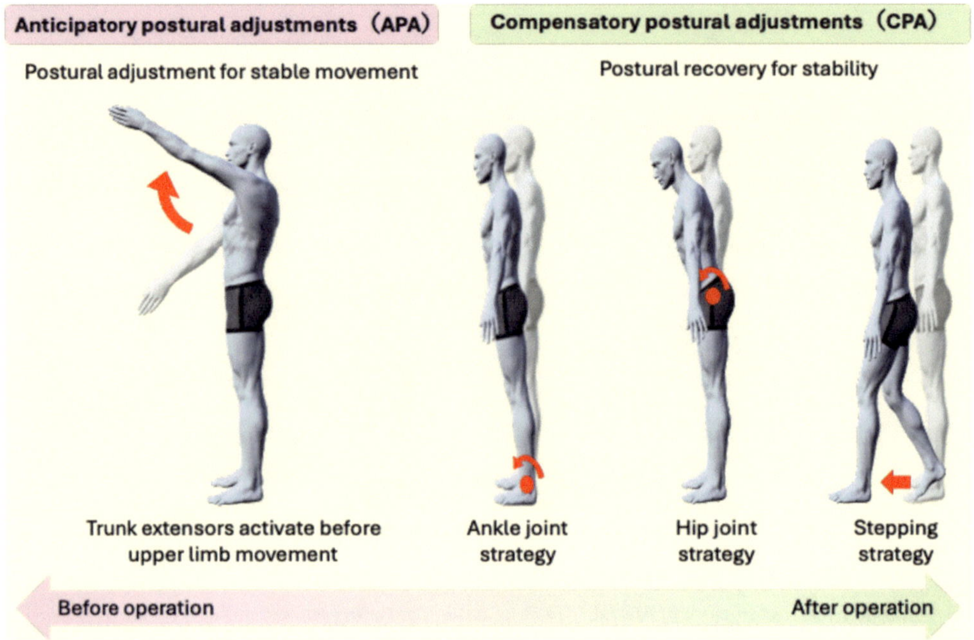

Figure 3.
Difference in the roles of anticipatory postural adjustments and compensatory postural adjustments. This figure illustrates how APA prepares the body for an intended movement before it occurs, whereas CPA restores stability after an unexpected perturbation. Understanding the temporal distinction between these two strategies enables clinicians to interpret which phase of postural control is impaired in individual patients.

APA is a control mechanism that occurs before an intended movement, whereas CPA is a control function that occurs after the movement. Although these functions differ temporally, both contribute to postural control and are interdependent. When APA is appropriately prepared, and CPA is effectively triggered in response to postural disturbances, the entire movement becomes stable (**Figure 3**).

3. Age-related changes

Postural control functions generally decline in older adults, making this a significant internal factor contributing to falls. Furthermore, physiological changes in the sensory, neurological, and musculoskeletal systems with aging affect standing balance ability. A summary of these changes is shown in **Figure 4**, and the main changes are listed below.

3.1 Changes in sensory function

With advancing age, the sensitivity of the visual, vestibular, and somatosensory systems—essential for maintaining balance—generally declines. Furthermore, somatosensory function shows significant deterioration in joint position and vibration sense. Older adults exhibit reduced sensitivity to changes in ankle angle and subtle vibratory stimuli [10]. Additionally, peripheral tactile sensitivity also declines, with a decrease in the density of Merkel discs and Meissner corpuscles, the tactile receptors in the sole [11].

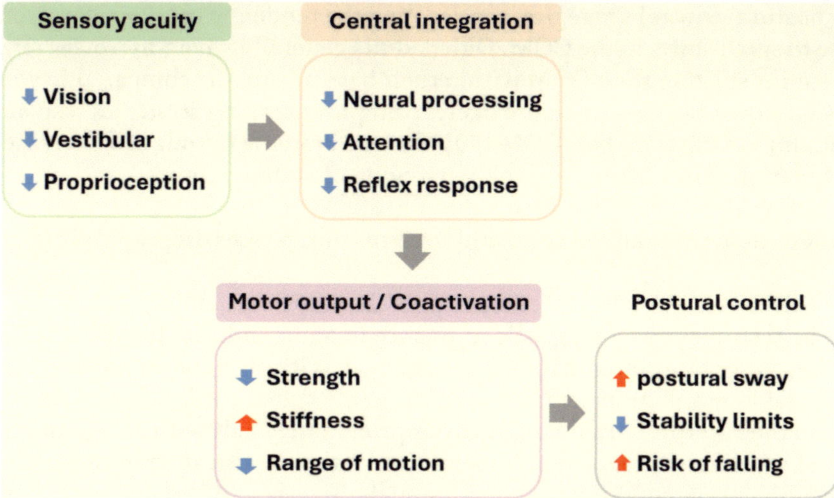

Figure 4.
Integrated model of age-related physiological mechanisms underlying postural control. This figure summarizes the age-related physiological mechanisms that contribute to impaired postural control in older adults. By visualizing these relationships, clinicians can advocate for the need to evaluate not only the musculoskeletal system but also the sensory and nervous systems in rehabilitation aimed at restoring postural stability.

Vestibular function is also significantly affected by aging. Hair cells in the sensory epithelium of the inner ear's balance organs (semicircular canals and otolith organs) decrease with age. Human autopsy studies report that the number of sensory cells in the balance organs decreases by approximately 40% in individuals aged >70 years [12]. This decline in vestibular sensitivity can cause dizziness and balance disorders in older adults. Aging impairs visual function—reducing visual acuity, depth perception, contrast sensitivity, and delayed dark adaptation—which can compromise balance in dimly lit or visually complex environments. Overall, the decline in proprioceptive acuity causes older adults to rely more on vision compared to younger individuals [13, 14]. In particular, the decline in the sensitivity of the proprioceptive sense in the elderly results in insufficient information necessary for postural control.

3.2 Changes in the musculoskeletal system

Decreased muscle strength and reduced range of motion are also major age-related changes. Skeletal muscle mass and strength decline markedly with aging—a condition known as sarcopenia—with muscle atrophy accelerating particularly after 50 years of age and being particularly pronounced in the lower limbs [15]. Changes in muscle fiber composition are characterized by a reduction in the diameter and number of fast-twitch (Type II) fibers, leading to a decrease in overall muscle explosive power and maximum output [16]. This selective atrophy of Type II fibers may result in difficulty generating explosive muscle force in older individuals. Muscle weakness with aging is most pronounced in the small muscles of the fingers and the muscles surrounding the foot and ankle. Specifically, the plantar flexors of the ankle joint show a significantly greater selective decline compared to the dorsiflexors [17, 18]. The ankle plantar flexors are the key antigravity muscles active during ankle strategy in the standing position, and their weakness directly contributes to sway during static standing [19]. Declines in musculoskeletal elements also impact the ability to execute postural control strategies, accelerating the tendency to take a step even in response to small shifts in the COM. Older adults generally have a narrower range of movement for shifting their COM within their base of support compared to younger adults. Consequently, they are more likely to employ stepping strategies to avoid falls even with minor shifts in their COM [20]. Reduced muscle output and decreased joint range of motion can contribute to this narrowing of stability limits.

3.3 Changes in neurotransmission and information processing capabilities

Aging also affects the central and peripheral nervous system function. Longitudinal studies using magnetic resonance imaging indicate that cerebral cortex volume decreases by approximately 0.5% per year, with atrophy primarily observed in the frontal lobe and hippocampus [21, 22]. In the spinal cord, the number of motor neurons in the anterior horn decreases by approximately half with aging, and the number of myelinated fibers in peripheral nerves also significantly declines [23]. Consequently, nerve conduction velocities, including those of brainstem and spinal reflexes, generally slow down. Collectively, these anatomical changes lead to reduced central information processing speed and prolonged motor response latency in older adults. For example, even a slight delay in postural reactions significantly increases the risk of falling in older adults, such as when the ankle collapses or when extending limbs to recover from a stumble, compared to younger individuals. Age-related changes in higher-level brain functions such as attention and judgment cannot be ignored. Furthermore, older adults are more prone to a further decline in postural control ability during dual tasking, such as performing cognitive tasks while walking [24]. This stems from the limited attentional resources and reduced information processing, leading to posture destabilization when attention to the environment is compromised. These neurological changes interact synergistically, resulting in a general decline in the timing and accuracy of sensory input, central processing, and motor output required for postural control in older adults. Consequently, postural sway is greater in older adults than in younger individuals, and responses to sudden postural disturbances are often delayed and inadequate. This creates a physical state prone to falls, significantly impacting independence and safety in activities of daily living. Accurately assessing age-related declines in postural control function and reducing fall risk through the appropriate interventions represent critical challenges in a super-aged society.

4. Current status of the evaluation methods for standing postural control

Accurate assessment of standing balance ability in older adults is critical for stratifying fall risk and determining the effectiveness of interventions [25]. This chapter outlines the assessment methods widely used in clinical practice, categorizing them into screening assessments and diagnostic and quantitative assessments (**Table 1**).

4.1 Screening assessments

Tests that can quickly and easily evaluate balance function in older adults are widely used in daily clinical practice, including outpatient clinics and group health examinations. These screening assessments are characterized by their simplicity and

DOI: http://dx.doi.org/10.5772/intechopen.1014303

Purpose	Assessments	Approx. time	Reliability (ICC)	Cutoff thresholds
Screening	One-leg standing time	<1 min	0.78–0.82	<20 s associated with fall risk
	Functional reach test (FRT)	<1 min	0.89–0.98	<15 cm associated with fall risk
	Timed up and go test (TUG)	1–2 min	0.80	≥9–13.5 s associated with fall risk
	Five-times sit-to-stand test (FTSST)	<1 min	0.94	≥10–14 s associated with fall risk
Diagnostic	Berg balance scale (BBS)	10–20 min	>0.95	<45 points associated with fall risk
	Mini-BESTest	15 min	0.91–0.98	<16 points associated with fall risk
Quantitative	Index of Postural Stability (IPS)	5 min	Clinical validity is limited	No cutoff value

This table summarizes commonly used assessments, their reliability, and representative cutoff values. Clinically, the table enables practitioners to select appropriate tools depending on the purpose—rapid screening, detailed diagnostic evaluation, or quantitative monitoring—and to interpret whether a patient's score indicates elevated fall risk.

Table 1.
Clinical framework for balance assessment in older adults.

short administration time, making them suitable for large-scale community checkups and for the initial evaluation of older patients. Representative examples include the One-Leg Standing Time measurement, the Functional Reach Test (FRT), and the Timed Up and Go (TUG). These tools can be administered quickly and allow clinicians to stratify fall risk at a population level with the minimal resources. However, they cannot identify the precise mechanisms underlying balance dysfunction or localize the impaired physiological systems.

The One-Leg Standing Time measures the time a participant can stand on one leg with the eyes open [26]. The individual is instructed to cross both arms in front of the chest and lift one leg off the floor, maintaining the position for as long as possible. Measurements are typically performed on either the left or right leg, selecting the side that can be held longer, with an upper time limit of 30 or 60 seconds. This test reflects multiple components of balance, including lower limb strength and COM sway. Older adults who cannot maintain this posture for more than a few seconds are at a significantly higher risk of falls [27]. Nevertheless, participants with musculoskeletal pain, dizziness, or other health conditions may find it difficult to perform the test safely, and therefore, support and safety measures are essential.

The FRT is another simple test that evaluates dynamic balance ability and stability limits by measuring maximum forward reach [28]. The participant stands with feet in a predetermined position, raises one arm horizontally to shoulder height, and is instructed to reach forward as far as possible without moving the feet. The distance reached by the tip of the hand is then recorded. The reach distance decreases with age. Values of ≥25 cm generally indicate good balance, whereas values ≤15 cm indicate significant limitation and high fall risk [29]. However, the FRT cannot evaluate lateral or backward stability and is influenced by individual physical characteristics, such as height and arm length.

In addition, the TUG and the Five-Times Sit-to-Stand tests are convenient measures of balance and functional mobility [30, 31]. Their feasibility makes them particularly suitable for community-based health screenings, where many participants are evaluated simultaneously. Nonetheless, these screening assessments provide only a broad overview and cannot specify which the aspects of balance control are impaired. Therefore, they should be integrated with more comprehensive diagnostic and quantitative assessments to obtain a more accurate and clinically meaningful evaluation of balance function.

4.2 Diagnostic and quantitative assessments

In contrast to screening assessments, diagnostic and quantitative assessments are designed to capture the mechanisms of balance control and identify risk factors comprehensibly. These assessments provide detailed information that can be utilized in developing individualized intervention plans. Representative examples include the Mini-Balance Evaluation Systems Test (Mini-BESTest), comprehensive balance scales such as the Berg Balance Scale (BBS), and instrument-based assessments that quantify postural sway and COP dynamics. Quantitative assessment using these tools helps generate accurate and objective data, enabling clinicians to individualize rehabilitation strategies based on specific impairments. However, their reliance on specialized equipment and trained personnel may limit widespread adoption in all clinical settings.

The BBS is one of the most widely used comprehensive balance evaluation tools. It comprises 14 items scored on a 0–4 scale, with a maximum total of 56 points [32]. It is highly reliable and reproducible, and BBS scores are often used to stratify fall risk in older adults [33]. Meanwhile, the Mini-BESTest comprises 14 items grouped into four domains—anticipatory postural adjustments, reactive postural control, sensory orientation, and dynamic gait—each scored from 0 to 2 points, with a maximum score of 28 [34]. Despite the smaller number of items, the Mini-BESTest is valued for its ability to assess qualitative aspects of postural control. For example, Yingyongyudha et al. [35] reported an area under the receiver operating characteristic curve of 0.84 for identifying fall history in a cohort of 200 older adults with a mean age of 70 years using the Mini-BESTest, which was higher than both the BBS and the TUG tests (area under the curve = 0.69). However, despite its strengths, the Mini-BESTest also presents several important trade-offs when compared with the BBS. The Mini-BESTest is highly sensitive to qualitative changes in postural control—including reactive balance, sensory reweighting, and dynamic gait—and shows minimal ceiling effects, making it particularly valuable for evaluating higher-functioning older adults. In contrast, the BBS provides broader coverage of basic daily activities such as standing up, reaching, and turning, allowing clinicians to assess the balance impairments that directly relate to ADL performance. These differences imply that the Mini-BESTest excels in detecting subtle deficits in advanced postural control mechanisms, whereas the BBS offers stronger comprehensiveness and safety for lower-functioning individuals or those requiring assistance. Moreover, although the Mini-BESTest enables domain-specific interpretation across its four subcomponents, the BBS remains easier to interpret clinically due to its straightforward total score and extensive evidence base across diverse populations. Therefore, the choice between the two measures should be guided by the patient's functional level, safety considerations, and whether the clinical goal is to detect high-level balance deficits or to evaluate ADL-oriented fall risk. As each tool has unique strengths and limitations, clinical best practice often involves combining multiple assessments. A stepwise approach is frequently recommended—for example, applying simple screening tests such as one-leg standing or the FRT initially, and then conducting more comprehensive evaluations with the BBS or Mini-BESTest if abnormalities are detected.

Beyond clinical scales, instrument-based quantitative evaluations provide objective and highly sensitive data. A common method is the use of a COP sway meter to record COP trajectories, while participants maintain a standing posture under various conditions [36]. One important extension of such measurements is the Index of Postural Stability (IPS), which captures both the stability of quiet standing and range over which an individual can voluntarily shift their COP [37]. The IPS is calculated by combining the area of intentional COP excursions in multiple directions with the baseline sway area during quiet standing, providing a logarithmic index that reflects the balance between postural stability and mobility (**Figure 5**) [38]. However, despite its conceptual utility, the IPS faces several methodological constraints. It has not yet been standardized across measurement devices, and its reproducibility may vary depending on foot placement, task instructions, and stabilometer resolution. Evidence linking IPS values to real-world fall events remains limited compared with the established force-plate metrics. Moreover, no clinically validated cutoff values have been proposed to date, limiting its application for diagnostic decision-making in routine practice. Therefore, future research should aim to establish clinically meaningful cutoff thresholds that can reliably stratify fall risk in older adults. Until such validation is achieved, the IPS should be interpreted as a supplementary rather than a standalone indicator of postural stability.

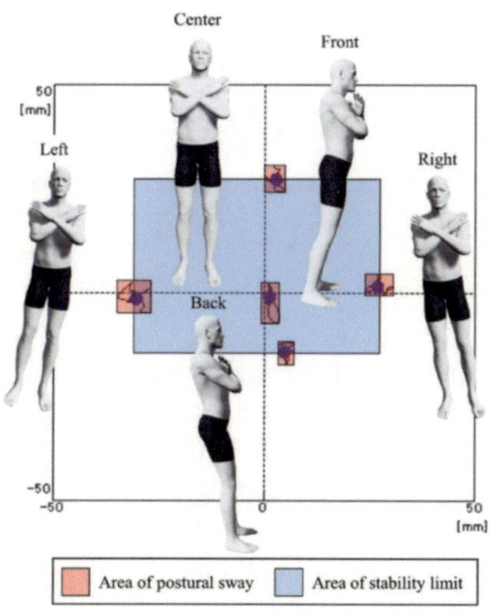

$$\text{IPS} = \log \frac{\text{Area of stability limit} + \text{Area of postural sway}}{\text{Area of postural sway}}$$

Figure 5.
Calculation method for Index of Postural Stability. Participants first undergo the measurement of COP sway at the central position. Next, they maintain postures with the COP shifted to the maximum extent forward, backward, right, and left. Postural sway area and stability threshold area are calculated from the five-direction COP sway data, and the Index of Postural Stability is calculated using the mentioned formula. The IPS provides a quantitative indicator of both stability and mobility, enabling clinicians to objectively monitor subtle balance impairments and track rehabilitation progress over time. Reproduced from Sawai et al. [38] Licensed under CC BY.

5. Technical advances in postural control assessments

In recent years, new methods utilizing cutting-edge technologies for assessing postural control abilities in older adults have emerged in medical and research fields. This chapter outlines three topics from among these: utilizing the light touch contact effect, utilizing virtual reality (VR) and augmented reality (AR) technologies, and measurement using wearable devices.

5.1 Virtual light-touch effect (StA^{2}BLE)

Conventional posturography assesses physical function by recording the magnitude and patterns of postural sway, but directly measuring sensory function has been difficult. In contrast, the recently developed standing assessment device StA^{2}BLE can simultaneously evaluate both "physical function" and "sensory function" in postural control (**Figure 6**) [39]. The light-touch phenomenon refers to the reduction in COM sway when a person lightly touches an object with their fingertip, demonstrating that tactile and mechanoreceptor input significantly contributes to postural stability [40]. StA^{2}BLE involves attaching a device that delivers a weak vibratory stimulus to an individual's dominant index finger. While the stimulus is applied, posture stabilizes through tactile and vibratory sensation. However, abruptly stopping this stimulus causes a momentary loss of balance and an increase in postural sway. The device records this change in conjunction with COP, enabling detailed analysis of the magnitude of sway and the time required for recovery. This mechanism allows quantification of "sensory system vulnerability," such as the stability and reaction speed of tactile input, alongside the body's compensatory control capabilities. This evaluation method quantifies sensory function decline and potential fall risks that are difficult to detect in daily life. It may also reveal "hidden instability" in older adults that is often overlooked by conventional simple sway measurements alone, enabling earlier intervention for fall prevention. Consequently, StA^{2}BLE could be a valuable screening tool in preventive care programs and health checkups for community-dwelling older adults. Furthermore, in research, analyzing bodily responses to changes in sensory input can also aid in evaluating age-related declines in sensory integration function and neuroplasticity.

5.2 VR and AR technologies

VR and AR are rapidly evolving as the novel frameworks for evaluating postural control in older adults. VR enables the manipulation of visual stimuli and dynamic environments within a virtual space, facilitating assessments of visual dependence and multisensory integration capabilities, which were challenging to assess using conventional posturography. For example, presenting floor inclines or background movement, followed by analyzing COP trajectories and spectral components, can quantify the stimulus intensity required to disrupt posture and adaptation speed achieved through repeated exposure [41]. Nonetheless, specific challenges have been reported, including the fact that VR sickness occurs in approximately 30% of older adults.

Recent attempts have been made to simultaneously measure electroencephalography, electromyography, and COP in VR environments and use machine learning to distinguish conditions or groups are advancing. This enables more multifaceted

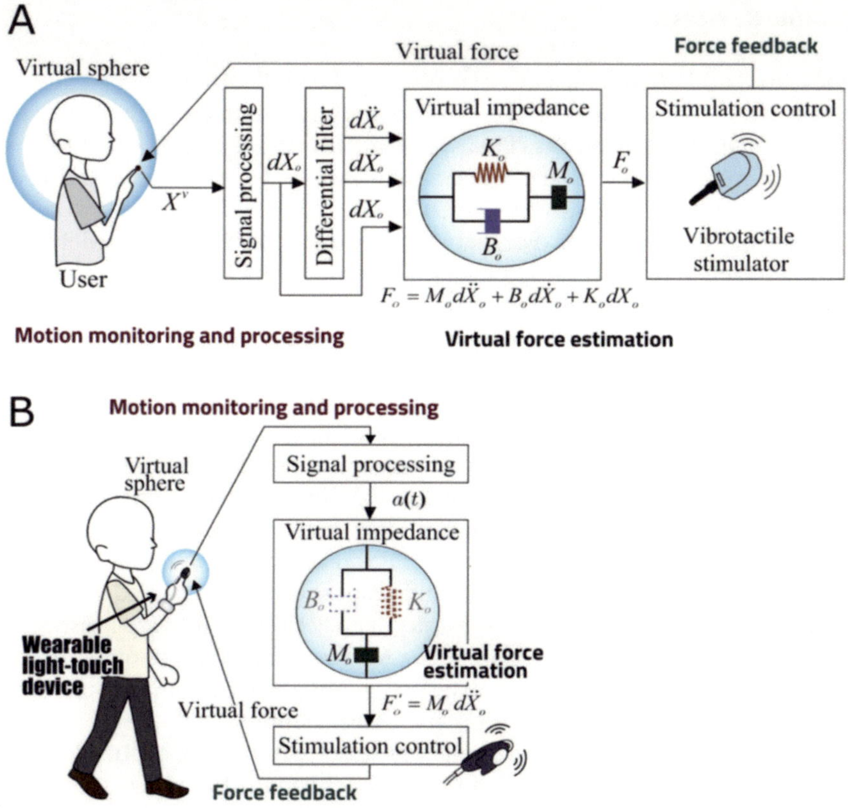

Figure 6.
Overview of the virtual light touch (VLT) system. (A) Basic system architecture. The user's finger position is tracked within a defined "virtual sphere" using three-dimensional motion capture. The displacement signal is processed and converted into a virtual force through a virtual impedance model consisting of mass, spring, and damping elements. The estimated virtual force is then delivered to the fingertip as vibrotactile feedback via *a stimulator, thereby providing a sensation equivalent to light-touch without physical contact. (B) Wearable configuration. A simplified system employing a lightweight accelerometer attached to the finger replaces full 3D motion capture. The virtual force is estimated based only on acceleration information, and vibrotactile stimulation is provided accordingly. This wearable version enables the practical application of VLT during daily activities and walking tasks. The VLT system allows safe and sensitive evaluation of tactile contribution to postural control, offering new possibilities for early detection of sensory deficits and for training balance in older adults. Reproduced from Shima et al. [39]. Licensed under CC BY-NC 4.0.*

evaluations, such as reaction latencies and frequency characteristics during sensory input loss, which were previously difficult to observe [42]. Additionally, validation studies comparing VR headset position data with force plate measurements have demonstrated the effectiveness of VR devices as low-cost balance assessment tools [43].

Meanwhile, AR technology overlays virtual information onto the real environment, enabling posture assessment in settings closer to daily life. For example, efforts are underway to assess fall risk in real-life environments by virtually projecting steps or obstacles and analyzing stepping-over actions or step reactions [44].

Overall, VR and AR technologies are increasingly recognized as powerful tools for safely simulating diverse sensory conditions and task environments, enabling more precise balance assessments than previously possible.

5.3 Wearable devices

Home-based and on-site measurements using inertial measurement units (IMU), smartphones, and plantar pressure sensors are rapidly gaining popularity for postural control assessment in older adults. Their primary advantage is low cost and high portability compared to stationary equipment like force plates while enabling quantification of body sway (approximate COM/COP metrics) and reaction characteristics during static and dynamic tasks. For example, a framework is being implemented where IMUs attached to the lumbar or sacral region extract features such as RMS, velocity, trajectory distance, and frequency components from time series data obtained during standing tasks (closed-base, single-leg, tandem). These features are used to identify fall-risk groups. The feasibility of implementing an IMU prototype for older adults has been demonstrated, with increases in sway corresponding to task difficulty, supporting its validity as a clinical screening tool [45].

Research using smartphone-embedded accelerometers has validated standing postural stability in terms of both mechanical validity and discriminative ability. These devices show moderate-to-high correlation with force plate measurements and can stratify fall risk among older adults [46]. For reactive postural control assessment, wearable disturbance devices quantify responses to unexpected mechanical disturbances. Tasks measuring outcomes such as reaction latency, step response, and stabilization time are under evaluation, and improvements in immediate reaction ability and lateral stability have been observed, highlighting their potential for clinical application that integrates rehabilitation and assessment [47].

The introduction of advanced technologies is revolutionizing postural control assessment for older adults. StA^{2}BLE simultaneously quantifies sensory system vulnerability and motor control ability by manipulating subtle tactile inputs, thereby visualizing potential fall risk. VR/AR enables the reproduction of diverse tasks and sensory conditions within a safe virtual environment, facilitating the assessment of dynamic characteristics such as visual dependence and adaptation speed. Furthermore, wearables like IMUs, smartphones, and plantar pressure sensors enable continuous monitoring and immediate feedback in daily environments, capturing fluctuations difficult to detect on a clinical scale.

However, addressing VR sickness, standardizing equipment and wearing conditions, and validating compatibility with force plates and clinical indicators remain future challenges. By integrating these technologies with traditional manual assessments, clinicians can more precisely understand balance ability and develop individualized fall prevention strategies. As technology advances and standardization progresses, it may significantly contribute to supporting the independence of older adults.

Moreover, several of these technologies, particularly wearable sensors and smartphone-based balance assessments, can be feasibly implemented in low-resource or telehealth settings. Their portability, affordability, and capacity for remote data collection make them valuable tools for extending postural control evaluation beyond traditional clinical environments.

6. Conclusions

Age-related declines in sensory, neural, and musculoskeletal systems interact to impair postural control. Clinical assessments capture the functional consequences of these deficits, whereas emerging technologies—such as light-touch devices, VR/AR systems, and wearable sensors—offer insights into the underlying mechanisms not detectable by the traditional tools. An integrative framework that links physiological mechanisms, clinical functional scales, and technology-based measurements is therefore essential for individualized fall-risk evaluation.

Key research priorities remain. Standardization and validation of technology-based assessments, including VR-induced perturbations, wearable sensor metrics, and indices such as the IPS, are necessary for broader clinical adoption. Establishing clinically meaningful cutoff values, improving reproducibility across devices, and developing multimodal diagnostic algorithms represent critical next steps. Advancing these areas will help build a comprehensive, scalable framework for evaluating postural control in aging populations.

Acknowledgements

This work was supported by JSPS KAKENHI grant [grant numbers: JP23K10417 and JP 25KJ2198].

Conflict of interest

The authors declare no conflict of interest.

Author details

Takato Nishida[1,2], Shin Murata[1], Shun Sawai[1,3], Shoya Fujikawa[1,4], Ryosuke Yamamoto[1,5], Yusuke Shizuka[1,4], Naoki Shimizu[1,4] and Hideki Nakano[1*]

1 Graduate School of Health Sciences, Kyoto Tachibana University, Kyoto, Japan

2 Faculty of Rehabilitation and Care, Seijoh University, Aichi, Japan

3 Japan Society for the Promotion of Science (JSPS), Tokyo, Japan

4 Department of Rehabilitation, Kyoto Kuno Hospital, Kyoto, Japan

5 Department of Rehabilitation, Tesseikai Neurosurgical Hospital, Osaka, Japan

*Address all correspondence to: nakano-h@tachibana-u.ac.jp

References

[1] Salari N, Darvishi N, Ahmadipanah M, Shohaimi S, Mohammadi M. Global prevalence of falls in the older adults: A comprehensive systematic review and meta-analysis. Journal of Orthopaedic Surgery and Research. 2022;**17**(1):334. DOI: 10.1186/s13018-022-03222-1

[2] World Health Organization. Falls – Key Facts. WHO Fact Sheets [Internet]. 2021. Available from: https://www.who.int/news-room/fact-sheets/detail/falls

[3] Centers for Disease Control and Prevention (CDC). Important Facts about Falls [Internet]. 2024. Available from: https://www.cdc.gov/falls/data-research/facts-stats/index.html

[4] Takakusaki K. Functional neuroanatomy for posture and gait control. Journal of Movement Disorders. 2017;**10**(1):1-17. DOI: 10.14802/jmd.16062

[5] Peterka RJ. Sensorimotor integration in human postural control. Journal of Neurophysiology. 2002;**88**(3):1097-1118. DOI: 10.1152/jn.2002.88.3.1097

[6] Horak F. Postural orientation and equilibrium: What do we need to know about neural control of balance to prevent falls? Age and Ageing. 2006;**35**(Suppl 2):ii7-ii11. DOI: 10.1093/ageing/afl077

[7] Santos MJ, Kanekar N, Aruin AS. The role of anticipatory postural adjustments in compensatory control of posture: 1. Electromyographic analysis. Journal of Electromyography and Kinesiology. 2010;**20**(3):388-397. DOI: 10.1016/j.jelekin.2009.06.006

[8] Santos MJ, Kanekar N, Aruin AS. The role of anticipatory postural adjustments in compensatory control of posture: 2. Biomechanical analysis. Journal of Electromyography and Kinesiology. 2010;**20**(3):398-405. DOI: 10.1016/j.jelekin.2010.01.002

[9] Wang Y, Watanabe K, Asaka T. Anticipatory and compensatory postural adjustments in response to dynamic platform perturbation during a forward step. Journal of Motor Behavior. 2023;**55**(1):31-38. DOI: 10.1080/00222895.2022.2092440

[10] Kanemitsu M, Nakasa T, Ikuta Y, Adachi N. Decreased joint position sense of the ankle joint is a risk factor for falls in the elderly. Cureus. 2023;**15**(12):e51084. DOI: 10.7759/cureus.51084

[11] García-Piqueras J, García-Mesa Y, Cárcaba L, Feito J, Torres-Parejo I, Martín-Biedma B, et al. Ageing of the somatosensory system at the periphery: Age-related changes in cutaneous mechanoreceptors. Journal of Anatomy. 2019;**234**(6):839-852. DOI: 10.1111/joa.12983

[12] Harada S, Koyama Y, Kobayashi Y, Imai T, Takimoto Y, Kobayashi H, et al. Efficacy of the silicon based agent for age related decline in vestibular function. Scientific Reports. 2025;**15**(1):29790. DOI: 10.1038/s41598-025-14302-7

[13] Whitson HE, Cronin-Golomb A, Cruickshanks KJ, Gilmore GC, Owsley C, Peelle JE, et al. American Geriatrics Society and National Institute on Aging bench-to-bedside conference: Sensory impairment and cognitive decline in older adults. Journal of the American Geriatrics Society. 2018;**66**(11):2052-2058. DOI: 10.1111/jgs.15506

[14] Billig AR, Feng NC, Behforuzi H, McFeeley BM, Nicastri CM, Daffner KR. Capacity-limited resources are used for managing sensory degradation and cognitive demands: Implications for age-related cognitive decline and dementia. Cortex. 2020;**133**:277-294. DOI: 10.1016/j.cortex.2020.09.005

[15] Cruz-Jentoft AJ, Sayer AA. Sarcopenia. Lancet. 2019;**393**(10191):2636-2646. DOI: 10.1016/S0140-6736(19)31138-9

[16] Serrano N, Colenso-Semple LM, Lazauskus KK, Siu JW, Bagley JR, Lockie RG, et al. Extraordinary fast-twitch fiber abundance in elite weightlifters. PLoS One. 2019;**14**(3):e0207975. DOI: 10.1371/journal.pone.0207975

[17] Simoneau E, Martin A, Van Hoecke J. Muscular performances at the ankle joint in young and elderly men. The Journals of Gerontology. Series A, Biological Sciences and Medical Sciences. 2005;**60**(4):439-447. DOI: 10.1093/gerona/60.4.439

[18] Tracy BL. Force control is impaired in the ankle plantarflexors of elderly adults. European Journal of Applied Physiology. 2007;**101**(5):629-636. DOI: 10.1007/s00421-007-0538-0

[19] Hernández-Guillén D, Tolsada-Velasco C, Roig-Casasús S, Costa-Moreno E, Borja-de-Fuentes I, Blasco JM. Association ankle function and balance in community-dwelling older adults. PLoS One. 2021;**16**(3):e0247885. DOI: 10.1371/journal.pone.0247885

[20] Si B, Zhu H, Wei X, Li S, Wu X. The mechanism of static postural control in the impact of lower limb muscle strength asymmetry on gait performance in the elderly. PeerJ. 2024;**12**:e17626. DOI: 10.7717/peerj.17626

[21] Fjell AM, Walhovd KB, Fennema-Notestine C, McEvoy LK, Hagler DJ, Holland D, et al. One-year brain atrophy evident in healthy aging. The Journal of Neuroscience. 2009;**29**(48):15223-15231. DOI: 10.1523/JNEUROSCI.3252-09.2009

[22] Gorbach T, Pudas S, Lundquist A, Orädd G, Josefsson M, Salami A, et al. Longitudinal association between hippocampus atrophy and episodic-memory decline. Neurobiology of Aging. 2017;**51**:167-176. DOI: 10.1016/j.neurobiolaging.2016.12.002

[23] Piekarz KM, Bhaskaran S, Sataranatarajan K, Street K, Premkumar P, Saunders D, et al. Molecular changes associated with spinal cord aging. Geroscience. 2020;**42**(2):765-784. DOI: 10.1007/s11357-020-00172-6

[24] Li KZH, Bherer L, Mirelman A, Maidan I, Hausdorff JM. Cognitive involvement in balance, gait and dual-tasking in aging: A focused review from a neuroscience of aging perspective. Frontiers in Neurology. 2018;**9**:913. DOI: 10.3389/fneur.2018.00913

[25] Lafontant K, Blount A, Suarez JRM, Fukuda DH, Stout JR, Trahan EM, et al. Comparing sensitivity, specificity, and accuracy of fall risk assessments in community-dwelling older adults. Clinical Interventions in Aging. 2024;**19**:581-588. DOI: 10.2147/CIA.S453966

[26] Kobayashi T, Morimoto T, Shimanoe C, Ono R, Otani K, Mawatari M. A simplified screening tool for the one-leg standing test to determine the severity of locomotive syndrome. Life (Basel). 2023;**13**(5):1190. DOI: 10.3390/life13051190

[27] Blodgett JM, Ventre JP, Mills R, Hardy R, Cooper R. A systematic review of one-legged balance performance

and falls risk in community-dwelling adults. Ageing Research Reviews. 2022;**73**:101501. DOI: 10.1016/j.arr.2021.101501

[28] Duncan PW, Weiner DK, Chandler J, Studenski S. Functional reach: A new clinical measure of balance. Journal of Gerontology. 1990;**45**(6):M192-M197. DOI: 10.1093/geronj/45.6.m192

[29] Francisco L, Duarte J, Albuquerque C, Albuquerque D, Pires IM, Coelho PJ. Mobile data gathering and preliminary analysis for the functional reach test. Sensors (Basel). 2024;**24**(4):1301. DOI: 10.3390/s24041301

[30] Podsiadlo D, Richardson S. The timed "up & go": A test of basic functional mobility for frail elderly persons. Journal of the American Geriatrics Society. 1991;**39**(2):142-148. DOI: 10.1111/j.1532-5415.1991.tb01616.x

[31] Grgic J, Schoenfeld BJ, Maier AB, Pedisic Z. Reference values for the five-times-sit-to-stand test: A pooled analysis including 45,470 participants from 14 countries. Geroscience. 2025. DOI: 10.1007/s11357-025-01863-8

[32] Kornetti D, Fritz S, Chiu Y, Light K, Velozo C. Rating scale analysis of the berg balance scale. Archives of Physical Medicine and Rehabilitation. 2004;**85**(7):1128-1135. DOI: 10.1016/j.apmr.2003.11.019

[33] Viveiro LAP, Gomes GCV, Bacha JMR, Carvas Junior N, Kallas ME, Reis M, et al. Reliability, validity, and ability to identify fall status of the berg balance scale, balance evaluation systems test (BESTest), mini-BESTest, and brief-BESTest in older adults who live in nursing homes. Journal of Geriatric Physical Therapy (2001). 2019;**42**(4):E45-E54. DOI: 10.1519/JPT.0000000000000215

[34] Jacobs JV, Kasser SL, Padgett PK. Clarification on the scoring of the mini-BESTest. Physical Therapy. 2013;**93**(6):860. DOI: 10.2522/ptj.2013.93.6.860

[35] Yingyongyudha A, Saengsirisuwan V, Panichaporn W, Boonsinsukh R. The mini-balance evaluation systems test (mini-BESTest) demonstrates higher accuracy in identifying older adult participants with history of falls than do the BESTest, berg balance scale, or timed up and go test. Journal of Geriatric Physical Therapy (2001). 2016;**39**(2):64-70. DOI: 10.1519/JPT.0000000000000050

[36] Quijoux F, Nicolaï A, Chairi I, Bargiotas I, Ricard D, Yelnik A, et al. A review of center of pressure (COP) variables to quantify standing balance in elderly people: Algorithms and open-access code. Physiological Reports. 2021;**9**:e15067. DOI: 10.14814/phy2.15067

[37] Suzuki Y, Yatoh S, Suzuki H, Tanabe Y, Shimizu Y, Hada Y, et al. Age-dependent changes in dynamic standing-balance ability evaluated quantitatively using a stabilometer. Journal of Physical Therapy Science. 2018;**30**(1):86-91. DOI: 10.1589/jpts.30.86

[38] Sawai S, Murata S, Sakano Y, Fujikawa S, Yamamoto R, Shizuka Y, et al. Dominance of attentional focus: A comparative study on its impact on standing postural control in healthy younger and older adults. Frontiers in Human Neuroscience. 2024;**18**:1384305. DOI: 10.3389/fnhum.2024.1384305

[39] Shima K, Shimatani K, Sakata M. A wearable light-touch contact device for human balance support. Scientific

Reports. 2021;**11**(1):7324. DOI: 10.1038/s41598-021-85687-4

[40] Baccini M, Rinaldi LA, Federighi G, Vannucchi L, Paci M, Masotti G. Effectiveness of fingertip light contact in reducing postural sway in older people. Age and Ageing. 2007;**36**(1):30-35. DOI: 10.1093/ageing/afl072

[41] Älmqvist Nae J, Nyström A, Luccini F, Magnusson M, Ekvall HE. Video exposure through virtual reality can improve older people's ability to manage postural instability caused by distortive visual environments. PLoS One. 2024;**19**(8):e0306834. DOI: 10.1371/journal.pone.0306834

[42] Stehle SA, Aubonnet R, Hassan M, Recenti M, Jacob D, Petersen H, et al. Predicting postural control adaptation measuring EEG, EMG, and center of pressure changes: BioVRSea paradigm. Frontiers in Human Neuroscience. 2022;**16**:1038976. DOI: 10.3389/fnhum.2022.1038976

[43] Sylcott B, Lin CC, Williams K, Hinderaker M. Investigating the use of virtual reality headsets for postural control assessment: Instrument validation study. JMIR Rehabilitation and Assistive Technologies. 2021;**8**(4):e24950. DOI: 10.2196/24950

[44] Araújo HAGO, Souza RJ, da Silva TCO, Nascimento TS, Terra MB, Smaili SM. Immediate effect of augmented reality, virtual reality, and neurofunctional physiotherapy on postural control and executive function of individuals with Parkinson's disease. Games for Health Journal. 2023;**12**(3):211-219. DOI: 10.1089/g4h.2021.0222

[45] Kongsawasdi S, Bunjan P, Wongjak M, Saenmueng W, Wantanajittikul K. Evaluating postural sway in the elderly using inertial measurement units: A study on center of mass measurements via accelerometers and gyroscopes. Journal of Clinical Medical Research. 2025;**17**(4):200-207. DOI: 10.14740/jocmr6184

[46] Hsieh KL, Roach KL, Wajda DA, Sosnoff JJ. Smartphone technology can measure postural stability and discriminate fall risk in older adults. Gait & Posture. 2019;**67**:160-165. DOI: 10.1016/j.gaitpost.2018.10.005

[47] Yamamoto M, Shimatani K, Yoshikawa D, Washida T, Takemura H. Perturbation-based balance exercise using a wearable device to improve reactive postural control. IEEE Journal of Translational Engineering in Health and Medicine. 2023;**11**:515-522. DOI: 10.1109/JTEHM.2023.3310503

Chapter 6

Challenges in Assessing Cognitive Frailty and the Implications for Dementia Prevention in a Super-Aging Society

Shoya Fujikawa, Shin Murata, Shun Sawai, Takato Nishida, Ryosuke Yamamoto, Yusuke Shizuka, Naoki Shimizu and Hideki Nakano

Abstract

As global populations age, dementia has emerged as a pressing public health concern, making its prevention and early detection increasingly important. Mild cognitive impairment (MCI), a transitional stage between normal aging and dementia, is characterized by cognitive decline with preserved daily functioning and is recognized as a high-risk factor for dementia onset. Of particular interest is "cognitive frailty," a condition marked by the coexistence of MCI and physical frailty, which is associated with an elevated risk of both dementia and mortality. Despite its significance, standardized evaluation and diagnostic criteria for cognitive frailty remain undeveloped, highlighting the need for effective early detection methods. Recent studies suggest a strong relationship between cognitive and physical function, raising the possibility that physical performance assessments could serve as the early indicators of cognitive frailty. This section explores the current approaches for assessing cognitive frailty, examines the potential of incorporating physical function into such evaluations, and discusses the key challenges involved in developing a new, reliable framework for cognitive frailty assessment.

Keywords: older adult, cognitive frailty, dementia, mild cognitive impairment, finger movement

1. Introduction

Global aging represents one of the most important demographic changes of the twenty-first century. By 2050, the world's population aged 60 years and older is projected to exceed 2 billion [1]. With this rapid aging, dementia has become a major public health issue.

Dementia refers to a syndrome characterized by progressive cognitive decline that interferes with the performance of activities of daily living [2]. According to estimates by the World Health Organization, the number of people with dementia worldwide reached approximately 55 million in 2019 and is projected to increase to 152 million by 2050 [3]. In particular, Alzheimer's disease is the most common cause of dementia, accounting for 60–70% of all cases [4]. In Japan, which has the most advanced aging population, the prevalence of dementia reaches approximately 15% among older adults aged 65 years and above [5], and this percentage increases rapidly with age. The global cost of dementia in 2019 was estimated at US$1.3 trillion [6], highlighting the enormous socioeconomic burden associated with the disease. Additionally, the current medical and nursing care systems face many challenges in responding to the increasing number of patients with dementia. First, access to specialized diagnosis and treatment remains limited. In many countries, a shortage of dementia specialists has resulted in missed opportunities for early diagnosis [7]. Second, the sustainability of long-term care systems is under threat. Although many patients with dementia eventually require facility-based care, securing sufficient capacity and personnel to provide high-quality care remains difficult [8]. These challenges underscore the importance of prevention and early intervention as the crucial strategies for mitigating the social impact of dementia. In particular, early detection is crucial for maintaining the quality of life for patients and reducing the burden of care. Addressing the growing impact of dementia in aging societies requires the establishment of a comprehensive approach centered on early detection. Developing a community-based dementia screening system and promoting integrated measures focused on early detection and early intervention are essential steps toward achieving a sustainable dementia care system [9].

A strong emphasis must be placed on identifying pre-dementia stages. In particular, recognizing cognitive frailty—a condition involving both cognitive decline and physical frailty—as a key target for early intervention is essential. Later sections discuss methods for assessing cognitive frailty and explore its potential in the early detection and prevention of dementia.

2. Overview of mild cognitive impairment

Early detection and prevention of dementia are critical, and understanding mild cognitive impairment (MCI) is essential in this context. MCI represents an intermediate stage between normal cognitive function and dementia and is recognized as a condition with a high risk of progression to dementia. However, progression from MCI to dementia does not occur in all cases; appropriate intervention during this reversible stage may help maintain or even improve cognitive function. Therefore, early detection and appropriate assessment of MCI play vital roles in dementia prevention strategies. This section first provides an overview of the definition and clinical characteristics of MCI and summarizes basic information, including diagnostic criteria, classification, and prevalence. Following this, findings on the risk of transition from MCI to dementia are presented, along with a discussion of cognitive function assessments, imaging tests, and motor function assessments, which have recently gained attention for predicting progression. Integration of these findings offers a foundation for developing a comprehensive understanding of MCI and for designing effective evaluation strategies.

2.1 Definition and characteristics of MCI

MCI refers to a state of cognitive decline situated between normal cognitive function and dementia [10]. This condition is defined as a decline in memory or other cognitive domains beyond what is expected for age, whereas the ability to perform activities of daily living remains intact [11]. Recognizing this stage plays a crucial role in identifying pre-dementia conditions and creating opportunities for early intervention.

The most widely used diagnostic framework for MCI is Petersen's criteria, which includes five elements: (1) reports of cognitive decline by the individual or an informant, (2) objective evidence of cognitive impairment, (3) preservation of overall cognitive function, (4) maintenance of basic activities of daily living, and (5) absence of dementia diagnosis [12]. Additionally, MCI can also be diagnosed as Mild Neurocognitive Disorder. This diagnosis utilizes the Diagnostic and Statistical Manual of Mental Disorders, 5th edition (DSM-5), which assesses cognitive function across six domains: Complex attention, Executive function, Learning and memory, Language, Perceptual–motor function, and Social cognition [13]. This assessment includes observational evaluations by the individual, family, and clinician, along with standardized neuropsychological testing. A diagnosis of Mild Neurocognitive Disorder is made when impairment is observed in one or more cognitive domains, despite the individual maintaining their daily living activities. These criteria distinguish MCI from dementia by emphasizing the preservation of functional independence.

MCI is categorized into amnestic and non-amnestic subtypes based on clinical characteristics [14]. Amnestic MCI primarily involves memory impairment and carries a high risk of progression to Alzheimer's disease. Conversely, non-amnestic MCI affects cognitive domains other than memory, such as executive function, language, and visuospatial cognition, and may be associated with progression to dementia with Lewy bodies or frontotemporal dementia. Further classification divides MCI into single-domain and multi-domain types, depending on the number of affected cognitive domains. Although estimates of MCI prevalence vary by study, approximately 10–20% of older adults aged 65 years or older are affected. Among those aged 85 years or older, the reported prevalence exceeds 30% [15].

In neuropsychological assessments, MCI is defined as a decline of 1.5 standard deviations or more from age- and education-adjusted norms in specific cognitive domains [16]. Amnestic MCI is characterized by poor performance on delayed recall tasks. Mild deficits in executive function and slowed processing speed may also be observed. These cognitive impairments do not significantly interfere with daily functioning. Imaging tests often reveal atrophy in the hippocampus and medial temporal lobe in individuals with MCI [17]. Such structural changes exceed those typically associated with aging and are less severe than those observed in Alzheimer's disease.

Although MCI carries a high risk of progression to dementia, not all cases follow this trajectory. According to the longitudinal study, approximately 10–15% of individuals with MCI progress to dementia within a year, whereas approximately 10–20% maintain stable cognitive function, and some recover to the normal levels [18]. These findings highlight the presence of MCI cases with stable or reversible symptoms, emphasizing the importance of early detection and the implementation of appropriate preventive interventions.

2.2 Risk of transition to dementia in MCI

The risk of transitioning to dementia among patients with MCI is significantly higher than in the general aging population, with an annual transition rate estimated at 10–15% [18]. This transition risk varies significantly depending on the subtype of MCI, the severity of cognitive impairment, and the presence of comorbid risk factors. Among the cognitive function assessments, the severity of episodic memory impairment serves as the strongest predictor of progression [19]. In particular, impaired delayed recall performance on story memory tests or word list learning tests is strongly associated with the transition to Alzheimer's disease. Additionally, an increase in the Clinical Dementia Rating (CDR) Sum of Boxes score and prolonged completion time on the Trail Making Test Part B is also associated with the transition risk [20]. Structural imaging, particularly magnetic resonance imaging, plays a critical role in risk prediction. Measurement of hippocampal volume has shown that individuals with an annual atrophy rate exceeding approximately 2% face a significantly increased the risk of progression [21]. Moreover, amyloid positron emission tomography positivity is observed in approximately 50–60% of patients with MCI, and the risk of dementia progression is significantly higher in positive individuals compared to negative individuals [22].

In recent years, repetitive finger movement assessments have emerged as promising tools for predicting dementia risk [23]. Sugioka et al. reported that changes in the velocity of finger tapping movements are associated with medial temporal lobe atrophy [24]. Given that medial temporal lobe atrophy is an early pathological change in Alzheimer's disease [25], finger tapping movement assessments may offer a simple and clinically useful method for identifying individuals at higher risk of progression from MCI to dementia. Cognitive function tests and neuroimaging findings provide high-sensitivity indicators for predicting MCI progression. Meanwhile, physical function assessments offer practical advantages for community-based, large-scale screening due to their simplicity and non-invasiveness. An integrated assessment approach using cognitive, imaging, and physical measures may facilitate participant stratification by dementia risk, guide the selection of participants for early intervention, and support the efficient allocation of healthcare resources.

3. The concept and significance of cognitive frailty

MCI provides a framework for assessing the risk of dementia from the perspective of cognitive function. However, the onset of dementia in older adults is also closely related to physical decline. In recent years, the concept of "cognitive frailty" has gained attention for its comprehensive approach for evaluating dementia risk from both cognitive and physical perspectives. Cognitive frailty refers to a condition characterized by the coexistence of physical frailty and cognitive decline. Studies have demonstrated that the risk of transition to dementia is significantly higher when both conditions are present simultaneously than when either exists in isolation. This concept holds particular importance because physical and cognitive functions interact and reinforce one another, creating a vicious cycle that accelerates cognitive deterioration. Traditionally, physical and cognitive functions have been evaluated and addressed separately; however, the concept of cognitive frailty highlights the need for an integrated understanding of both and the development of more effective preventive strategies.

In this section, we first describe the definition and clinical significance of cognitive frailty, and then outline the mechanisms underlying the interaction between physical frailty and cognitive decline. This section will clarify that cognitive frailty is an important target for dementia prevention.

3.1 Definition of cognitive frailty

Cognitive frailty is defined as a condition in which physical frailty and cognitive impairment coexist [26]. A joint consensus by the International Association of Gerontology and Geriatrics (IAGG) and the International Association of Nutrition and Aging (IANA) describes cognitive frailty as "a decline in cognitive function (CDR = 0.5) caused by physical or brain disease, or accelerated brain aging in the absence of obvious brain disease" [27]. This definition requires the presence of both physical frailty and mild cognitive impairment. Compared to either condition alone, cognitive frailty has been associated with a poorer prognosis [28]. A meta-analysis revealed that the risk of dementia among frail older adults with cognitive impairment is approximately 2.5 to 5 times higher than among older adults without cognitive impairment [29, 30]. Furthermore, the 5-year cumulative incidence rate of dementia in the cognitive frailty group has been reported to reach approximately 30–40%.

3.2 Interaction between physical frailty and cognitive decline

Physical frailty and cognitive decline, which constitute cognitive frailty, have a complex bidirectional relationship [31]. Physical frailty is defined as "a medical syndrome caused by multiple causes and triggers, characterized by a decline in muscle strength and endurance and a decrease in physiological function, with an increased vulnerability to requiring care or death" [32]. Physical frailty increases the risk of cognitive decline, whereas cognitive decline simultaneously accelerates the progression of physical frailty. Common pathological mechanisms and synergistic effects can explain this interaction. One proposed mechanism by which physical frailty influences cognitive function involves increased inflammatory cytokines associated with muscle mass loss. These cytokines may induce neuroinflammation, contributing to cognitive decline [33]. Additionally, brain-derived neurotrophic factors play a crucial role in maintaining neuroplasticity and cognitive function. However, decreased physical activity may reduce the production of brain-derived neurotrophic factors and contribute to cognitive decline [34]. Moreover, decreased cardiovascular function has been suggested to reduce cerebral blood flow, further impairing cognitive function [35].

Conversely, the impact of cognitive decline on physical frailty holds similar importance. Cognitive decline makes it difficult to plan and execute daily activities, leading to a decrease in physical activity. Older adults with cognitive decline frequently demonstrate slower gait velocity than cognitively healthy peers [36]. Moreover, a high prevalence of malnutrition among cognitively impaired individuals has been reported [37], with poor nutrition contributing to weight and muscle loss. Furthermore, cognitive decline increases the risk of falls [38]. Falls limit activity and accelerate the progression of physical frailty.

Based on the aforesaid, physical frailty leads to social isolation, and a decrease in external stimuli accelerates cognitive decline. This vicious cycle promotes the progression of cognitive frailty to dementia, underscoring the critical importance of early detection and preventive interventions.

4. Assessment of cognitive frailty

Cognitive frailty is a condition in which the risk of transition to dementia is significantly increased due to the interaction between physical frailty and cognitive decline. Detecting cognitive frailty at an early stage and providing appropriate intervention requires the establishment of reliable and valid assessments. However, current assessments have many issues and may not fully capture the essence of cognitive frailty. In particular, conventional assessment approaches independently evaluate physical and cognitive functions and do not adequately reflect the dynamic interaction between these two domains. Additionally, the lack of standardized assessment tools continues to hinder both research advancement and clinical application. Overcoming these challenges and developing more comprehensive and practical assessment methods remains critically important for the early detection of cognitive frailty and the implementation of effective preventive interventions.

This section first summarizes the issues associated with currently used cognitive frailty assessments and then discusses the potential of physical function evaluation, particularly finger movement assessment, as a comprehensive assessment index for assessing cognitive frailty. This discussion aims to clarify the direction for developing a novel assessment approach.

4.1 Current assessment methods and issues in cognitive frailty

The primary challenge in assessing cognitive frailty is the lack of established assessment methods and diagnostic criteria [39]. Although definitions have been provided through the joint consensus of the IAGG and IANA, considerable variation exists among researchers regarding the actual assessment procedures. This lack of uniformity impedes research progress on cognitive frailty and limits its clinical applicability, as evidenced in several areas. Various tools are used to assess physical frailty, including the Fried criteria, the Frailty Index, the FRAIL scale, and the Clinical Frailty Scale [40]. Fried's criteria capture the "phenotype of frailty" through five items: weight loss, fatigue, reduced grip strength, decreased walking speed, and reduced physical activity. This criterion classifies individuals with three or more items as frail, those with one to two items as pre-frail, and those with zero items as robust. The Frailty Index is calculated based on the concept of accumulated health impairment. It is derived as the ratio of the number of deficient items to the total number of items, using a diverse set of health indicators (symptoms, diseases, functional impairments, abnormal test values, etc.), ranging from 30 to 70 items. A higher score indicates a more severe degree of frailty. The Clinical Frailty Scale is a visual scale that assesses frailty on a 9-point scale from 1 (very healthy) to 9 (terminal), based on a clinical overall picture including the activities of daily living and cognitive function. On this scale, a score of 5 or higher is classified as frail. In other words, Fried's criteria represent a phenotype focused on physical function, the Frailty Index demonstrates health impairment using a cumulative deficit model, and the Clinical Frailty Scale provides an assessment based on clinical judgment. On the other hand, cognitive function assessments utilize tests such as the Mini-Mental State Examination (MMSE), Montreal Cognitive Assessment (MoCA), CDR, and neuropsychological test batteries [40]. The MMSE and MoCA serve as screening tests that quantify cognitive domains, including orientation, memory, attention, language, and visuospatial cognition. In contrast, the CDR is a clinical rating scale that evaluates six domains: memory, orientation, judgment and problem solving, social adjustment, domestic situation, and care situation. It assesses severity on a scale from 0 (normal) to 3 (severe dementia). Neuropsychological test batteries aim to accurately assess detailed functions within each cognitive domain. Thus, these evaluation methods assess cognitive function from different perspectives. Whether cognitive frailty, as diagnosed through these disparate tools, represents the same condition remains unclear. Therefore, the reliability and validity of current assessments are insufficient. Additionally, conventional assessments evaluate physical and cognitive functions independently, without integrating the interaction between them [41]. However, as cognitive frailty arises from complex interactions between both functions, this assessment approach may not fully capture the essence of the condition. Furthermore, independent evaluation of each domain makes the detection of subtle changes—especially during preclinical or transitional phases—extremely difficult. This limitation increases the risk of overlooking frailty at reversible stages, which may delay preventive intervention.

To address these challenges, the development of more sensitive indicators and the establishment of internationally standardized cognitive frailty assessments are urgently needed. Particularly, new assessment approaches that reflect the interaction between physical and cognitive functions are expected to improve early detection efforts.

4.2 The importance of physical function assessment in cognitive frailty

Conventional cognitive frailty assessments evaluate the physical and cognitive functions independently without adequately considering the interaction between them. However, recent studies have revealed that changes in physical function reflect the status of cognitive function [42]. This evidence suggests that physical function assessment may serve as an alternative indicator of cognitive function. In other words, cognitive frailty can be comprehensively evaluated through a new approach that indirectly assesses cognitive status using physical function measures.

Previous studies have shown that gait velocity, balance ability, and muscle strength are related to cognitive function and are useful for predicting cognitive decline [43]. However, these physical functions are related to overall cognitive function, making it difficult to evaluate specific aspects (executive function, motor programming, temporal perception, etc.) in detail. Moreover, older adults with mobility limitations or who use wheelchairs often face difficulties undergoing these evaluations. Among upper limb functions, finger dexterity holds particular promise for assessing cognitive function. Carment et al. proposed a conceptual diagram presenting a qualitative model of finger dexterity tasks and the complex cognitive functions involved (**Figure 1**) [44]. In this conceptual diagram, force tracking tasks demand real-time adjustment of motor output using sensory feedback, indicating stronger involvement of the sensory cortex, premotor cortex, and primary motor cortex. Meanwhile, tasks involving cognitive factors, such as finger tapping and multi-finger tapping, activate the prefrontal cortex and hippocampus. The pegboard test, which assesses attention and sensorimotor processing, has also been associated with cognitive decline in community-dwelling older adults [45]. Furthermore, finger tapping movements decline with age [46]. Notably, deterioration in movement variability and rhythmic control are the early indicators of cognitive decline [47]. Based on these findings, the

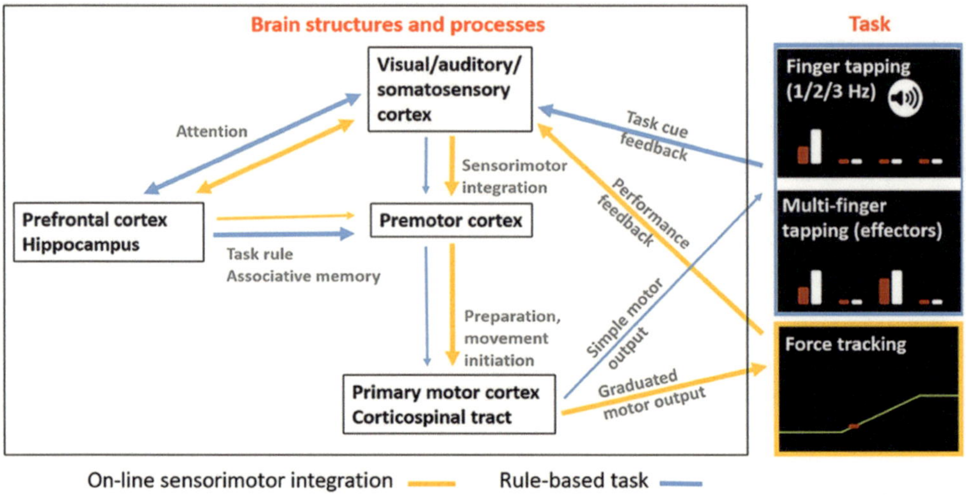

Figure 1.
A conceptual overview of how different brain regions contribute to tasks involving manual dexterity, depending on the degree to which cognitive rule formation and sensorimotor processing are required [44]. The thickness of the arrows reflects the relative involvement of each brain region in a given task. This hypothesis proposes that the neural mechanisms underlying finger dexterity vary according to two task-dependent components: (i) online sensorimotor integration (yellow arrows) for adapting movements based on feedback and (ii) rule-based association (blue arrows) for generating performance predictions and adapting those predictions during movement. Force tracking requires real-time adjustment of motor output using sensory feedback, with stronger involvement of the sensory cortex, premotor cortex, and primary motor cortex. In contrast, tasks like finger tapping or multi-finger tapping, which involve cognitive factors based on task rules (stored in working memory), show greater involvement of the prefrontal cortex and hippocampus. For clarity, the basal ganglia and cerebellum are not depicted in this diagram [44].

next section proposes finger movement assessment as an integrated indicator of both physical and cognitive function in the evaluation of cognitive frailty.

5. Possibility of a new cognitive frailty assessment

The previous sections outlined the fundamental issues in current cognitive frailty assessments, including the absence of unified standards and the failure to capture the interaction between physical and cognitive functions. To resolve these issues, a new approach that can assess both functions in an integrated manner is needed. The finger movement assessment described in the latter half of the previous sections holds potential as a new indicator for cognitive frailty assessment, as it reflects the complex aspects of cognitive function and allows for objective and quantitative assessment. In particular, finger tapping movements, although simple in execution, require cognitive processes such as attention, executive function, and motor programming. These movements also relate closely to physical frailty, making them well suited for comprehensive assessment of cognitive frailty.

This section proposes a specific assessment approach utilizing finger tapping movements and presents its scientific basis and advantages. Additionally, this section summarizes the key issues that must be addressed for the practical implementation of this new assessment method and outlines future research directions. These steps aim to establish an assessment strategy capable of enabling early detection of cognitive frailty and guiding effective interventions.

5.1 Proposal of an evaluation approach using finger movements

This section proposes the use of finger movements as an indicator for the integrated assessment of physical and cognitive functions. Specifically, measuring finger tapping movements with a magnetic sensor-type finger tapping device allows for the accurate quantification of multifaceted parameters such as movement velocity, rhythm, and phase coordination between both hands (**Figure 2**) [46, 48, 49]. In relation to cognitive function, previous studies have reported correlations between cognitive decline and a reduced number of taps [50], altered movement velocity [24], and diminished rhythm regularity [48, 51]. These parameters reflect complex cognitive processes, including attention, executive function, and motor programming. Regarding physical frailty, a study by Fujikawa et al. involving community-dwelling older adults revealed that physically frail older adults exhibited a significant reduction in movement during the two-hand tapping exercise [52]. Finger tapping movements offer an objective and quantitative means of assessment using magnetic sensor technology. This method can be easily administered in a seated position and completed in a short period, making it accessible for older populations. Given that both cognitive decline and physical frailty are associated with impairments in finger tapping, integrating these characteristics may enable a comprehensive assessment of cognitive frailty. Finger tapping assessment offers a simultaneous evaluation of cognitive and physical functions, addressing the limitations of conventional approaches that evaluate each independently. This method presents a promising tool for early detection and severity assessment of cognitive frailty by capturing the interaction between cognitive and physical domains.

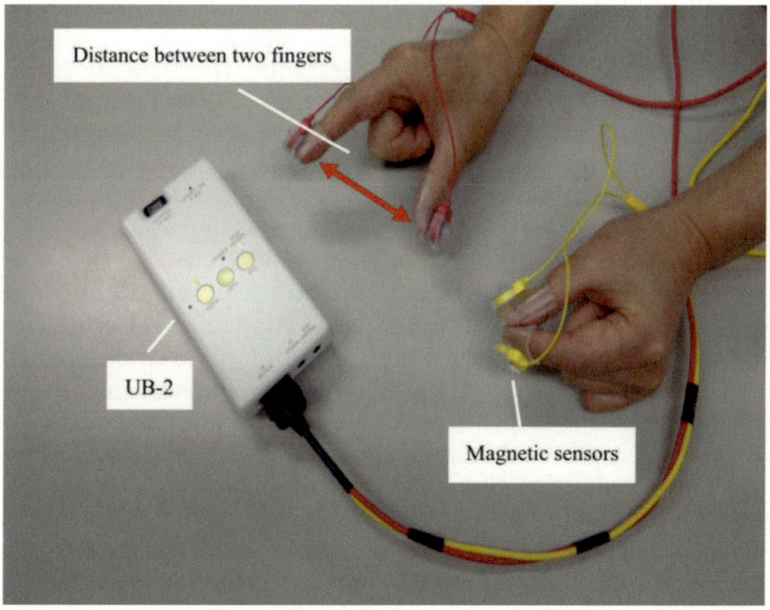

Figure 2.
Magnetic sensor-type finger tapping device (UB-2, Maxell Ltd., Tokyo, Japan) [47, 48]. The yellow cable is attached to the thumb and index finger of the left hand, and the red cable is attached to the thumb and index finger of the right hand. When the main unit is connected to a computer, the waveform of the finger tapping can be confirmed on the computer screen. The UB-2 is lightweight and portable.

5.2 Organization of issues for establishing cognitive frailty assessment using finger movements

Several challenges must be addressed to establish cognitive frailty assessments based on finger tapping movements for practical application. The first challenge involves standardizing assessment criteria. Although previous studies have described finger tapping characteristics associated with cognitive decline and physical frailty, specific characteristics of cognitive frailty remain unclear, and no evaluation criteria have been defined. Establishing standard values that account for age, sex, and educational background, along with cutoff values aligned with the severity of cognitive frailty, will be essential.

Next, we need to build evidence through longitudinal studies to enhance the predictive value of bilateral hand tapping. Current findings are primarily validated based on cross-sectional studies. However, for the early detection of cognitive frailty, it is crucial to clarify whether changes in finger tapping performance can predict symptom progression. Therefore, it is necessary to validate changes in finger tapping performance through long-term follow-up studies.

By addressing these challenges, it is expected that the evaluation method using finger tapping exercises will contribute to the early detection of cognitive frailty and the promotion of effective preventive interventions, leading to its establishment as a standardized objective evaluation method.

6. Conclusions

This work discussed the importance of cognitive frailty in the early detection of dementia and outlined the new possibilities for assessment methods. With the global aging of the population, dementia has emerged as a serious public health concern. Early detection of MCI and cognitive frailty, which are pre-stages of dementia, plays a crucial role in dementia prevention. Cognitive frailty, defined as the coexistence of physical frailty and cognitive decline, represents a condition in which both domains interact and mutually reinforce one another. Compared to physical frailty or cognitive impairment alone, cognitive frailty carries a 2.5 to 5 times higher risk of progression to dementia, making it a key target for early intervention. Conventional assessment methods typically evaluate physical and cognitive functions separately, failing to capture the interactive nature of cognitive frailty. Additionally, the lack of unified evaluation criteria has hindered the comparability of studies and the translation of findings into clinical practice. To address these limitations, this chapter proposed a novel assessment approach using finger tapping movements. Finger movements offer insight into complex cognitive functions and correlate with indicators of physical frailty. The use of a magnetic sensor-type finger tapping device enables accurate, objective, and quantitative measurement of movement velocity, rhythm, and bilateral coordination. This method can be easily performed in a seated position and is less affected by differences in cultural and educational backgrounds.

Moving forward, it is necessary to standardize evaluation criteria for finger tapping movements specifically targeting cognitive frailty and to accumulate evidence through follow-up studies. Through these efforts, finger tapping movement assessment has the potential to be applied as a standardized evaluation method for the early detection of cognitive frailty and for preventive interventions. The practical application of this new assessment method will likely contribute to dementia prevention and the maintenance of quality of life among older adults.

Acknowledgements

This work was supported by JSPS KAKENHI Grant Numbers JP23K10417 and JP 25KJ2198, as well as by the Yuumi Memorial Foundation for Home Health Care.

Conflict of interest

The authors declare no conflict of interest.

Appendices and nomenclature

MCI	mild cognitive impairment
CDR	clinical dementia rating
MMSE	mini-mental state examination
MoCA	Montreal Cognitive Assessment
IAGG	International Association of Gerontology and Geriatrics
IANA	International Academy of Nutrition and Aging

Author details

Shoya Fujikawa[1,2], Shin Murata[1], Shun Sawai[1,3], Takato Nishida[1,4], Ryosuke Yamamoto[1,5], Yusuke Shizuka[1,2], Naoki Shimizu[1,2] and Hideki Nakano[1*]

1 Graduate School of Health Sciences, Kyoto Tachibana University, Kyoto, Japan

2 Department of Rehabilitation, Kyoto Kuno Hospital, Kyoto, Japan

3 Society for the Promotion of Science (JSPS), Research Fellow (DC), Japan

4 Faculty of Rehabilitation and Care, Seijoh University, Aichi, Japan

5 Department of Rehabilitation, Tesseikai Neurosurgical Hospital, Osaka, Japan

*Address all correspondence to: nakano-h@tachibana-u.ac.jp

References

[1] United Nations. World Population Ageing 2019: Highlights. New York: United Nations; 2019. DOI: 10.18356/9df3caed-en

[2] McKhann GM, Knopman DS, Chertkow H, et al. The diagnosis of dementia due to Alzheimer's disease: Recommendations from the National Institute on Aging-Alzheimer's Association workgroups on diagnostic guidelines for Alzheimer's disease. Alzheimer's & Dementia. 2011;**7**(3):263-269. DOI: 10.1016/j.jalz.2011.03.005

[3] World Health Organization. Global Status Report on the Public Health Response to Dementia. Geneva: World Health Organization; 2021. DOI: 10.2471/BLT.21.287144

[4] Alzheimer's Disease International. World Alzheimer Report 2021: Journey through the Diagnosis of Dementia. London: Alzheimer's Disease International; 2021. DOI: 10.1002/alz.12328

[5] Ohara T, Hata J, Yoshida D, et al. Trends in dementia prevalence, incidence, and survival rate in a Japanese community. Neurology. 2017;**88**(20):1925-1932. DOI: 10.1212/WNL.0000000000003932

[6] Wimo A, Seeher K, Cataldi R, et al. The worldwide costs of dementia in 2019. Alzheimer's & Dementia. 2023;**19**(7):2865-2873. DOI: 10.1002/alz.12901

[7] Prince M, Comas-Herrera A, Knapp M, et al. World Alzheimer Report 2016: Improving Healthcare for People Living with Dementia. London: Alzheimer's Disease International; 2016. DOI: 10.13140/RG.2.2.22580.04483

[8] Wittenberg R, Hu B, Barraza-Araiza L, et al. Projections of Older People with Dementia and Costs of Dementia Care in the United Kingdom, 2019-2040. London, UK: Care Policy and Evaluation Centre, London School of Economics and Political Science; 2019. DOI: 10.21953/lse.5mqce2t01q5s

[9] Livingston G, Huntley J, Sommerlad A, et al. Dementia prevention, intervention, and care: 2020 report of the lancet commission. Lancet. 2020;**396**(10248):413-446. DOI: 10.1016/S0140-6736(20)30367-6. Epub 2020 Jul 30. Erratum in: Lancet. 2023 Sep 30;402(10408):1132. doi: 10.1016/S0140-6736(23)02043-3

[10] Petersen RC. Mild cognitive impairment as a diagnostic entity. Journal of Internal Medicine. 2004;**256**(3):183-194. DOI: 10.1111/j.1365-2796.2004.01388.x

[11] Winblad B, Palmer K, Kivipelto M, et al. Mild cognitive impairment–beyond controversies, towards a consensus: Report of the international working group on mild cognitive impairment. Journal of Internal Medicine. 2004;**256**(3):240-246. DOI: 10.1111/j.1365-2796.2004.01380.x

[12] Petersen RC, Caracciolo B, Brayne C, et al. Mild cognitive impairment: A concept in evolution. Journal of Internal Medicine. 2014;**275**(3):214-228. DOI: 10.1111/joim.12190

[13] American Psychiatric Association. Diagnostic and Statistical Manual of Mental Disorders. 5th ed. Washington, DC: APA Publishing; 2013. DOI: 10.1176/appi.books.9780890425596

[14] Petersen RC, Roberts RO, Knopman DS, et al. Mild cognitive

impairment: Ten years later. Archives of Neurology. 2009;**66**(12):1447-1455. DOI: 10.1001/archneurol.2009.266

[15] Ward A, Arrighi HM, Michels S, et al. Mild cognitive impairment: Disparity of incidence and prevalence estimates. Alzheimer's & Dementia. 2012;**8**(1):14-21. DOI: 10.1016/j.jalz.2011.01.002

[16] Jak AJ, Bondi MW, Delano-Wood L, et al. Quantification of five neuropsychological approaches to defining mild cognitive impairment. The American Journal of Geriatric Psychiatry. 2009;**17**(5):368-375. DOI: 10.1097/JGP.0b013e31819431d5

[17] Jack CR Jr, Petersen RC, Xu YC, et al. Prediction of AD with MRI-based hippocampal volume in mild cognitive impairment. Neurology. 1999;**52**(7):1397-1403. DOI: 10.1212/wnl.52.7.1397

[18] Ganguli M, Dodge HH, Shen C, et al. Mild cognitive impairment, amnestic type: An epidemiologic study. Neurology. 2004;**63**(1):115-121. DOI: 10.1212/01.wnl.0000132523.27540.81

[19] Belleville S, Fouquet C, Hudon C, et al. Neuropsychological measures that predict progression from mild cognitive impairment to Alzheimer's type dementia in older adults: A systematic review and meta-analysis. Neuropsychology Review. 2017;**27**(4):328-353. DOI: 10.1007/s11065-017-9361-5

[20] O'Bryant SE, Waring SC, Cullum CM, et al. Staging dementia using clinical dementia rating scale sum of boxes scores: A Texas Alzheimer's research consortium study. Archives of Neurology. 2008;**65**(8):1091-1095. DOI: 10.1001/archneur.65.8.1091

[21] Jack CR Jr, Shiung MM, Weigand SD, et al. Brain atrophy rates predict subsequent clinical conversion in normal elderly and amnestic MCI. Neurology. 2005;**65**(8):1227-1231. DOI: 10.1212/01.wnl.0000180958.22678.91

[22] Okello A, Koivunen J, Edison P, et al. Conversion of amyloid positive and negative MCI to AD over 3 years: An 11C-PIB PET study. Neurology. 2009;**73**(10):754-760. DOI: 10.1212/WNL.0b013e3181b23564

[23] Bangert AS, Balota DA. Keep up the pace: Declines in simple repetitive timing differentiate healthy aging from the earliest stages of Alzheimer's disease. Journal of the International Neuropsychological Society. 2012;**18**(6):1052-1063. DOI: 10.1017/S1355617712000860

[24] Sugioka J, Suzumura S, Kuno K, Kizuka S, Sakurai H, Kanada Y, et al. Relationship between finger movement characteristics and brain voxel-based morphometry. PLoS One. 2022;**17**(10):e0269351. DOI: 10.1371/journal.pone.0269351

[25] Scheltens P, Leys D, Barkhof F, Huglo D, Weinstein HC, Vermersch P, et al. Atrophy of medial temporal lobes on MRI in "probable" Alzheimer's disease and normal ageing: Diagnostic value and neuropsychological correlates. Journal of Neurology, Neurosurgery, and Psychiatry. 1992;**55**(10):967-972. DOI: 10.1136/jnnp.55.10.967

[26] Kelaiditi E, Cesari M, Canevelli M, et al. Cognitive frailty: Rational and definition from an (I.A.G.G./I.A.N.A.) International Consensus Group. The Journal of Nutrition, Health & Aging. 2013;**17**(9):726-734. DOI: 10.1007/s12603-013-0367-2

[27] Morley JE, Morris JC, Berg-Weger M, et al. Brain health: The importance of recognizing cognitive impairment: An IAGG consensus conference. Journal

of the American Medical Directors Association. 2015;**16**(9):731-739. DOI: 10.1016/j.jamda.2015.06.017

[28] Feng L, Nyunt MS, Gao Q, et al. Cognitive frailty and adverse health outcomes: Findings from the Singapore Longitudinal Ageing Studies (SLAS). Journal of the American Medical Directors Association. 2017;**18**(3):252-258. DOI: 10.1016/j.jamda.2016.09.015

[29] Panza F, Lozupone M, Solfrizzi V, et al. Different cognitive frailty models and health- and cognitive-related outcomes in older age: From epidemiology to prevention. Journal of Alzheimer's Disease. 2018;**62**(3):993-1012. DOI: 10.3233/JAD-170963

[30] Grande G, Haaksma ML, Rizzuto D, et al. Co-occurrence of cognitive impairment and physical frailty, and incidence of dementia: Systematic review and meta-analysis. Neuroscience and Biobehavioral Reviews. 2019;**107**:96-103. DOI: 10.1016/j.neubiorev.2019.09.001

[31] Robertson DA, Savva GM, Kenny RA. Frailty and cognitive impairment–A review of the evidence and causal mechanisms. Ageing Research Reviews. 2013;**12**(4):840-851. DOI: 10.1016/j.arr.2013.06.004

[32] Morley JE, Vellas B, van Kan GA, et al. Frailty consensus: A call to action. Journal of the American Medical Directors Association. 2013 Jun;**14**(6):392-397. DOI: 10.1016/j.jamda.2013.03.022

[33] Sathyan S, Barzilai N, Atzmon G, Milman S, Ayers E, Verghese J. Association of anti-inflammatory cytokine IL10 polymorphisms with motoric cognitive risk syndrome in an Ashkenazi Jewish population. Neurobiology of Aging. Oct 2017;**58**:238.e1-238.e8. DOI: 10.1016/j.neurobiolaging.2017.06.006. Epub 2017 Jun 19

[34] Erickson KI, Weinstein AM, Lopez OL. Physical activity, brain plasticity, and Alzheimer's disease. Archives of Medical Research. 2012;**43**(8):615-621. DOI: 10.1016/j.arcmed.2012.09.008

[35] de la Torre JC. Cardiovascular risk factors promote brain hypoperfusion leading to cognitive decline and dementia. Cardiovascular Psychiatry and Neurology. 2012;**2012**:367516. DOI: 10.1155/2012/367516

[36] Kostic E, Kwak K, Kim D. Changes in sensory, postural stability and gait functions depending on cognitive decline, and possible markers for detection of cognitive status. BMC Medical Informatics and Decision Making. 2022;**22**(Suppl. 5):252. DOI: 10.1186/s12911-022-01955-x

[37] Kiesswetter E, Pohlhausen S, Uhlig K, et al. Malnutrition is related to functional impairment in older adults receiving home care. The Journal of Nutrition, Health & Aging. 2013;**17**(4):345-350. DOI: 10.1007/s12603-012-0409-1

[38] Muir SW, Gopaul K, Montero Odasso MM. The role of cognitive impairment in fall risk among older adults: A systematic review and meta-analysis. Age and Ageing. 2012;**41**(3):299-308. DOI: 10.1093/ageing/afs012

[39] Arai H, Satake S, Kozaki K. Cognitive frailty in geriatrics. Clinics in Geriatric Medicine. 2018;**34**(4):667-675. DOI: 10.1016/j.cger.2018.06.011

[40] Facal D, Maseda A, Pereiro AX, et al. Cognitive frailty: A conceptual systematic review and an operational proposal for future research. Maturitas. 2019;**121**:48-56. DOI: 10.1016/j.maturitas.2018.12.006

[41] Malek Rivan NF, Shahar S, Rajab NF, Singh DKA, Din NC, Hazlina M, et al. Cognitive frailty among Malaysian older adults: Baseline findings from the LRGS TUA cohort study. Clinical Interventions in Aging. 2019;**14**:1343-1352. DOI: 10.2147/CIA.S211027

[42] Kueper JK, Speechley M, Lingum NR, et al. Motor function and incident dementia: A systematic review and meta-analysis. Age and Ageing. 2017;**46**(5):729-738. DOI: 10.1093/ageing/afx084

[43] Clouston SA, Brewster P, Kuh D, Richards M, Cooper R, Hardy R, et al. The dynamic relationship between physical function and cognition in longitudinal aging cohorts. Epidemiologic Reviews. 2013;**35**(1):33-50. DOI: 10.1093/epirev/mxs004. Epub 2013 Jan 24

[44] Carment L, Abdellatif A, Lafuente-Lafuente C, Pariel S, Maier MA, Belmin J, et al. Manual dexterity and aging: A pilot study disentangling sensorimotor from cognitive decline. Frontiers in Neurology. 2018;**9**:910. DOI: 10.3389/fneur.2018.00910

[45] Kobayashi-Cuya KE, Sakurai R, Suzuki H, Ogawa S, Takebayashi T, Fujiwara Y. Observational evidence of the association between handgrip strength, hand dexterity, and cognitive performance in community-dwelling older adults: A systematic review. Journal of Epidemiology. 2018;**28**(9):373-381. DOI: 10.2188/jea.JE20170041. Epub 2018 Mar 10

[46] Shizuka Y, Murata S, Goda A, Sawai S, Fujikawa S, Yamamoto R, et al. Aging-related changes in bimanual coordination as a screening tool for healthy aging. Geriatrics (Basel). 2025;**10**(2):45. DOI: 10.3390/geriatrics10020045

[47] Rabinowitz I, Lavner Y. Association between finger tapping, attention, memory, and cognitive diagnosis in elderly patients. Perceptual and Motor Skills. 2014;**119**(1):259-278. DOI: 10.2466/10.22.PMS.119c12z3. Epub 2014 Jun 24

[48] Suzumura S, Kanada Y, Osawa A, Sugioka J, Maeda N, Nagahama T, et al. Assessment of finger motor function that reflects the severity of cognitive function. Fujita Medical Journal. 2021;7(4):122-129. DOI: 10.20407/fmj.2020-013. Epub 2020 Dec 16

[49] Shima K, Tsuji T, Kan E, Kandori A, Yokoe M, Sakoda S. Measurement and evaluation of finger tapping movements using magnetic sensors. Annual International Conference of the IEEE Engineering in Medicine and Biology Society. 2008;**2008**:5628-5631. DOI: 10.1109/IEMBS.2008.4650490

[50] Tomita Y, Tanaka S, Takahashi S, Takeuchi N. Detecting cognitive decline in community-dwelling older adults using simple cognitive and motor performance tests. Geriatrics & Gerontology International. 2020;**20**(3):212-217. DOI: 10.1111/ggi.13863. Epub 2020 Jan 9

[51] Sugioka J, Suzumura S, Kawahara Y, Osawa A, Maeda N, Ito M, et al. Assessment of finger movement characteristics in dementia patients using a magnetic sensing finger-tap device. Japanese Journal of Comprehensive Rehabilitation Science. 2020;**11**:91-94. DOI: 10.11336/jjcrs.11.91

[52] Fujikawa S, Murata S, Goda A, Sawai S, Yamamoto R, Shizuka Y, et al. Comparison of characteristics of bimanual coordinated movements in older adults with frailty, pre-frailty, and robust health. Frontiers in Aging. 2025;**6**:1519129. DOI: 10.3389/fragi.2025.1519129

Section 3

Musculoskeletal Rehabilitation and Integrative Care

Chapter 7

Comparing Myofascial Release and Muscle Energy Technique for Hamstring Muscle Tightness in Symptomatic University Students

Chijindu-Orji Iseh-Ntah

Abstract

Hamstring muscle tightness is a common musculoskeletal issue, particularly among students, due to prolonged sitting and physical inactivity. This study compares the effects of two manual therapies, myofascial release (MFR) and muscle energy technique (MET), on hamstring muscle tightness, pain, and flexibility in symptomatic students at the University of Calabar. A total of 60 students were randomly assigned to MFR or MET groups. Both groups underwent 12 therapy sessions over 4 weeks. Pain, flexibility, and tightness were assessed using the numerical pain rating scale (NPRS), active knee extension test (AKET), and sit and reach test (SRT). Both interventions led to significant improvements ($p < 0.05$). However, only MET showed statistically superior results in reducing hamstring tightness ($p = 0.003$).

Keywords: hamstring tightness, myofascial release, muscle energy technique, flexibility, muscle tightness, manual therapy, pain reduction

1. Introduction

The hamstring muscles are involved in a wide range of daily activities and physical movements, making them susceptible to overuse and injury [1]. Students, particularly those engaged in prolonged sitting or sedentary routines, face an increased risk of hamstring tightness due to physical inactivity and poor posture, which can cause the muscles to lose flexibility and subsequently restrict range of motion [2, 3]. Tight hamstrings can reduce physical performance and increase the risk of injuries such as hamstring strains and low back pain, and if left untreated, may worsen existing musculoskeletal issues like posterior pelvic tilting and reduced lumbar lordosis, ultimately impacting quality of life and functional independence [4, 5].

A wide range of interventions, such as cryotherapy, static stretching, and proprioceptive neuromuscular facilitation, have traditionally been employed to manage hamstring tightness; however, manual therapies like myofascial release (MFR) and muscle energy technique (MET) have gained popularity [6]. MFR uses sustained pressure and stretching to release fascial restrictions, potentially improving both muscle extensibility and overall tissue mobility [7, 8]. MET involves isometric muscle contractions followed by stretching, leveraging neuromuscular mechanisms like autogenic and reciprocal inhibition to restore function [9, 10].

Although these techniques are widely used, most studies evaluating their effectiveness have been conducted in Asia and focused on asymptomatic or athletic populations [1, 11]. There is a lack of comparative evidence from African contexts, particularly involving symptomatic student populations. This study addresses that gap by comparing the effects of MFR and MET on hamstring tightness, pain, and flexibility among university students in Nigeria.

2. Literature review

2.1 Anatomy and function of the hamstrings

Hamstring muscles, comprising the semimembranosus, semitendinosus, and biceps femoris, form the posterior compartment of the thigh; they cross both the hip and knee joints, acting primarily to extend the hip and flex the knee, and play a critical role in locomotion such as walking, running, and climbing stairs [12, 13]. Due to their dual function and anatomical location, the hamstrings are particularly susceptible to tightness, especially in individuals with sedentary lifestyles or those who engage in vigorous physical activity without sufficient stretching [2].

The hamstrings are innervated by the sciatic nerve and originate from the ischial tuberosity, with distal insertions on the tibia and fibula. Their long tendons and overlapping muscle bellies facilitate force transmission, but this structure also contributes to their vulnerability to strain and shortening [14]. An imbalance in their activation or flexibility can significantly affect pelvic alignment, resulting in postural dysfunctions like posterior pelvic tilt and decreased lumbar lordosis [15, 16].

2.2 Assessment of hamstring flexibility

Clinical tools such as the active knee extension test (AKET), sit and reach test (SRT), and the numeric pain rating scale (NPRS) are widely used to assess hamstring tightness, flexibility, and related discomfort [17, 18]. These tools are validated for use in both clinical and academic settings.

2.3 Myofascial release (MFR)

MFR is a manual therapy technique involving sustained, gentle pressure to fascia and surrounding tissues to relieve tension and improve mobility [19]. It facilitates soft tissue extensibility and improves blood flow, making it effective for localized tightness and fascial restrictions [20]. Techniques such as cross-hand release and longitudinal plane release target various fascial planes to restore normal tissue function [7, 8].

2.4 Muscle energy technique (MET)

MET is an active therapy that utilizes isometric contractions followed by passive stretching to restore muscle length and joint range of motion, with its effects attributed to the underlying mechanisms of autogenic and reciprocal inhibition that facilitate muscle relaxation and neuromuscular re-education [9, 10].

2.5 Empirical evidence supporting myofascial release (MFR) and muscle energy technique (MET)

Several studies have evaluated the effects of myofascial release (MFR) and muscle energy technique (MET) on hamstring flexibility. One study found that both methods significantly improved hamstring flexibility in footballers, with no statistical difference between the groups [1]. Another study echoed these findings in a student population, suggesting comparable benefits of the two techniques [3]. A separate study observed that both MET and Active Release Technique (ART) produced significant improvements in flexibility and pain reduction, although ART was slightly more effective [21]. Similar trends were reported in another trial, which concluded that while both MET and ART were effective, ART yielded a superior immediate impact on flexibility [4].

3. Methodology

3.1 Research design

This study utilized a pretest–posttest experimental design. Participants were randomly assigned into two treatment groups: one receiving Myofascial Release (MFR) and the other receiving muscle energy technique (MET), with each group undergoing identical assessment procedures at baseline and post-intervention.

3.2 Population and sampling

The study population comprised male and female students of the University of Calabar, aged 18 to 35 years, presenting with unilateral hamstring muscle tightness and full passive knee extension range of motion. Exclusion criteria included acute hamstring injury, neurological deficits, systemic illness, or deformities. Simple random sampling was used to ensure equal representation. A total of 60 students were recruited for the study.

3.3 Data collection instrument

3.3.1 Data capture form

The data capture form was used to collect information on age, gender, level of study, height, weight and vital signs, as well as to record baseline health parameters and the outcome of the treatment administered to the participants.

3.3.2 Weighing scale

A floor-type weighing scale calibrated from 0 to 160 kg was used to measure participants' body weight in kilograms (kg).

3.3.3 Height meter

A height meter calibrated from 0 to 200 cm was used to measure participants' height in centimeters (cm).

3.3.4 Digital blood pressure monitor

A digital blood pressure monitor was used to measure systolic and diastolic blood pressure in millimeter mercury (mmHg) as well as the pulse rate in beats per minute (bpm).

3.3.5 Digital thermometer

The digital thermometer was used to measure body temperature in degree centigrade (°C).

3.3.6 Digital stop watch

The digital stopwatch was used to assess the respiratory rate in cycles per minute (cpm) following the rise and fall of the chest wall in 1 minute.

3.3.7 Measuring tape

A non-stretch tape measure calibrated in centimeters (0 to 150 cm) and inches (0 to 60 inches) was used to assess hamstring muscle flexibility in inches during the sit and reach test.

3.3.8 Goniometer

A 360-degree universal goniometer was used to measure the popliteal angle during the active knee extension test during the active knee extension test.

3.4 Outcome measures

3.4.1 Numerical pain rating scale (NPRS)

The Numerical Pain Rating Scale (NPRS) is a commonly used self-report instrument for assessing pain intensity, using an 11-point scale ranging from 0 (no pain) to 10 (worst imaginable pain) [22]. The scale is often categorized as follows: 0 indicates no pain, 1 to 3 represents mild pain, 4 to 6 indicates moderate pain, and 7 to 10 represents severe pain [23]. Participants are asked to rate their worst pain intensity over the past 24 hours on this scale [22].

The NPRS has demonstrated strong psychometric properties, including good to excellent test-retest reliability (intraclass correlation coefficient: 0.64–0.96) and strong correlation with the visual analog scale ($r = 0.79–0.95$), supporting its validity [24, 25]. Due to its simplicity, reliability, and sensitivity to clinical change, the NPRS is widely accepted in both clinical and research settings [24].

3.4.2 Active knee extension test

The popliteal angle is a common clinical indicator used to assess hamstring muscle tightness and is measured using the active knee extension (AKE) test, which evaluates hamstring muscle length based on the range of active knee extension when the hip is flexed to 90 degrees [26]. During the test, the participant lies supine on a plinth with the non-tested leg extended and stabilized, while the tested limb is flexed at the hip to

90 degrees and the participant is instructed to actively extend the knee as far as possible [27]. A lag of up to 20 degrees from full extension is generally considered normal, while an angle greater than 20 degrees is indicative of hamstring tightness [26].

The knee extension angle is measured using a universal goniometer, with the fulcrum aligned with the lateral femoral epicondyle, the stationary arm pointing toward the greater trochanter, and the movable arm aligned with the fibula toward the lateral malleolus [27]. The active knee extension (AKE) test has demonstrated high inter-rater and intra-rater reliability, with intraclass correlation coefficients (ICCs) ranging from 0.87 to 0.99 and has been validated against radiographic assessments and other clinical measures for evaluating hamstring flexibility [28].

3.4.3 Sit and reach test

The sit-and-reach test is a widely used method for assessing hamstring muscle flexibility, and in its V sit-and-reach variation, a baseline is marked on the floor with a measuring ruler placed perpendicular to it intersecting at the 15-inch mark; the participant sits with heels aligned to the baseline, feet 12 inches apart, and legs extended, then slowly bends forward as far as possible while keeping the knees straight, holds the position for 2 seconds, and the furthest reach is recorded across three trials, with the best score taken [29].

This test demonstrates moderate criterion-related validity for estimating hamstring flexibility, with population-corrected correlation coefficients ranging from 0.46 to 0.67 [30], and it shows high test-retest reliability, with intraclass correlation coefficients typically exceeding 0.80 [31].

3.5 Ethical considerations

Ethical approval was obtained from the Health, Research and Ethics Committee of the Department of Physiotherapy, University of Calabar. Written informed consent was obtained from each participant. Anonymity and confidentiality were ensured throughout the study.

3.6 Intervention protocol

Participants went through a series of pre-treatment assessment using the numerical pain rating scale (NPRS), active knee extension test (AKET), and sit and reach test (SRT). These pre-treatment assessments established a baseline for each participant, which was later compared to post-treatment measurements using the same assessment tools. Following the pre-treatment assessments, participants received treatments based on their allocated groups three times per week for 4 weeks, totaling 12 sessions.

For Group A, participants received Myofascial Release (MFR) using the cross-hand release technique. The participant lay in a prone position with legs extended, while the researcher, positioned beside the affected limb, placed one hand on the posterior thigh near the knee and the other just below the ischial tuberosity; firm pressure was applied into the tissue barrier and maintained for 30 seconds, with the technique repeated five times to complete the session [19].

Group B participants received muscle energy technique (MET) using the post isometric relaxation approach. The participant lay in a supine position and was instructed to fully flex the hip on the affected side; the researcher, positioned beside the treatment bed, extended the knee to the point of resistance and rested the participant's calf over their shoulder, using one hand to stabilize the unaffected leg and the other to support the affected thigh, then guided the participant to perform a 20% hamstring contraction held for 10 seconds against resistance, followed by a 5-second relaxation and further knee extension, repeating the sequence five times [9, 10].

Both groups were reassessed post-treatment using NPRS, AKET, and SRT to evaluate the effectiveness of each intervention.

3.7 Data analysis

Data were analyzed using IBM SPSS Statistics version 27. Descriptive statistics summarized demographic and clinical characteristics. Analysis of Covariance (ANCOVA) was employed to compare post-intervention outcomes between MFR and MET groups, using pre-intervention scores as covariates. Statistical significance threshold was set at $p \leq 0.05$.

4. Results and discussion

4.1 Participant demographic, physical, and clinical profile

A total of 60 symptomatic university students participated in the study, with equal allocation to the myofascial release (MFR) group (n = 30) and the muscle energy technique (MET) group (n = 30). The sociodemographic characteristics showed that the majority of participants were aged 21–25 years (55%) and female (56.7%). Most participants were in their 300 level of study (28.3%), and the right thigh was identified as the dominant side affected by hamstring tightness in 68.3% of cases. BMI classification showed that 48.3% of participants were of normal weight, another 48.3% were overweight, and 3.3% were classified as obese. These details are summarized in **Table 1**.

Physical and clinical parameters revealed a mean age of 23.4 years (SD = 3.38), average BMI of 24.72 kg/m^2 (SD = 2.84), systolic BP of 111.6 mmHg (SD = 8.8), diastolic BP of 69.9 mmHg (SD = 6.1), and body temperature of 36.74°C (SD = 0.38). These details are summarized in **Table 2**.

4.2 Intervention effects: ANCOVA analysis

Post-intervention results showed improvements in pain intensity, hamstring extensibility, and flexibility for both groups. However, ANCOVA revealed statistically significant differences in favor of MET in the active knee extension test (AKET) ($F = 9.595$, $p = 0.003$), while other outcome measures did not differ significantly. These findings are presented in **Table 3** and visually illustrated in **Figure 1**, which compares the adjusted post-intervention mean scores across outcome measures for both groups.

These findings indicate that both techniques were effective, but MET produced superior gains in hamstring extensibility.

4.3 Gender variance analysis

Independent t-tests showed no significant differences between male and female participants across most parameters. An exception was BMI, which was

Variables	Frequency	Percent
Age group		
18–20 years	12	20.0
21–25 years	13	55.0
26–30 years	13	21.5
31–35 years	2	3.3
Gender		
Male	26	43.3
Female	34	56.7
Body mass index class		
Normal weight	29	48.3
Overweight	29	48.3
Obese	2	3.3
Level of study		
100 level	11	18.3
200 level	16	26.7
300 level	17	28.3
400 level	11	18.3
500 level	5	8.3
Affected thigh		
Left	19	31.7
Right	41	68.3
Treatment group		
Myofascial release (MFR)	30	50.0
Muscle energy technique (MET)	30	50.0

Table 1.
Frequency distribution of sociodemographic characteristics of Participants (n = 60).

Variables	Mean	SD	Minimum	Maximum
Age (years)	23.40	3.38	18	32
Weight (kilogram)	69.35	8.46	54	87
Height (meters)	1.68	0.09	1.51	1.85
Body mass index (kg/m^2)	24.72	2.84	19.30	35.30
Systolic blood pressure (mmHg)	111.58	8.84	92	123
Diastolic blood pressure (mmHg)	69.95	6.11	62	84
Respiratory rate (cycles per minute)	15.90	1.67	12	18
Pulse rate (beats per minute)	66.33	3.10	62	73
Temperature (degree centigrade)	36.74	0.38	35.80	38.50

Keys: mmHg - millimeter mercury; kg/m^2 - kilogram per meter square; SD - Standard Deviation.

Table 2.
Descriptive statistics of mean ± SD of physical and clinical characteristics of participants (n = 60).

Variables	MFR (30) Adjusted Mean ± SD	MET (30) Adjusted Mean ± SD	F	p-value
Numerical Pain rating after intervention	4.03 ± 1.47	4.20 ± 1.38	0.242	0.625[NS]
Active knee extension test after intervention (°)	35.70 ± 8.73	32.67 ± 8.43	9.595	0.003**
Sit and reach test after intervention (inches)	19.43 ± 3.01	19.90 ± 2.72	0.455	0.503[NS]

*Keys: ** - highly significant; NS - not significant; MFR - myofascial release; MET - muscle energy technique; ° - degree; SD - Standard Deviation.*

Table 3.
Analysis of covariance results for the effect of myofascial release versus muscle energy technique.

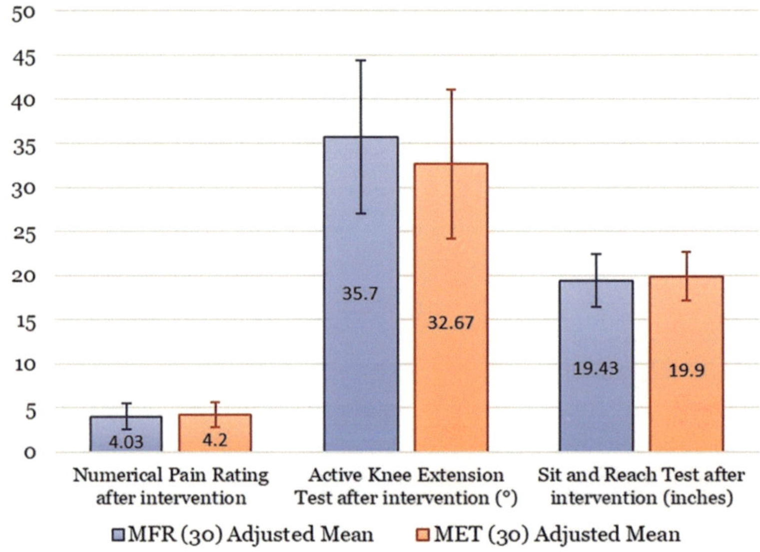

Figure 1.
Adjusted post-intervention mean scores of NPRS, AKET, and SRT between MFR and MET groups. Keys: *MFR - myofascial release; MET - muscle energy technique; ° - degree; SD - standard deviation.*

significantly higher among females (p = 0.042). No gender-based differences were observed in post-intervention NPRS, AKET, or SRT scores. These details are summarized in **Table 4**.

4.4 Discussion

The findings of this study demonstrate that both MFR and MET are effective interventions for reducing hamstring pain and tightness and improving flexibility. The greater efficacy of MET in improving popliteal angle supports the neuromuscular basis of the technique, which leverages autogenic and reciprocal inhibition to facilitate muscle lengthening [9, 10].

These findings align with the results of the studies in Refs. [1, 3], which found both MFR and MET effective in improving hamstring flexibility. The current results also echo the study in Ref. [4], which concluded that both MET and Active Release

Variables	Male (26) Mean ± SD	Female (34) Mean ± SD	t-value	p-value
Age (years)	23.77 ± 3.24	23.12 ± 3.50	.738	0.463
Weight (kilogram)	68.00 ± 8.89	70.38 ± 8.10	−1.082	0.284
Height (meters)	1.69 ± .10	1.66 ± .07	1.243	0.219
Body mass index (kg/m^2)	23.87 ± 3.60	25.37 ± 1.91	−2.079	0.042
Systolic Blood pressure (mmHg)	110.54 ± 8.99	112.38 ± 8.78	−.798	0.428
Diastolic blood pressure (mmHg)	70.04 ± 6.19	69.88 ± 6.14	.097	0.923
Respiratory rate (cycles per minute)	15.69 ± 1.57	16.06 ± 1.74	−.843	0.403
Pulse rate (beats per minute)	66.42 ± 3.58	66.26 ± 2.73	.194	0.847
Temperature (°C)	36.68 ± .20	36.78 ± .47	−1.031	0.307
NPRS before treatment	6.00 ± 1.50	6.12 ± 1.57	−.293	0.770
NPRS after treatment	3.92 ± 1.06	4.27 ± 1.64	−.925	0.359
AKET before treatment (°)	42.89 ± 9.55	47.15 ± 9.64	−1.704	0.094
AKET after treatment (°)	32.00 ± 8.21	35.85 ± 8.71	−1.740	0.087
SRT before treatment (inches)	16.58 ± 2.63	15.71 ± 2.37	1.347	0.183
SRT after treatment (inches)	19.89 ± 3.04	19.50 ± 2.74	.514	0.609

Keys: NPRS - numerical pain rating scale; AKET - active knee extension test; SRT - sit and reach test; kg/m^2 - kilogram per meter square; °C - degree centigrade; mmHg - millimeter mercury; ° - degree.

Table 4.
Gender variance in age, anthropometric measurements, cardiorespiratory parameters, body temperature, pain, active knee extension test, and sit and reach test.

Technique significantly improved flexibility, though ART was slightly more effective. Moreover, the study in Ref. [2] emphasized that sedentary habits among students predispose them to hamstring tightness, reinforcing the relevance of these findings.

Interestingly, while MET was superior in AKET results, pain (NPRS) and flexibility (SRT) scores did not significantly differ between interventions. This suggests that both techniques offer holistic benefits, and selection can be individualized based on patient preference or practitioner expertise.

5. Conclusion

This study compared the effectiveness of myofascial release (MFR) and muscle energy technique (MET) in the treatment of hamstring muscle tightness among symptomatic university students. The findings confirmed that both interventions were effective in reducing pain (as measured by NPRS), increasing flexibility (*via* SRT), and enhancing hamstring extensibility (*via* AKET). However, MET demonstrated a statistically significant advantage in improving hamstring extensibility, as indicated by superior AKET outcomes ($p = 0.003$).

These results reinforce previous research affirming the clinical value of both MFR and MET [1, 3], while highlighting MET's potential superiority in muscle length restoration. The outcomes also emphasize the importance of incorporating targeted manual therapies into physiotherapy regimens for student populations affected by musculoskeletal limitations due to sedentary behavior.

Appendixes

Data capture form

a. *Demographic and Physical Characteristics*

Code:
Age (years):
Gender:
Level of study:
Height (m):
Weight (kg):

b. *Clinical Parameters*

Heart rate (bpm):
Blood pressure (mmHg):
Temperature (°C):
Respiratory rate (cpm):

c. *Health status*

Presenting condition:

d. *Intervention*

Treatment group:
Affected thigh:

e. *Numerical pain rating scale*

Baseline:
After intervention:

f. *Active knee extension test*

Baseline (°):
After intervention (°):

g. *Sit and reach test*

Baseline (inches):
After intervention (inches):

Author details

Chijindu-Orji Iseh-Ntah
University of Calabar, Calabar, Nigeria

*Address all correspondence to: chijipeters1@gmail.com

References

[1] Patel N, Patel A, Patel M. Immediate effects of muscle energy technique versus myofascial release techniques on hamstring flexibility in footballers: A comparative study. International Journal of Science and Research. 2023;**12**(7):240-245. DOI: 10.21275/SR23703123353

[2] Chellapillai FM, Wijayalath WP, Dayarathna WM, Safinaz ZM, Ihsan AN, Neranjan EP, et al. Predisposing factors for hamstring tightness among university students. Journal of Physiotherapy and Physical Rehabilitation. 2019;**4**(2):1-3

[3] Balasubramaniam A, Gandhi MV, Kumar PR, Vasanthi RK, Purushothaman VK. Myofascial release therapy versus muscle energy technique on hamstring flexibility in physically inactive students - a randomized controlled trial. Universal Journal of Public Health. 2022;**10**(4):299-303. DOI: 10.13189/ujph.2022.100403

[4] Khan S, Patel B, Limbani B. Immediate effect of active release technique versus muscle energy technique in subjects with hamstring tightness: A randomized clinical trial. Indian Journal of Physiotherapy and Occupational Therapy. 2021;**15**(2):59. DOI: 10.37506/ijpot.v15i2.14514

[5] Akinpelu A, Bakare U, Adegoke B. Influence of age on hamstring tightness in apparently healthy Nigerians. Journal of the Nigeria Society of Physiotherapy. 2005;**15**(2):35-41

[6] Gayathri K, Senthil P, Swathi S, Neelam N, Nainar M, Haribabu L. Effectiveness of myofascial release technique and muscle energy technique on pain and physical function among smartphone users with trapezitis. Chettinad Health City Medical Journal. 2022;**11**(4):37-41. DOI: 10.24321/2278.2044.202238

[7] Bradbury-Squires DJ, Noftall JC, Sullivan KM, Behm DG, Power KE. Roller-massager application to the quadriceps and knee-joint range of motion and neuromuscular efficiency during a lunge. Journal of Athletic Training. 2015;**50**(2):133-140

[8] Wong KK, Chai HM, Chen YJ, Wang CL, Shau YW, Wang SF. Mechanical deformation of posterior thoracolumbar fascia after myofascial release in healthy men: A study of dynamic ultrasound imaging. Musculoskeletal Science and Practice. 2017;**27**:124-130. DOI: 10.1016/j.math.2016.10.011

[9] Chaitow L, Crenshaw K. Muscle energy techniques. 3rd ed. Edinburgh: Elsevier Churchill Livingstone; 2006

[10] Gibbons J. Muscle Energy Technique: A Practical Guide for Physical Therapists. 2nd ed. Oxford: Bodymaster Method; 2022. ISBN: 978-1905367238

[11] Raza A, Ijaz A, Saqib MS, Zahoor IA, Ahmed I, Abid N. Effectiveness of hamstring stretching versus muscle energy technique on hamstring flexibility in patients with non-specific knee pain: A randomized clinical trial. The Healer Journal. 2023;**3**(7):671. DOI: 10.55735/hjprs.v3i7.187

[12] Grujičić R. Biceps Femoris Muscle. Leipzig, Germany: Kenhub Library; 2023. Available from: https://www.kenhub.com/en/library/anatomy/biceps-femoris-muscle [Accessed: March 26, 2025]

[13] Moore KL, Dalley AF, Agur AM. Clinically Oriented Anatomy. 7th ed.

Philadelphia: Lippincott Williams & Wilkins; 2014

[14] Linklater J, Hamilton B, Carmichael J, Orchard J, Wood D. Hamstring injuries: Anatomy, imaging, and intervention. Seminars in Musculoskeletal Radiology. 2010;**14**(2):131-161

[15] Fatima G, Qamar M, Hassan J, Basharat A. Extended sitting can cause hamstring tightness. Saudi Journal of Sports Medicine. 2017;**17**(2):110-114. DOI: 10.4103/sjsm.sjsm_5_17

[16] Kanishka GK, Sandamali H, Weerasinghe I, Binduhewa L, Dilshara C, DeSilva C, et al. Prevalence of hamstring tightness and associated factors among sewing machine operators. Ceylon Journal of Medical Science. 2019;**56**(1):24-31. DOI: 10.4038/cjms.v56i1.4957

[17] Hamid M, Ali M, Yusof A. Interrater and intrarater reliability of the active knee extension (AKE) test among healthy adults. Journal of Physical Therapy Science. 2013;**25**(8):957-961. DOI: 10.1589/jpts.25.957

[18] Ferraz M, Quaresma M, Aquino L, Atra E, Tugwell P, Goldsmith C. Reliability of pain scales in the assessment of literate and illiterate patients with rheumatoid arthritis. Journal of Rheumatology. 1990;**17**:1022-1024

[19] Duncan RA. Myofascial Release. United States: Versa Press; 2014. ISBN: 978-1450444576

[20] Beardsley C, Karabot J. Effects of self-myofascial release: A systematic review. Journal of Bodywork and Movement Therapies. 2015;**19**(4):747-758. DOI: 10.1016/j.jbmt.2015.08.007

[21] Sheth R, Rizvi S. The immediate effect of muscle energy technique versus active release technique on hamstring tightness in footballers. International Journal of Science and Healthcare Research. 2022;**7**(2):282-294. DOI: 10.52403/ijshr.20220440

[22] Farrar JT, Young JP Jr, LaMoreaux L, Werth JL, Poole RM. Clinical importance of changes in chronic pain intensity measured on an 11-point numerical pain rating scale. Pain. 2001;**94**(2):149-158

[23] Childs JD, Piva SR, Fritz JM. Responsiveness of the numeric pain rating scale in patients with low back pain. Spine. 2005;**30**(11):1331-1334

[24] Salaffi F, Stancati A, Silvestri CA, Ciapetti A, Grassi W. Minimal clinically important changes in chronic musculoskeletal pain intensity measured on a numerical rating scale. European Journal of Pain. 2004;**8**(4):283-291

[25] Williamson A, Hoggart B. Pain: A review of three commonly used pain rating scales. Journal of Clinical Nursing. 2005;**14**(7):798-804

[26] Davis DS, Quinn RO, Whiteman CT, Williams JD, Young CR. Concurrent validity of four clinical tests used to measure hamstring flexibility. Journal of Strength and Conditioning Research. 2008;**22**(2):583-586

[27] Gajdosik RL, Lusin G. Hamstring muscle tightness: Reliability of an active-knee-extension test. Physical Therapy. 1983;**63**(7):1085-1090

[28] Bandy WD, Irion JM, Briggler M. The effect of time and frequency of static stretching on flexibility of the hamstring muscles. Physical Therapy. 1997;**77**(10):1090-1096

[29] Mayorga-Vega D, Merino-Marban R, Viciana J. Criterion-related validity of sit-and-reach tests for estimating

hamstring and lumbar extensibility: A meta-analysis. Journal of Sports Science and Medicine. 2014;**13**(1):1-14

[30] Ayala F, Sainz de Baranda P, de Ste CM, Santonja F. Reproducibility and criterion-related validity of the sit-and-reach and toe-touch tests for estimating hamstring flexibility in recreationally active young adults. Physical Therapy in Sport. 2012;**13**(4):219-226

[31] Baltaci G, Tunay V, Besler A, Gerçeker G. Absolute reliability of modified sit-and-reach and back-saver sit-and-reach tests for estimating hamstring flexibility in futsal players. Apunts Medicina de l'Esport. 2011;**46**(170):81-88

Chapter 8

Integrative Treatment for Arthritis

Stefka Stoilova

Abstract

Integrative medicine is a holistic approach that focuses on the patient (the person as a whole) rather than the disease; it combines methods of conventional evidence-based medicine with complementary therapies to improve all aspects of health, including physical, mental and spiritual well-being. Leading global organizations recommend the use of both pharmacological and non-pharmacological treatments in the management of arthritis, with the participation of a multidisciplinary team. Recommendations include both medical and non-medical interventions provided by healthcare professionals – nurses, physical therapists (PTs) and occupational therapists (OTs). The implementation of integrative interventions for arthritis management, such as exercise, rehabilitation and diet, as well as the assessment of educational needs, provision of psychosocial support and encouragement of self-management, complement pharmacological treatment and involve patients in shared decision-making in arthritis care.

Keywords: non-pharmacological treatment, arthritis, rheumatic and musculoskeletal diseases (RMD), integrative treatment, complementary and alternative medicine (CAM)

1. Introduction

Arthritis is a chronic disease spread throughout the world. It is characterized by pain, joint stiffness, swelling and structural changes that can lead to impairment and limitation in the function of the musculoskeletal system. There are over 100 different types of arthritis, but the most common is osteoarthritis or degenerative arthritis, which is a non-inflammatory arthritis. Inflammatory arthritis can be caused by autoimmune diseases (rheumatoid arthritis, psoriatic arthritis, ankylosing spondylitis, etc.) or accompany other autoimmune diseases (systemic lupus erythematosus, Sjogren's syndrome, scleroderma, myositis, inflammatory bowel disease, celiac disease, etc.) and can also occur with gout or infections [1]. According to the Global RA Network (2021), more than 350 million people worldwide suffer from some form of arthritis [2]. In the United States, arthritis affects one in four people, and it is estimated that 78 million adults will have arthritis [3]. According to the World Health Organization (2021), about 14 million people worldwide suffer from rheumatoid arthritis [4], and up to 3% of the world's population has psoriatic arthritis [5]. Osteoarthritis is the most common joint disease in the United States, with more than 32.5 million adults estimated to have osteoarthritis, and a significant proportion of the world's population, about 42 million people, has gout [6]. The disease is increasingly burdening society economically and socially. In order to meet the complex needs of patients, multi-sectoral, integrated strategies for the treatment and support of those affected, with an emphasis on interdisciplinary care, are recommended. Modern management of rheumatic diseases is largely oriented toward pharmacological treatment with the aim of optimally reducing disease activity or achieving remission. However, the effect of the applied standard treatment is not always satisfactory, which is why some of the needs of patients remain unmet, and this is a reason to search for other options such as unconventional therapeutic agents, both pharmacological and non-pharmacological. As an integral part of the treatment of arthritis, informing patients about the possibilities for changing lifestyle or behavior aimed at improving symptoms and preventing disease progression is also considered.

Principles and recommendations from leading world organizations for the treatment of arthritis emphasize the multidisciplinary approach in the implementation of integrative interventions for the management of arthritis – the use of exercise, rehabilitation, diet and additional integrative interventions that complement pharmacological treatment, as well as the need to engage patients for shared decision-making in the provision of care for people with arthritis.

2. Integrative medicine and non-pharmacological integrative therapies

Integrated medicine, also known as integrative medicine [1], combines complementary and alternative medicine (CAM) procedures with conventional diagnostic and treatment methods to increase therapeutic efficacy and effectiveness based on the individual's specific needs [2]. Currently, there is no single generally accepted definition of CAM, and the concept is changing over time. The National Center for Complementary and Integrative Health (NCCIH) defines complementary and alternative medicine as the application of practices and products that are not part of standard medicine [3]. Patients with rheumatic diseases report frequent use of CAM – between 22 and 95% [4]. However, the prevalence and use of different types of CAM varies significantly between different parts of the world. Data obtained from a study in the United States indicated that 92% of patients with rheumatic diseases used CAM methods [5], and a study in Australia showed that 95% of patients with ankylosing spondylitis reported CAM use [6]. Other studies in North America reported chiropractic as the most commonly used CAM (31 to 59%) for rheumatic diseases, while acupuncture and homeopathy are less common [7]. In their publication, Eardley et al. [8] reported that musculoskeletal problems are the most common condition treated with CAM [9]. It has also been reported that patients with non-inflammatory rheumatic diseases use CAM more often than those with inflammatory diseases [10, 11], most likely due to the increasing prevalence and use of effective pharmacological therapies for inflammatory rheumatic diseases, as well as concern about potential interactions between conventional medical therapies and CAM therapies. Furthermore, it is assumed that complementary and alternative medicine is based on the notion that the human body is capable of self-healing [12].

3. Evidence-based CAM (EBCAM) therapies

Integrative medicine is an approach that strives to provide the best care for the patient by taking into account the needs of the individual as a whole (body, mind and spirit) and considering all aspects of lifestyle [13]; it places the patient at the center of the impact of a range of factors – physical, emotional, mental, social, spiritual and environmental – that influence person's health [14].

Written evidence of complementary and alternative medicine systems dates back to before 200 BC, with versions of traditional medicine being presented in China, Korea, Japan, India and Vietnam, but many practices predate written records and have been passed down orally for over 3000 years [15–17].

Historically, CAM emerged from culturally-based practices and beliefs. Subsequently, a dramatic increase in the use of CAM has been observed in countries where healthcare is based on Western scientific methods and evidence-based medicine [18].

"Alternative medicine" is defined as a set of products, practices, and theories that are not evidence-based or scientifically established, and therefore are not considered part of standard medical care. In the 1970s, these practices were rejected by Western medicine and even called "quackery", but in the 1990s, the use of alternative medicine began to be promoted [19], with the term complementary medicine being introduced, as it is seen as working alongside conventional medicine, rather than in opposition to it [20]. Alternative therapies are considered to be those used instead of conventional/allopathic therapies. Complementary therapies are those CAMs that are used alongside conventional treatment [21]. Currently, not all modalities included in CAM are subject to professional regulation. This depends largely on state regulation and the region where these practices are practiced. For example, in the United Kingdom, there is no statutory regulation of complementary and alternative treatments other than chiropractic. Acupuncture was legalized in the United States in the 1970s [22]. In addition, chiropractic and massage therapy are also licensed in most states, while naturopathy and homeopathy are permitted in fewer states [23].

Nowadays, evidence-based medicine (EBM) applies the scientific method to medical practice, requiring health professionals to make conscientious, explicit and judicious use of the best current evidence in making decisions about the provision of patient care [24]. At the same time, EBM empowers patients to make informed choices about the health care they receive and the use of their preferred technique [25].

Evidence-based CAM (EBCAM) therapies have shown success in treating a wide range of conditions. Literature data indicate that patients prefer to use conventional medical services together with complementary medicine [26]. EBCAM therapies in fact emphasize the need to integrate CAM and conventional medicine in terms of evidence-based knowledge [27].

These reasons have encouraged various internationally recognized organizations to develop guidelines for the methods, techniques and treatments used in the field of integrative medicine.

The French Collaborative university platform for Evaluating Health Prevention and Supportive care Programs (CEPS) defines non-pharmacological interventions (NPI) as scientifically based and non-invasive interventions for human health aimed at preventing or treating health problems. They can include products, methods, programs or services such as psychological, physical, nutritional, digital or other health interventions. According to CEPS, non-pharmacological interventions (NPI) can be called by different names: preventive actions, behavioral interventions, alternative and complementary medicines, Chinese medicine, complementary medicine, behavioral medicine, alternative medicine, natural medicine, unconventional care practices, natural health products, health services, adjuvant care, supportive care, non-traditional care, integrated care, non-pharmacological therapies, unconventional therapies, complementary therapies, etc. [28]. In Europe, an estimated 10 to 40% of the population uses some form of complementary NPI [29].

Another European project, CAMbrella, defines Complementary and Alternative Medicine (CAM) as "a set of different medical systems and therapies based on knowledge, skills and practices derived from theories, philosophies and experience, used to maintain and improve health, and to prevent, diagnose, alleviate or treat physical and mental illness" [30].

CAM is usually used as a complement to biomedical care, but it can also be an expression of a preference for more personalized and holistic care over biomedical practice due to unsatisfactory results from it or due to dissatisfaction with the doctor-patient relationship [31].

In 1978, the First International Conference on Primary Health Care (Alma Ata) in Russia made the first recommendations on the application of integrative and complementary interventions to the practices of traditional medicine [32]. Decades later, leading organizations on rheumatic and musculoskeletal diseases (RMD) also provide their guidelines on the application of non-pharmacological treatment, including lifestyle, for these diseases.

4. Position of CAM in international recommendation for treatment of people with joint diseases

4.1 ACR (American College of Rheumatology) recommendations for the use of non-pharmacological and pharmacological therapies for hand, hip and knee osteoarthritis (2012)

The report offers both "strong" and "provisional" recommendations for the management of OA. It recommends the use of non-pharmacological interventions such as aerobic exercise combined with manual therapies and the use of supplements and topical aids, strength training and weight management to achieve therapeutic and psychosocial benefits for people with arthritis [33].

4.2 European league against rheumatism (EULAR) recommendations for non-pharmacological primary treatment of hip and knee osteoarthritis: 2023 update

A multidisciplinary team updated the 2013 recommendations by describing recommendations for optimal management of hip and knee OA and clarifying the definition of primary non-pharmacological management. The results largely focus on the impacts on pain and physical function. The recommendation regarding information, education and self-management has the highest priority for implementation in order to ensure a better life for patients with OA as well as support for physical activity [34].

4.3 EULAR (European Alliance of rheumatology associations) recommendations for physical activity in people with inflammatory arthritis and osteoarthritis (2018)

In order to enhance the health benefits of physical activity (PA), recommendations have been developed to provide guidance in the development, conduct and evaluation of PA in daily clinical practice for the following conditions: Inflammatory arthritis (IA) including rheumatoid arthritis (RA) and spondyloarthritis (SpA) and osteoarthritis (OA) including hip/knee OA (HOA/KOA). The recommendations should be implemented in accordance with individual needs and national health systems [35].

A recent study by Lin et al. [36] provided a comprehensive evaluation of the evidence regarding lifestyle medicine and integrative therapies in inflammatory arthritis (IA). The study examines the impact and effect of a number of interventions such as acupuncture, diet, exercise, herbal medicine, nutritional supplements and mind-body therapies on the following diseases: rheumatoid arthritis, spondyloarthritis and gout. Exercise has been shown to be beneficial for rheumatoid arthritis and spondyloarthritis; however, the effects of Chinese herbal medicine, acupuncture, yoga and anti-inflammatory diets have not been thoroughly studied, and there is also uncertainty regarding other lifestyle recommendations for RA and gout. There is also insufficient available evidence regarding the high level of usage of integrative therapies in the specific chronic arthritis population due to the absence of a thorough study focused on integrative therapies for CIA [36].

Because there is no specific treatment for OA, non-pharmacological approaches are considered the primary treatment for hip and knee OA to prevent or slow disease progression, relieve symptoms and improve or maintain physical function.

The ACR strongly recommends aerobic exercise and/or strength training, weight loss (if overweight), tai chi and a variety of pharmacological and non-pharmacological methods for the treatment of osteoarthritis (OA) of the knee, hi or hand. The guidelines tentatively recommend balance exercises, yoga, acupuncture and other non-pharmacological approaches, such as self-management programs and walking aids, for the management of knee OA [37]. All management guidelines strongly support the use of non-pharmacological therapy not only at the onset but also throughout the course of the disease as adjunctive treatment for OA [38].

Exercise (strengthening exercises and aerobic exercises) is recommended as beneficial for reducing pain, improving joint mobility and strengthening the muscles around the joints [39].

The main non-pharmacological complementary and integrative health treatments for OA include mind-body practices such as acupuncture, deep breathing, yoga, tai chi, meditation, massage and relaxation techniques [40]. Some studies have been published supporting the use of acupuncture, tai chi and yoga in OA [41–43]. A 2018 *Journal of Pain Research* report [44] also describes the use of acupuncture as an adjunctive therapy for osteoarthritis pain, and although the effectiveness of acupuncture varies, it is considered to provide pain relief in some patients and may be recommended as a suitable treatment for patients with OA of the hand, knee or hip [41].

The effects of omega-3 supplements on OA remain inconclusive [45], and alternative medicine treatments such as heat therapy and therapeutic ultrasound have also been shown to have little effect on reducing pain in patients with OA [46]. Glucosamine and chondroitin are popular, commonly used supplements for arthritis patients. The ACR notes that the evidence for their effectiveness is inconclusive [36, 41, 47].

Current OA treatment guidelines also recommend that CAMs, such as acupuncture, nutritional supplements, massage, meditation, and Tai Chi, be used in conjunction with conventional therapies, such as physiotherapy, NSAIDs and corticosteroid injections [33].

In combination with lifestyle factors, assistive devices may offer another type of non-pharmacological treatment for patients. The use of assistive devices, such as braces or splints, is recommended for pain management, but their effectiveness is still controversial, and they are not always well-implemented [48]. The use of appropriate interventions, such as canes, braces and some orthoses (especially for the hand), should be guided by a physiotherapist.

Maintaining physical activity and weight management are major trends in the management of OA [41]. Physical activity improves pain, stiffness and range of motion, and weight loss can help relieve OA symptoms and slow down structural damage, while obesity or being overweight has been associated with the development and progression of knee OA [49]. Lifestyle changes are an integral part of the overall management of arthritis pain. To reduce inflammation and pain in arthritis, weight loss (if appropriate) is recommended to reduce the burden on joints, as well as the inclusion of anti-inflammatory foods such as fruits, vegetables and omega-3 fatty acids. Weight loss counseling is a key component of successfully managing overweight patients. Counseling can be provided through motivational interviewing by a healthcare provider, providing good advice to help the patient and referring them to program resources and education [50].

The US Centers for Disease Control and Prevention (CDC) and the American Physical Therapy Association (APTA) support the use of arthritis management programs and other related chronic conditions [51]. An example of good practice is the Arthritis-Appropriate, Evidence-Based Interventions (AAEBIs) programs in the United States, which provide effective strategies for the prevention and management of arthritis:

- Physical activity programs – cover a variety of endurance-building activities, relaxation techniques and include health education topics leading to improved functional ability and reduced stress and depression. They are individually designed and include aerobic, strengthening and flexibility exercises [52].

- Self-management education programs – educational programs that offer training in coping with the impact of arthritis and promote healthy behaviors [53]. Self-management programs in combination with pain control through medications, acupuncture, aquatic therapy, etc. support patients with pain management strategies, provide social support and self-care opportunities, which contribute to improving pain and physical function with the ability to maintain an active and fulfilling life [40]. The treatment of OA requires the development and implementation of a multifaceted and individualized plan that provides improved sleep, support for coping skills and mental health and social support [54]. The potential of mind-body techniques such as meditation, yoga and tai chi to affect arthritis pain is increasingly recognized. They can contribute to increasing muscle strength, improving flexibility and balance, improving physical function and mood and reducing stress. They contribute to improvements in pain, fatigue, stiffness and helplessness [55]. Evidence in the literature recommends the use of tai chi in patients with OA of the hip and knee [46]. A publication by Haaz S and colleagues reports that in patients with knee OA, yoga can help increase flexibility and strength, as well as develop breathing and relaxation techniques [56].

The above statements are also confirmed by the Arthritis Foundation (AF), which states that "Yoga can help improve joint flexibility and range of motion, while promoting relaxation and stress relief" [57].

DOI: http://dx.doi.org/10.5772/intechopen.1009694

4.4 EULAR recommendations on lifestyle behaviors and work participation to prevent the progression of rheumatic and musculoskeletal diseases (RMD) 2021

An EULAR workgroup of health professionals have summarized the available evidence and have developed new advice by assessing six lifestyle factors in group RMD. As a result, five overarching principles and 18 recommendations have been developed to support healthy lifestyle choices; they also serve to prevent RMD progression and encourage work participation. Exercise recommendations demonstrate the safety and benefits of physical activity on pain, particularly in osteoarthritis or axial spondyloarthritis. Dietary recommendations stress the importance of a healthy and balanced diet for people with RMD. Lifestyle improvements are measured by achieving a higher quality of life and better disease outcomes, but the need for education about the benefits in lifestyle change is also noted [58].

Integrative medicine recognizes the positive impact of health behaviors on chronic musculoskeletal (MSK) pain in patients with rheumatic diseases (RD). Smoking cessation and increased physical activity have been shown to be associated with pain reduction in patients with RD, and incorporating behavioral health (BH) interventions into rheumatology practices may be key to maintaining desired health behaviors leading to improved patient outcomes [59].

Studies by other authors have evaluated the effectiveness of physical activity on quality of life (QoL) and self-rated function in patients with RA, spondyloarthritis (SpA) and psoriatic arthritis (PsA) [60], as well as in patients with OA [61].

Previous EULAR (2021) recommendations for lifestyle changes in people with rheumatic and musculoskeletal diseases, including rheumatoid arthritis, are supported by new evidence and emphasize the need to maintain a healthy lifestyle, as well as the importance of adhering to a whole plant-based diet, physical activity and stress management to limit disease activity in the long term [62].

4.5 ACR guidelines for exercise, rehabilitation, diet and complementary integrative interventions for rheumatoid arthritis (2022)

The recommendations appear to supplement the existing pharmacological treatment guidelines, rather than replacing them with disease-modifying anti-rheumatic drugs (DMARDs) and are based on a shared decision-making approach between patients and clinicians. The significance of multidisciplinary treatment teams, that guarantee the implementation of these recommendations, is emphasized as an opportunity to provide optimal care for individuals with RA. The integration of the recommendations in the overall management of RA seeks to increase patients' and clinicians' awareness of these interventions by providing additional evidence to assist shared decision-making, as well as improving access to recommended interventions [63].

Integrative medicine for RA patients uses a combination of conventional treatments with complementary therapies to address the physical symptoms and emotional and psychological aspects of the disease.

The ACR strongly recommends, as part of non-pharmacological treatment for RA, ongoing engagement in exercise. Exercise should be personalized for each patient and adapted to their current health status, abilities and access to resources. Tentative recommendations include the use of aerobic exercise, aquatic exercise, resistance exercise, mind-body exercises (yoga), tai chi and qigong used as adjuncts to conventional treatment plans, which have been shown to have a positive impact on patients' functional status [64, 65].

Regarding the use of rehabilitation, the ACR tentatively recommends a comprehensive program of occupational therapy (OT) and physical therapy (PT) in rheumatoid arthritis for pain management.

Exercise is considered to have proven value and is therefore widely accepted as part of a comprehensive treatment program for patients with arthritis, with proven benefits for physical and mental health.

There is a mixed opinion regarding the role of dietary interventions in the treatment of patients with chronic inflammatory or autoimmune musculoskeletal disease. However, the ACR tentatively recommends adherence to a Mediterranean diet, but does not recommend adherence to other diets and the use or excessive addition of nutritional supplements and the use of herbal therapies [63]. The Mediterranean-style diet refers to the consumption of low-fat dairy products, fish, whole grains, vegetables, fruits, nuts/seeds and olive oil and limits the intake of processed foods, added sugars, saturated fats and refined carbohydrates. The Mediterranean diet derives fewer calories from animal fat and includes consumption of less red meat and processed foods, focusing more on poultry, fish, fruits, vegetables, whole grains, olive oil, peas and beans, nuts and seeds. The evidence evaluating anti-inflammatory diets (e.g., the Mediterranean) is approaching clinical relevance [66].

As additional integrative interventions for RA, with low-level evidence and few harms, the ACR tentatively recommends the use of:

- Standardized self-management program.
- Cognitive-behavioral therapy and/or mind–body approaches.
- Therapeutic massage.
- Acupuncture – the existing evidence is of very low certainty and conflicting evidence for the benefits of different acupuncture methods, and the results are largely not clinically meaningful [67].
- Heat treatments.

The ACR tentatively recommends against the use of chiropractic and electrotherapy [63].

A limited number of studies suggest that tai chi may improve mood and quality of life in people with rheumatoid arthritis when used in conjunction with other treatments. Following an anti-inflammatory diet and taking targeted herbal and nutrient supplements such as boswellia, turmeric, borage oil and green tea may have positive effects on the gut and microbiome to balance inflammation [68], but further research is needed to demonstrate their beneficial effects in reducing inflammation in RA.

Very limited evidence is available for the purported benefits of quercetin and omega-3 and omega-6 fatty acids and evidence for other therapies has been assessed as clinically inconclusive [66].

Ayurveda: A variety of products and practices are used. Some Ayurvedic blends have been studied in osteoarthritis and rheumatoid arthritis, but there is insufficient evidence of efficacy.

DOI: http://dx.doi.org/10.5772/intechopen.1009694

Cannabis and cannabinoids. Their use for chronic pain is controversial, with a high rate of side effects and concerns about standardization of dosage.

5. Treatment of acute and recurrent gout: ACR clinical practice guidelines

Clinical guidelines have been developed to provide guidance for the treatment of acute and recurrent gout in adults. The review evaluates non-pharmacological interventions: dietary regimen, lifestyle changes, hydration and pharmacological interventions: anti-inflammatory drugs, colchicine and urate-lowering drugs alone or in combinations [69].

According to Chan and colleagues, it is not uncommon for patients with gout to use complementary and alternative medicine, although it is less common than for other rheumatic diseases [70]. Traditional Chinese Medicine (TCM) has been known for thousands of years for its therapeutic effects in the treatment of gout. Today, it is successfully used in combination with modern medical approaches for the prevention and treatment of gouty arthritis (GA) [71]. Numerous studies have reported the efficacy of traditional Chinese medicines, Western herbal therapies, nutritional supplements and dietary strategies for the prevention and/or treatment of hyperuricemia and/or gout [72]. Despite the lack of sufficient evidence regarding the effectiveness of Western herbal medicine for the treatment of gout, some benefits to patients from herbal treatment have been reported [73]. There is also no strong evidence to provide clinical guidelines for the efficacy and safety of natural product dietary supplements (NPDS) for the treatment of gout [74]. Numerous publications have reported the use of traditional Chinese herbal medicines in the form of decoctions, herbal powders, capsules, tablets, herbal teas, tinctures, alcoholic beverages, herbal soaps, ointments and creams [75] in East Asia for the treatment of gout, but evidence such as a systematic review is lacking [76].

According to a study published in *Medicine* [77], traditional Chinese medicine decoction (TCMD) may be an acceptable complementary and alternative therapy for the treatment of patients with gout, although there are few evidence-based results on the efficacy and safety of TCMD for GA.

In 2016, the ACR developed a guideline for clinical recommendations on the treatment of gout. The report reviewed pharmacological and non-pharmacological interventions and combinations of pharmacological and dietary or alternative treatments. Non-pharmacological management of gout focuses on dietary and lifestyle changes such as weight loss and exercise:

- dietary interventions: low-purine diet, tart cherry juice, dairy products and vegetables, Mediterranean diet and DASH [Dietary Approaches to Stop Hypertension] diet); restriction of fructose, other carbohydrates, ethanol;

- lifestyle measures (smoking cessation, exercise and hydration) and nutritional supplements and alternative treatments (vitamin C supplementation and traditional Chinese medicine such as herbs and acupuncture), but these have a low level of evidence.

It has also been reported that dietary modification approaches (such as reducing intake of red meat, shellfish and yeast-rich foods and increasing intake of low-fat dairy products, vegetables and cherries) are no more effective than general dietary advice (encouraging weight loss and reducing alcohol intake) in reducing serum urate levels in patients with gout, so there is insufficient evidence to recommend them [69]. However, data are available for patients with gout in whom consumption of specific foods and beverages identified as risk factors has been shown to influence the course of the disease.

Homeopathy: Few studies have investigated the effectiveness of specific homeopathic therapies.

There is very low certainty of evidence regarding the use of acupuncture for patients with gouty arthritis as an alternative or complementary treatment [78].

5.1 ASAS-EULAR recommendations for the treatment of axial spondyloarthritis: 2022 update

The latest update of the Assessment of SpondyloArthritis International Society (ASAS)-EULAR recommendations for the management of axSpA states that the treatment of patients with axSpA includes both pharmacological and non-pharmacological interventions (Overarching principle "C"). It also emphasizes that non-pharmacological treatment is an integral part of the optimal management of axSpA and is of paramount importance. Recommendation 4 of the same report specifies that patients should perform regular exercise and physiotherapy, and also draws attention to smoking as a risk factor and emphasizes the benefits of quitting [79]. Ankylosing spondylitis (AS) is part of the axSpA group. The most important component of care for patients with AS is exercise and physiotherapy, and natural products and mind-body therapies are usually the most commonly used among patients with rheumatic diseases.

The European League Against Rheumatism (EULAR) guidelines encourage regular exercise and recommend a combination of aerobic and resistance exercise to improve functional status. Physical therapy includes physical modalities such as exercise, heat, cold and electrotherapy, which aim to maintain and/or improve the individual's comfort, independence, social integration and quality of life [40].

A Cochrane review (2008) investigated the positive effects of individualized home exercise programs in AS on spinal mobility and physical function [80].

There are a number of reports of significant use of CAM by patients with arthritis (such as RA and AS) to relieve pain and increase mobility [10], although current evidence is less supportive of the use of CAM in axial spondyloarthritis [40].

A study by Kocyigit and colleagues summarizes the types of CAM used to relieve pain in patients with AS:

Pilates – improves physical capacity in patients with AS [81–84] and helps manage symptoms of spondylitis.

Massage – favorable clinical results [85] indicate its use to relieve muscle tension, improve blood circulation, thereby suppressing pain.

Balneotherapy – limits disease activity and improves quality of life and functionality in the short term [86–88].

Yoga practices – applicable and acceptable in AS [89] through a combination of physical postures, breathing exercises and meditation, help to improve flexibility and strength, reduce pain and improve mental well-being.

Tai Chi – has a positive effect on disease activity and flexibility [90] by combining deep breathing and slow and controlled movements, to improve balance and overall health and helps to reduce pain and improve quality of life [91] and physical function.

Acupuncture – shows efficacy in patients with AS [92, 93].

Transcutaneous electrical nerve stimulation (TENS) – stimulates nerves to relieve pain and improve stiffness and fatigue [94].

A 2021 study shows that aerobic exercise can help improve AS symptoms and disease activity [95].

Meditation: helps reduce stress and promote relaxation, which in turn can reduce pain perception and lead to improved overall well-being.

Nutritional therapy – following a Mediterranean diet [96, 97] is recommended to improve symptoms and reduce inflammation in AS, including foods rich in omega-3 fatty acids, antioxidants and fiber, vitamin D and turmeric, which has been shown to have anti-inflammatory properties; maintaining a healthy gut microbiome, but the evidence is currently very uncertain about the benefits of interventions such as diet and nutritional supplements.

Hypnotherapy – There is insufficient evidence to assess the efficacy of hypnotherapy in AS [98], however, clinical hypnosis may be used to manage chronic pain by changing the way the brain processes pain signals.

Music therapy: The emotional relief of listening to music can reduce the perception of pain through distraction and relaxation.

Dance therapy: Used to improve physical fitness and emotional well-being.

Relaxation therapies: Using techniques such as progressive muscle relaxation and guided imagery can help reduce muscle tension and relieve pain.

Chiropractic treatment: Doctors do not recommend this treatment for AS.

Medical marijuana treatment – used in shared decision-making.

6. CAM modalities

The National Center for Complementary and Alternative Medicine (NCCAM) (2000) [99] divides CAM modalities into five categories:

1. Alternative medical systems – exist independently of or in parallel with allopathic (conventional) medicine. Some may be practiced by individual cultures around the world. These include traditional Chinese medicine (TCM, including acupuncture, Chinese herbs, tui na massage, tai chi and chi kung), Ayurveda, homeopathy and naturopathy.

2. Mind-body interventions – use the power of thought and emotions to positively influence health and well-being. Mind-body therapies (MBTs) include meditation, relaxation, hypnosis, biofeedback, prayer, expressive therapies (dance, art and music) and breathing.

3. Biologically based treatment – defined as the use of "substances found in nature" and includes specialized diets, the use of plant products, animal extracts, vitamins, minerals, herbal products and other natural products.

4. Manipulative and body-based methods – movement of one or more parts of the body with a focus on bones and joints, soft tissues and the circulatory and lymphatic systems. Includes osteopathic manipulation, chiropractic, massage and reflexology.

5. Energy therapies, which involve the manipulation and application of energy fields to the body. There are two types:

- Biofield therapies: Energy fields penetrate the human body by applying direct or indirect pressure to these fields – qigong, reiki, healing touch and therapeutic touch.

- Bioelectromagnetic therapies: Electromagnetic fields are used – pulsed magnetic fields and alternating or direct current fields [21].

CAM modalities include traditional Chinese or Tibetan medicine, acupuncture, Ayurveda, herbal medicine, homeopathy, naturopathy, osteopathy and chiropractic.

It can be said that the original sources of modern integrative medicine are Ayurvedic medicine and traditional Chinese medicine and nowadays homeopathy and naturopathy (naturopathic medicine) /Naturopathy/exist as more modern systems of treatment [16].

Ayurveda means "science of life", originated in India and has both preventive and curative aspects related to the observance of hygiene, the use of exercise, herbs, yoga, physiotherapy and diet to achieve physical, mental and spiritual health and well-being.

Traditional Chinese medicine (TCM) is based on the balance of yin and yang by directing the natural flow of Qi. /qi/ – life energy, to keep the body healthy. Practices used in TCM include acupuncture and acupressure, herbal medicine, nutrition, massage – tui na, exercises – tai chi/tai chi/ and qi gong/qi gong/ combined with meditation [17].

Moxibustion – burning a stick made of ground mugwort leaves on acupuncture points above the skin to improve the flow of qi.

Acupuncture – a method in which very thin needles are inserted through acupuncture points into the skin, which is believed to regulate qi along the energy pathways in the human body. The World Health Organization (WHO 2002) [100] recognizes acupuncture for the treatment of a number of diseases.

Herbal medicine – also called phytomedicine or phytotherapy – refers to the use of seeds, fruits, roots, leaves, bark or flowers of plants for medicinal purposes. In TCM, herbs and herbal decoctions are used, and some are recognized as nutritional sources, others as medicinal.

Dietary therapy – refers to the selection of foods that provide balance to the body and the avoidance of foods that can cause imbalance. TCM defines nutritional therapy as the first line of treatment.

Tui Na massage– means "pressing grip" and is also used to improve the flow of qi.

Tai chi exercises – slow movements of the Qigong principles of breathing, meditation, strength and balance.

Qi gong – means "cultivation of life force energy," contains elements of meditation by using deep breathing techniques along with performing certain movements, some of which imitate animals in nature. Correct posture and diaphragmatic breathing are also applied.

Tai Chi and Qigong are part of Mind-body therapies (MBT).

Meditation is a state of constant self-observation or observation of all experiences related to the body, feelings, mind and phenomena [17].

Tibetan medicine, Sowa Rigpa ("the science of healing"), is based on the mind-body concept and Buddhist psychology. It emphasizes lifestyle and dietary changes, uses herbal and mineral remedies and physical therapies to treat diseases [101].

Chiropractic – is most often used to treat neuromuscular and skeletal complaints such as back pain, neck pain, joint pain in the arms or legs and headaches. Chiropractic is the spinal manipulation of the spine, known as spinal adjustment, to correct spinal abnormalities.

Osteopathy – is based on the theory that the body can heal itself under normal, healthy structural relationships, environmental conditions and nutrition. Treatment is based on the relationship between individual structure (anatomy) and body function (physiology) and is patient-centered, not disease-centered. A major component of osteopathy is its attention to body mechanics and manual methods.

Yoga – the practice of physical exercise combined with controlled breathing, relaxation, dietary control, positive thinking and meditation, aimed at developing harmony in the body, mind and environment [101].

Homeopathy is the oldest form of complementary and alternative medicine and is the longest-established CAM in Europe. It was founded by Samuel Hahnemann. Homeopathy is based on the "principle of similars" and the "Law of the Minimum Dose" and aims to stimulate the body's own healing mechanisms, believing that a disease can be cured by natural substances that, when given to a healthy person, will cause similar symptoms of the same disease, but to a lesser extent. The treatment process in homeopathy begins with a long consultation, discussing all aspects of the patient's illness and life and selecting the appropriate treatment. In homeopathy, remedies are obtained by diluting substances, as it is believed that the efficacy of the medicine increases with its dilution [102]. Naturopathy emphasizes the prevention of disease by focusing on the patient's overall condition, rather than on individual symptoms, using natural treatment methods such as water, fresh air, diet and herbs [103]. Naturopathy uses herbal medicines, vitamins and minerals, homeopathy, aromatherapy, massage and other natural products and therapies. It emphasizes disease prevention by focusing on the overall condition of the patient rather than on individual symptoms, using natural healing methods such as water, fresh air, diet and herbs [104]. All of these medical systems are based on the idea that the body has the power to heal itself using a variety of techniques involving the mind, body and spirit.

According to the WHO Global Report on Traditional and Complementary Medicine (2019), various systems of traditional medicine used around the world include acupuncture, herbal medicine, indigenous traditional medicine, homeopathy, traditional Chinese medicine, naturopathy, chiropractic, osteopathy, Ayurveda and Unani medicine [105]. It is essential that the practices used in integrative medicine have been scientifically proven to be safe and effective [106].

6.1 Application of integrated care in the treatment of arthritis

Integration is a concept that includes a wide range of definitions. Integrated care can be understood as the overall organization of health care delivery with the aim of optimizing patient care through better coordination of services provided [107, 108].

Integrated care is an approach that aims to simultaneously improve the quality of care provided and improve patient outcomes. The patient with rheumatic disease requires a multifaceted treatment approach to overcome the consequences of the disease, achieve better management of comorbidities and improve quality and duration of life. As a result, integration and coordinated person-centered care dominate health and care policy debates worldwide. Available reports in the literature indicate that many patients with some form of inflammatory arthritis (IA) use complementary and integrative therapies, such as 47% of RA patients worldwide use complementary therapies, but only 30% of them report this use to their doctor. For patients with ankylosing spondylitis, the use of integrative therapy is over 40%. There is even less evidence for the use of integrative therapy in gout – 23.9%, despite the limitations of the available studies [95].

6.2 Types of integrative approaches

Integrative approaches can be categorized based on their method of delivery.

Nutritional approaches include special diets, nutritional supplements, herbs, probiotics and microbial therapies.

Psychological approaches include practices such as meditation, hypnosis, music therapy and relaxation therapies.

Physical approaches include techniques such as acupuncture, massage and spinal manipulation.

Flanagan S et al. reported the effects of integrated care interventions on improving quality of life (QoL) in patients with various chronic conditions [109]. Independently, Baxter S et al. also examined the effects of integrated care and concluded that integrated care models were associated with increased patient satisfaction, perceived quality of care and access to services. At the same time, it is considered that such models of care may be most appropriate for specific patient groups (such as those with complex needs) rather than for all patients in general [110].

In this context, Vodopivec V and colleagues analyzed integrated health models for rheumatoid arthritis, where they identified a priority for the implementation of strategies aimed at improving outcomes and patient satisfaction, noting that integrated care for rheumatoid arthritis is currently poorly developed [110].

This idea was further developed by Courel-Ibáñez and colleagues, who described the application of integrative non-pharmacological care for individuals at risk of developing rheumatoid arthritis. The study emphasized that the use of integrative interventions and multidisciplinary care strategies combining pharmacological treatment with non-pharmacological approaches – the implementation of modifiable lifestyle factors (e.g., smoking cessation, dental health, physical activity and diet) could possibly improve the prognosis of RA in individuals at risk, mainly through changes in epigenetics. In conclusion, it is suggested that an integrative, multifactorial intervention approach be offered to individuals at risk of developing and progressing RA [111].

Integrated care is viewed not only in light of patient benefit but also as an opportunity to improve cost-effectiveness in healthcare.

A study by Delft, E.V. and colleagues described a positive impact of integrating care networks on patient outcomes and was associated with cost-effectiveness by providing sustainable and comprehensive care for patients with arthralgia [112].

These and other reports in the literature demonstrate the benefit of implementing integrated care leading to improvements in clinical outcomes and quality of life in chronic diseases [113], such as rheumatic diseases.

An integrated engagement of the healthcare team for patients with rheumatic diseases is needed, working on programs aimed at meeting the need for comprehensive, coordinated management of these patients. One component of these programs includes access to CAM practitioners.

7. Health professionals providing integrative care for arthritis

There is currently an increasing demand for complementary therapies alongside conventional treatments, with patients preferring to be guided by health professionals when using them [114].

The integrative health professionals who work in integrative rheumatology centers are experts in their fields: rheumatologists, immunologists, physical and occupational therapists, oncology social workers, psychologists, psychiatrists and dietitians, music therapists, experts in epidemiology, exercise physiology, integrative medicine, nurses, nutritionists, occupational therapists, physiotherapists. They develop personalized treatment plans tailored to the individual needs of each patient, combining evidence-based therapies with a compassionate approach to improve quality of life.

A key principle in rheumatology is that the management of rheumatic and musculoskeletal diseases requires a coordinated, integrated, multidisciplinary and multiprofessional approach focused on the needs of the individual, with members of this team working closely together [115]. It is also recognized that collaboration between primary care providers and providers of non-pharmacological therapies can improve access to non-pharmacological treatments. For pain management in rheumatic patients, health care professionals may combine conventional treatments (anti-inflammatory drugs, immunosuppressants nd biologic agents) with integrative therapies (yoga, acupuncture, tai chi, etc.) aimed at restoring the balance of the immune system, suppressing inflammation and alleviating pain. Other complementary interventions include adherence to nutritional approaches (anti-inflammatory diet, targeted supplements) or maintenance of physical activity (implementation of a regular exercise regimen), as well as lifestyle changes tailored to the individual needs of each patient [116]. It is also emphasized the identification of barriers at the clinician level that hinder the implementation of these treatments, such as: insufficient knowledge of the efficacy and role of non-pharmacological treatments, limited practice opportunities and inadequate communication channels between providers [117]. In their work, Majnik and colleagues analyzed the role of various non-pharmacological treatments (NPT) in difficult-to-treat RA (D2TRA) covering a wide range of interventions, such as exercise, psychological interventions, physiotherapy and balneotherapy, dietary interventions and education, applied by various specialists, which can have a complex and synergistic effect together with the applied pharmacological therapies in D2TRA. The authors also recommend the development of an individual program for non-pharmacological therapy (NPT) for each individual patient under the supervision of a rheumatologist, psychologist and physiotherapist [118].

7.1 Contribution of nurses to integrative practices

Healthcare today is a team effort and nurses practicing integrative care are recognized as partners in the delivery of integrated health care [19]. According to Mortada, health care professionals (HCPs) should be aware of and apply all clinical options complementary to conventional medicine in order to achieve satisfaction in patients' preferences and requirements [27].

Due to the lack of a precise definition of terminology defining the use of non-pharmacological interventions complementary to biomedical practice, in their publication van der Heijden and colleagues use the terms "complementary non-pharmacological interventions" (NPIs) and "integrative nursing" (IN) to describe such interventions used in nursing practice [29].

A publication in the American Nurses Association's (ANA) Scope and Standards of Practice describes the competencies of advanced practice registered nurses that enable them to prescribe evidence-based traditional and integrative treatments, therapies and procedures that are compatible with the cultural preferences, norms and abilities of the client and that are consistent with the principles of integrated nursing [13].

In a recent publication, Indridadottir O and colleagues propose a new framework for holistic physical assessment in the hospital setting that focuses on the whole person, their background and experiences, based on the holistic nursing philosophy and integrative nursing principles [119].

Freitas and colleagues view caring as the foundation of the nursing profession. They conclude that incorporating Integrative and Complementary Practices (PICS) into standard care activities allows for greater interaction between nurses and patients [32].

Building on the theories of holism and humanism, Jasemi et al. [120] note that holistic care considers the "whole" person, within their context including family and social environment. Holistic care is characterized by "establishing a progressive relationship between nurse and patient that is based on openness, equality and reciprocity and aims to restore patients' power and responsibility and support their self-care practices" [121].

7.2 Integrative nursing

The growing impact of rheumatology worldwide requires an increasing involvement of specialist nurses in the care of patients with arthritis as part of a multidisciplinary team. Nurses are expected to provide a specialist service of the highest quality to meet complex care needs by applying specific knowledge and skills and initiating practices and strategies carried out in collaboration with other professionals. The role of nurses has changed significantly in recent years, with their activities in the management of patients with arthritis including not only disease monitoring and participation in treatment but also providing support for self-management and patient education. In practice, integrated nursing is a framework for providing care with the aim of improving the health and well-being of the whole person through care and relationships. The principles of integrated nursing care include the use of evidence-based complementary therapies, depending on need and context. Complementary therapies (CT) are characteristically practiced outside the health systems of Europe. In Europe, integrated nursing is relatively unknown, but it is consistent with the holistic and person-centered approach to nursing [114], as nurses consider the patient as a whole – the sum of physical, mental, emotional and spiritual well-being. In this way, the integration of all aspects of health forms the holistic foundation on which integrative medicine is based.

Six principles of integrative nursing define the framework within which nurses use evidence to select therapeutic strategies for the implementation of all possible interventions [13].

Principles:

1. Human beings are inseparable from and influenced by the environment.

2. Human beings have an innate capacity for health and well-being.

3. Integrative nursing is person-centered and relationship-based.

4. Nature has healing and restorative properties that contribute to health and well-being.

5. Integrative nursing is evidence-based and uses the full range of conventional and integrative approaches, using the least intensive intervention possible, depending on the need and context.

6. Integrative nursing focuses on the health and well-being of caregivers as well as those they serve [122].

The principles are a guide that makes it possible to provide purposeful, quality nursing care. Nurses who follow these principles do not simply "add" integrative interventions to their practice; they actually become the core of their practice, which does not mean that they reject biomedical interventions [13].

A qualitative study by Kreitzer and colleagues found that nurses can discuss with their patients the inclusion of complementary therapies and non-pharmacological interventions in the treatment plan [123].

Author details

Stefka Stoilova
Medical University, Plovdiv, Bulgaria

*Address all correspondence to: ef_i@abv.bg

References

[1] Senthelal S, Li J, Ardeshirzadeh S, et al. Arthritis. In: StatPearls [Internet]. Treasure Island (FL): StatPearls Publishing; 2024. [Online]. Available from: https://www.ncbi.nlm.nih.gov/books/NBK518992/ [Accessed: June 20, 2023]

[2] Global RA Network. About arthritis and RA. [Online]. Available from: https://globalranetwork.org/project/disease-info/

[3] Hootman JM, Helmick CG, Barbour KE, Theis KA, Boring MA. Updated projected prevalence of self-reported doctor-diagnosed arthritis and arthritis-attributable activity limitation among US adults, 2015-2040. Arthritis & Rhematology. 2016;**68**(7):1582-1587. DOI: 10.1002/art.39692

[4] WHO. World Health Statistics 2021: Monitoring Health for the SDGs, Sustainable Development Goals. World: OCHA website; 2021. [Online]. Available from: https://reliefweb.int/report/world/world-health-statistics-2021-monitoring-health-sdgs

[5] National Psoriasis Foundation (NPF)/USA. Psoriasis Statistics. [Online]. Available from: https://www.psoriasis.org/psoriasis-statistics/

[6] Jacobson A. Arthritis Statistics 2025. The Checkup by SyngleCare. [Online]. Available from: https://www.singlecare.com/blog/news/arthritis-statistics/

[7] Rees L. Integrated medicine. BMJ. 2001;**322**(7279):119-120. DOI: 10.1136/bmj.322.7279.119

[8] Castonguay LG, Eubanks CF, Goldfried MR, Muran JC, Lutz W. Research on psychotherapy integration: Building on the past, looking to the future. Psychotherapy Research. 2015;**25**(3):365-382. DOI: 10.1080/10503307.2015.1014010

[9] National Center for Complementary and Integrative Health. Complementary, Alternative, or Integrative Health: What's In a Name? U.S. Department of Health and Human Services, National Institutes of Health. [Online]. Available from: https://www.nccih.nih.gov/health/complementary-alternative-or-integrative-health-whats-in-a-name

[10] Department of Internal Medicine Nursing, University of Health Sciences Turkey, Gulhane Faculty of Nursing, Ankara, Turkey, et al. Use of complementary and alternative medicine in patients with ankylosing spondylitis. European Journal of Rheumatology. 2021;**8**(1):20-26. DOI: 10.5152/eurjrheum.2020.20111

[11] Sleath B, Callahan LF, Devellis RF, Beard A. Arthritis patients' perceptions of rheumatologists' participatory decision-making style and communication about complementary and alternative medicine. Arthritis Care and Research. 2008;**59**(3):416-421. DOI: 10.1002/art.23307

[12] Chatfield SM et al. Complementary and alternative medicines in ankylosing spondylitis: A cross-sectional study. Clinical Rheumatology. 2009;**28**(2):213-217. DOI: 10.1007/s10067-008-1029-3

[13] Kreitzer MJ, Koithan M, Weil A, editors. Integrative Nursing. 2nd ed. New York: Oxford University Press; 2018. DOI: 10.1093/med/9780190851040.001.0001

[14] Institute of Medicine (US). Summary. In: Integrative Medicine and

the Health of the Public: A Summary of the February 2009 Summit [Online]. Washington (DC): National Academies Press (US); 2009. Available from: https://www.ncbi.nlm.nih.gov/books/NBK219637/ [Accessed: March 15, 2025]

[15] Ng JY et al. The brief history of complementary, alternative, and integrative medicine terminology and the development and creation of an operational definition. Integrative Medicine Research. 2023;**12**(4):100978. DOI: 10.1016/j.imr.2023.100978

[16] Tabish SA. Complementary and Alternative Healthcare: Is it Evidence-based? International Journal of Health Sciences (Qassim). 2008;**2**(1):V-IX

[17] Marshall AC. Traditional Chinese medicine and clinical pharmacology. In: Hock FJ, Gralinski MR, editors. Drug Discovery and Evaluation: Methods in Clinical Pharmacology. Cham: Springer International Publishing; 2020. pp. 455-482. DOI: 10.1007/978-3-319-68864-0_60

[18] Coulter ID, Willis EM. The rise and rise of complementary and alternative medicine: A sociological perspective. The Medical Journal of Australia. 2004;**180**(11):587-589. DOI: 10.5694/j.1326-5377.2004.tb06099.x

[19] Lee G. Complementary and alternative medicine use in patients with chronic diseases in primary care is associated with perceived quality of care and cultural beliefs. Family Practice. 2004;**21**(6):654-660. DOI: 10.1093/fampra/cmh613

[20] Andrews GJ. Complementary and alternative medicine. In: Kitchin R, Thrift N, editors. International Encyclopedia of Human Geography. Oxford: Elsevier; 2009. pp. 234-238. DOI: 10.1016/B978-008044910-4.00325-4

[21] Koithan M. Introducing complementary and alternative therapies. The Journal for Nurse Practitioners. 2009;**5**(1):18-20. DOI: 10.1016/j.nurpra.2008.10.012

[22] NHS. Complementary and alternative medicine. [Online]. Available from: https://www.nhs.uk/conditions/complementary-and-alternative-medicine/

[23] Institute of Medicine (US) Committee on the Use of Complementary and Alternative Medicine by the American Public. Complementary and Alternative Medicine in the United States. Introduction. Vol. 1. Washington (DC): National Academies Press (US); 2005. [Online]. Available from: https://www.ncbi.nlm.nih.gov/books/NBK83804/

[24] Sackett DL, Rosenberg WMC, Gray JAM, Haynes RB, Richardson WS. Evidence based medicine: What it is and what it isn't. BMJ. 1996;**312**(7023):71-72. DOI: 10.1136/bmj.312.7023.71

[25] Akan H et al. Knowledge and attitudes towards complementary and alternative medicine among medical students in Turkey. BMC Complementary and Alternative Medicine. 2012;**12**(1):115. DOI: 10.1186/1472-6882-12-115

[26] Negahban A, Maleki M, Abbassian A. Elements of integrating traditional and complementary medicine into primary healthcare: A systematic review. Journal of Clinical and Diagnostic Research. 2018;**12**(12):IE05-IE11. DOI: 10.7860/JCDR/2018/36136.12417

[27] Mortada EM. Evidence-based complementary and alternative medicine in current medical practice. Cureus. 2024;**16**(1):e52041. DOI: 10.7759/cureus.52041

[28] Ninot G et al. La Plateforme CEPS : une structure universitaire de réflexion sur l'évaluation des interventions non médicamenteuses (INM). Hegel. 2017;**1**(1):53. DOI: 10.4267/2042/62022

[29] Van Der Heijden MJE, Busch M, Gunnarsdottir TJ, Lunde A, Falkenberg T, Van Dijk M. Educational courses on non-pharmacologic complementary interventions for nurses across Europe: The INES mapping pilot study. Nurse Education Today. 2022;**116**:105419. DOI: 10.1016/j.nedt.2022.105419

[30] Castellano-Tejedor C. Non-pharmacological interventions for the Management of Chronic Health Conditions and non-Communicable Diseases. International Journal of Environmental Research and Public Health. 2022;**19**(14):8536. DOI: 10.3390/ijerph19148536

[31] Kemppainen LM, Kemppainen TT, Reippainen JA, Salmenniemi ST, Vuolanto PH. Use of complementary and alternative medicine in Europe: Health-related and sociodemographic determinants. Scandinavian Journal of Public Health. 2018;**46**(4):448-455. DOI: 10.1177/1403494817733869

[32] Rodrigo De Freitas J, Da Silva AJ, Alves Da Silva JA, Ramos JRB, Da Mata Vasconcelos Silva F. A importância do enfermeiro nas práticas integrativas e complementares no sistema único de saúde. Saúde Coletiva Barueri. 2021;**11**(63):5376-5389. DOI: 10.36489/saudecoletiva.2021v11i63p5376-5389

[33] Prusak K, Prusak K, Mahoney J. An integrated mind–body approach to arthritis: A pilot study. Journal of Traditional and Complementary Medicine. 2014;**4**(2):99-107. DOI: 10.4103/2225-4110.124364

[34] Moseng T et al. EULAR recommendations for the non-pharmacological core management of hip and knee osteoarthritis: 2023 update. Annals of the Rheumatic Diseases. 2024;**83**(6):730-740. DOI: 10.1136/ard-2023-225041

[35] Rausch Osthoff A-K et al. 2018 EULAR recommendations for physical activity in people with inflammatory arthritis and osteoarthritis. Annals of the Rheumatic Diseases. 2018;**77**(9):1251-1260. DOI: 10.1136/annrheumdis-2018-213585

[36] Lin J et al. The effectiveness and safety of lifestyle medicine and integrative therapies in inflammatory arthritis: An umbrella review using a hierarchical evidence gathering approach. Frontiers in Medicine. 2024;**11**:1357914. DOI: 10.3389/fmed.2024.1357914

[37] National Center for Complementary and Integrative Health. Complementary health approaches for chronic pain: What the science says. 2022. [Online]. Available from: https://www.nccih.nih.gov/health/providers/digest/complementary-health-approaches-for-chronic-pain-science

[38] Osteoarthritis Action Alliance. Nonpharmacologic. Osteoarthritis Prevention & Management in Primary Care. [Online]. Available from: https://oaaction.unc.edu/oa-module/oa-treatment/nonpharmacolgic/ [Accessed: March 15, 2025]

[39] Mora JC, Przkora R, Cruz-Almeida Y. Knee osteoarthritis: Pathophysiology and current treatment modalities. Journal of Pain Research. 2018;**11**:2189-2196. DOI: 10.2147/JPR.S154002

[40] Spondylitis Association of America. Non-Medicinal Approaches to Treating Spondyloarthritis. Latest News. [Online]. Available from: https://

spondylitis.org/spondylitis-plus/non-medicinal-approaches-to-treating-spondyloarthritis/

[41] Kolasinski SL et al. 2019 American College of Rheumatology/Arthritis Foundation guideline for the Management of Osteoarthritis of the hand, hip, and knee. Arthritis & Rhematology. 2020;**72**(2):220-233. DOI: 10.1002/art.41142

[42] Phang JK et al. Complementary and alternative medicine for rheumatic diseases: A systematic review of randomized controlled trials. Complementary Therapies in Medicine. 2018;**37**:143-157. DOI: 10.1016/j.ctim.2018.03.003

[43] Manheimer E et al. Acupuncture for hip osteoarthritis. Cochrane Database of Systematic Reviews. 2018;**5**(5):CD013010. DOI: 10.1002/14651858.CD013010

[44] Yuan X-C et al. Electroacupuncture potentiates peripheral CB2 receptor-inhibited chronic pain in a mouse model of knee osteoarthritis. Journal of Pain Research. 2018;**11**:2797-2808. DOI: 10.2147/JPR.S171664

[45] Shawl M, Geetha T, Burnett D, Babu J. Omega-3 supplementation and its effects on osteoarthritis. Nutrients. 2024;**16**(11):1650. DOI: 10.3390/nu16111650

[46] Block JA. OA guidelines: Improving care or merely codifying practice? Nature Reviews Rheumatology. 2014;**10**(6):324-326. DOI: 10.1038/nrrheum.2014.61

[47] Jerosch J. Effects of glucosamine and chondroitin sulfate on cartilage metabolism in OA: Outlook on other nutrient partners especially Omega-3 fatty acids. International Journal of Rheumatology. 2011;**2011**:1-17. DOI: 10.1155/2011/969012

[48] Thomas S, Browne H, Mobasheri A, Rayman MP. What is the evidence for a role for diet and nutrition in osteoarthritis? Rheumatology. 2018;**57**(Suppl. 4):iv61-iv74. DOI: 10.1093/rheumatology/key011

[49] Messier SP. Obesity and osteoarthritis: Disease genesis and nonpharmacologic weight management. The Medical Clinics of North America. 2009;**93**(1):145-159. DOI: 10.1016/j.mcna.2008.09.011

[50] Rose SA, Poynter PS, Anderson JW, Noar SM, Conigliaro J. Physician weight loss advice and patient weight loss behavior change: A literature review and meta-analysis of survey data. International Journal of Obesity. 2013;**37**(1):118-128. DOI: 10.1038/ijo.2012.24

[51] American Physical Therapy Association, Centers for Disease Control, and and Prevention. Evidence-Based Community Programs: Physical Activity Programs at a Glance. Help Your Patients Take Charge. [Online]. Available from: https://www.apta.org/contentassets/8af7aa55337d4a94aad3aa1f64006f5f/arthritis-evidence-based-community-programs.pdf

[52] Osteoarthritis Action Alliance. Arthritis-appropriate, evidence-based interventions (AAEBI). In: Evidence-Based Programs that are Proven to Improve the Quality of Life for Adults with Arthritis. [Online]. Available from: https://oaaction.unc.edu/aaebi-2/ [Accessed: March 15, 2025]

[53] Murphy LB, Theis KA, Brady TJ, Sacks JJ. Supporting self-management education for arthritis: Evidence from the arthritis conditions and health effects survey on the influential role of health care providers. Chronic Illness. 2021;**17**(3):217-231. DOI: 10.1177/1742395319869431

[54] Hawker GA et al. A longitudinal study to explain the pain-depression link in older adults with osteoarthritis. Arthritis Care and Research. 2011;**63**(10):1382-1390. DOI: 10.1002/acr.20298

[55] Callahan LF, Cleveland RJ, Altpeter M, Hackney B. Evaluation of tai chi program effectiveness for people with arthritis in the community: A randomized controlled trial. Journal of Aging and Physical Activity. 2016;**24**(1):101-110. DOI: 10.1123/japa.2014-0211

[56] Haaz S, Bartlett SJ. Yoga for arthritis: A scoping review. Rheumatic Diseases Clinics of North America. 2011;**37**(1):33-46. DOI: 10.1016/j.rdc.2010.11.001

[57] The Arthritis Foundation. About Arthritis. Yoga Benefits for Arthritis. [Online]. Available from: https://www.arthritis.org/ [Accessed: March 15, 2025]

[58] Gwinnutt JM et al. 2021 EULAR recommendations regarding lifestyle behaviours and work participation to prevent progression of rheumatic and musculoskeletal diseases. Annals of the Rheumatic Diseases. 2023;**82**(1):48-56. DOI: 10.1136/annrheumdis-2021-222020

[59] Patterson D, Link-Malcolm J, Ghebranious M, Makris U. Integrated behavioral health services for patients with chronic musculoskeletal pain: Rheumatology provider perspectives [abstract]. Arthritis & Rhematology. 2022;**74**(Suppl. 9). [Online]. Available from: https://acrabstracts.org/abstract/integrated-behavioral-health-services-for-patients-with-chronic-musculoskeletal-pain-rheumatology-provider-perspectives/

[60] Björk M et al. Inflammatory arthritis and the effect of physical activity on quality of life and self-reported function: A systematic review and meta-analysis. Arthritis Care and Research. 2022;**74**(1):31-43. DOI: 10.1002/acr.24805

[61] Pelle T et al. Comparison of physical activity among different subsets of patients with knee or hip osteoarthritis and the general population. Rheumatology International. 2020;**40**(3):383-392. DOI: 10.1007/s00296-019-04507-1

[62] Wagenaar C et al. OP0330-HPR long-term effectiveness of a lifestyle intervention for rheumatoid arthritis: Two-year follow-up after the 'plants for joints' randomized clinical trial. Annals of the Rheumatic Diseases. 2024;**83**(Suppl. 1):203. DOI: 10.1136/annrheumdis-2024-eular.885

[63] England BR et al. 2022 American College of Rheumatology Guideline for exercise, rehabilitation, diet, and additional integrative interventions for rheumatoid arthritis. Arthritis Care and Research. 2023;**75**(8):1603-1615. DOI: 10.1002/acr.25117

[64] Mudano AS, Tugwell P, Wells GA, Singh JA. Tai Chi for rheumatoid arthritis. Cochrane Database of Systematic Reviews. 2019;**9**(9):CD004849. DOI: 10.1002/14651858.CD004849.pub2

[65] Wang Y et al. Integrative effect of yoga practice in patients with knee arthritis: A PRISMA-compliant meta-analysis. Medicine (Baltimore). 2018;**97**(31):e11742. DOI: 10.1097/MD.0000000000011742

[66] Chen L, Michalsen A. Management of chronic pain using complementary and integrative medicine. BMJ. 2017:j1284. DOI: 10.1136/bmj.j1284

[67] Ramos A, Domínguez J, Gutiérrez S. Acupuncture for rheumatoid arthritis.

Medwave. 2018;**18**(06):e7283-e7283. DOI: 10.5867/medwave.2018.06.7283

[68] Lester T. The role of lifestyle factors in autoimmune disease management. Autoimmune. [Online]. Available from: https://www.rupahealth.com/post/the-role-of-lifestyle-factors-in-autoimmune-disease-management [Accessed: March 15, 2025]

[69] Qaseem A, Harris RP, Forciea MA, for the Clinical Guidelines Committee of the American College of Physicians. Management of Acute and Recurrent Gout: A clinical practice guideline from the American College of Physicians. Annals of Internal Medicine. 2017;**166**(1):58. DOI: 10.7326/M16-0570

[70] Chan E, House ME, Petrie KJ, Horne A, Taylor WJ, Dalbeth N. Complementary and alternative medicine use in patients with gout: A longitudinal observational study. Journal of Clinical Rheumatology. 2014;**20**(1):16-20. DOI: 10.1097/RHU.0000000000000059

[71] Liang H et al. Advances in experimental and clinical research of the gouty arthritis treatment with traditional Chinese medicine. Evidence-based Complementary and Alternative Medicine. 2021;**2021**:1-15. DOI: 10.1155/2021/8698232

[72] Vu N, Nguyen TTT, Parmenter BH, Thouas GA. Safety, efficacy and tolerability of a combination micronutrient and polyherbal preparation (GoutFighter™) for gout: A single-arm open-label pilot study. Journal of Complementary and Integrative Medicine. 2021;**18**(1):113-121. DOI: 10.1515/jcim-2019-0074

[73] Corp N, Barbara P. The role of Western herbal medicine in the treatment of gout. Journal of Herbal Medicine. 2013;**3**:157-170. DOI: 10.1016/j.hermed.2013.08.002

[74] Yang J, Li G, Xiong D, Chon TY, Bauer BA. The impact of natural product dietary supplements on patients with gout: A systematic review and meta-analysis of randomized controlled trials. Evidence-based Complementary and Alternative Medicine. 2020;**2020**(1):7976130. DOI: 10.1155/2020/7976130

[75] Kumadoh D, Kwakye KO. Dosage forms of herbal medicinal products and their stability considerations - An overview. 2017. [Online]. Available from: https://api.semanticscholar.org/CorpusID:59420076

[76] Hwang JH, Song HS. External application of herbal medicine for gout: A protocol for systematic review and meta-analysis of randomized controlled trials. Medicine (Baltimore). 2021;**100**(16):e25649. DOI: 10.1097/MD.0000000000025649

[77] Qu P et al. Treatment of gouty arthritis with traditional Chinese medicine decoction: Meta-analysis, network pharmacology analysis, and molecular docking. Medicine (Baltimore). 2024;**103**(1):e36722. DOI: 10.1097/MD.0000000000036722

[78] Liang H et al. Efficacy and safety of acupuncture combined with herbal medicine in treating gouty arthritis: Meta-analysis of randomized controlled trials. Evidence-based Complementary and Alternative Medicine. 2021;**2021**:1-15. DOI: 10.1155/2021/8161731

[79] Ramiro S et al. ASAS-EULAR recommendations for the management of axial spondyloarthritis: 2022 update. Annals of the Rheumatic Diseases. 2023;**82**(1):19. DOI: 10.1136/ard-2022-223296

[80] Dagfinrud H, Hagen KB, Kvien TK. Physiotherapy interventions for ankylosing spondylitis. Cochrane Database of Systematic Reviews. 2009;**2**:2008. DOI: 10.1002/14651858. CD002822.pub3

[81] Altan L, Korkmaz N, Dizdar M, Yurtkuran M. Effect of Pilates training on people with ankylosing spondylitis. Rheumatology International. 2012;**32**(7):2093-2099. DOI: 10.1007/ s00296-011-1932-9

[82] Roşu MO, Ţopa I, Chirieac R, Ancuta C. Effects of Pilates, McKenzie and Heckscher training on disease activity, spinal motility and pulmonary function in patients with ankylosing spondylitis: A randomized controlled trial. Rheumatology International. 2014;**34**(3):367-372. DOI: 10.1007/ s00296-013-2869-y

[83] Oksüz S, Unal E. Comparison of the effects of aerobic training alone versus aerobic training combined with clinical Pilates exercises on the functional and psychosocial status of patients with ankylosing spondylitis: A randomized controlled trial. Physiotherapy Theory and Practice. 2023;**39**(1):61-71. DOI: 10.1080/09593985.2021.2005199

[84] Bağlan Yentür S et al. The effects of Pilates training on respiratory muscle strength in patients with ankylosing spondylitis. Physiotherapy Theory and Practice. 2024;**40**(1):31-41. DOI: 10.1080/09593985.2022.2109540

[85] Romanowski MW, Špiritović M, Rutkowski R, Dudek A, Samborski W, Straburzyńska-Lupa A. Comparison of deep tissue massage and therapeutic massage for lower back pain, disease activity, and functional capacity of ankylosing spondylitis patients: A randomized clinical pilot study. Evidence-based Complementary and Alternative Medicine. 2017;**2017**(1):9894128. DOI: 10.1155/2017/9894128

[86] Altan L, Bingöl Ü, Aslan M, Yurtkuran M. The effect of balneotherapy on patients with ankylosing spondylitis. Scandinavian Journal of Rheumatology. 2006;**35**(4):283-289. DOI: 10.1080/03009740500428806

[87] Bestaş E, Dündar Ü, Köken T, Koca B, Yeşil H. The comparison of effects of balneotherapy, water-based and land-based exercises on disease activity, symptoms, sleep quality, quality of life and serum sclerostin level in patients with ankylosing spondylitis: A prospective, randomized study. Archives of Rheumatology. 2022;**37**(2):159-168. DOI: 10.46497/ ArchRheumatol.2022.9024

[88] Forestier R, Bugnard A, Thomas T. Balneotherapy in spondyloarthropathy: A systematic review. Thérapie. 2022;**77**(6):723-730. DOI: 10.1016/j. therap.2022.02.006

[89] Singh J et al. Designing, validation, and feasibility of a yoga module for patients with ankylosing spondylitis. Journal of Ayurveda and Integrative Medicine. 2022;**13**(1):100479. DOI: 10.1016/j.jaim.2021.06.019

[90] Lee E-N, Kim Y-H, Chung WT, Lee MS. Tai chi for disease activity and flexibility in patients with ankylosing spondylitis—A controlled clinical trial. Evidence-based Complementary and Alternative Medicine. 2008;**5**(4):457-462. DOI: 10.1093/ecam/nem048

[91] Cetin SY, Calik BB, Ayan A, Kabul EG. The effectiveness of 10-tai chi movements in patients with ankylosing spondylitis receiving anti-tumor necrosis factor α therapy: A randomized

controlled trial. European Journal of Integrative Medicine. 2020;**39**:101208. DOI: 10.1016/j.eujim.2020.101208

[92] Dang S et al. Efficacy and safety of warm acupuncture in the treatment of ankylosing spondylitis: A protocol for systematic review and meta-analysis. Medicine (Baltimore). 2021;**100**(1):e24116. DOI: 10.1097/MD.0000000000024116

[93] Xuan Y, Huang H, Huang Y, Liu D, Hu X, Geng L. The efficacy and safety of simple-needling therapy for treating ankylosing spondylitis: A systematic review and meta-analysis of randomized controlled trials. Evidence-based Complementary and Alternative Medicine. 2020;**2020**(1):4276380. DOI: 10.1155/2020/4276380

[94] Chen F-C, Jin Z-L, Wang D-F. A retrospective study of transcutaneous electrical nerve stimulation for chronic pain following ankylosing spondylitis. Medicine (Baltimore). 2018;**97**(27):e11265. DOI: 10.1097/MD.0000000000011265

[95] Basakci Calik B et al. Investigation of the effectiveness of aerobic exercise training in individuals with ankylosing spondylitis: Randomized controlled study. Modern Rheumatology. 2021;**31**(2):442-450. DOI: 10.1080/14397595.2020.1745409

[96] Tel Adıgüzel K, Gül Yurdakul F, Seremet Kürklü N, Yaşar E, Bodur H. Relationship between diet, oxidative stress, and inflammation in ankylosing spondylitis. Archives of Rheumatology. 2022;**37**(1):1-10. DOI: 10.46497/ArchRheumatol.2022.9015

[97] Ometto F et al. Mediterranean diet in axial spondyloarthritis: An observational study in an Italian monocentric cohort. Arthritis Research & Therapy. 2021;**23**(1):219. DOI: 10.1186/s13075-021-02600-0

[98] Kocyigit BF, Sagtaganov Z, Yessirkepov M, Akyol A. Assessment of complementary and alternative medicine methods in the management of ankylosing spondylitis, rheumatoid arthritis, and fibromyalgia syndrome. Rheumatology International. 2022;**43**(4):617-625. DOI: 10.1007/s00296-022-05267-1

[99] US Department of Health and Human Services; US Department of Education; US Department of Justice. Report of the Surgeon General's Conference on Children's Mental Health: A National Action Agenda. Washington (DC): US Department of Health and Human Services; 2000

[100] World Health Organization. Acupuncture: Review and Analysis of Reports on Controlled Clinical Trials. World Health Organization; 2002

[101] EUROCAM. CAM modalities. [Online]. Available from: https://cam-europe.eu/cam-modalities/ [Accessed: March 15, 2025]

[102] Loudon I. A brief history of homeopathy. Journal of the Royal Society of Medicine. 2006;**99**(12):607-610. DOI: 10.1177/014107680609901206

[103] Fleming SA, Gutknecht NC. Naturopathy and the primary care practice. Primary Care: Clinics in Office Practice. 2010;**37**(1):119-136. DOI: 10.1016/j.pop.2009.09.002

[104] Pollock K. Alternative health therapies - Homeopathy and Naturopathy. [Online]. Available from: https://teara.govt.nz/en/alternative-health-therapies/page-3

[105] World Health Organization. WHO Global Report on Traditional

and Complementary Medicine 2019. [Online]. Available from: https://www.who.int/publications/i/item/978924151536

[106] Millstine D, Chen CY, Bauer B. Complementary and integrative medicine in the management of headache. BMJ. 2017:j1805. DOI: 10.1136/bmj.j1805

[107] Shaw S, Rosen R, Rumbold B. What Is Integrated Care? Nuffield Trust. [Online]. Available from: https://www.nuffieldtrust.org.uk/research/what-is-integrated-care [Accessed: March 15, 2025]

[108] Murtagh S et al. Integrating primary and secondary care to enhance chronic disease management: A scoping review. International Journal of Integrated Care. 2021;**21**(1):4. DOI: 10.5334/ijic.5508

[109] Flanagan S, Damery S, Combes G. The effectiveness of integrated care interventions in improving patient quality of life (QoL) for patients with chronic conditions. An overview of the systematic review evidence. Health and Quality of Life Outcomes. 2017;**15**(1):188. DOI: 10.1186/s12955-017-0765-y

[110] Baxter S, Johnson M, Chambers D, Sutton A, Goyder E, Booth A. The effects of integrated care: A systematic review of UK and international evidence. BMC Health Services Research. 2018;**18**(1):350. DOI: 10.1186/s12913-018-3161-3

[111] Courel-Ibáñez J et al. Integrative non-pharmacological care for individuals at risk of rheumatoid arthritis. Rheumatology International. 2024;**44**(3):413-423. DOI: 10.1007/s00296-023-05507-y

[112] Van Delft E, Han KH, Hazes J, Lopes Barreto D, Weel A. FRI0512 integrated care network As a building stone for sustainable and comprehensive care for patients with arthralgia. Annals of the Rheumatic Diseases. 2020;**79**(Suppl. 1):855. DOI: 10.1136/annrheumdis-2020-eular.2323

[113] Spezia N, Barello S, Torri C, Celano A, Graffigna G. Patient experience of integrated care: Findings from a cross-sectional study involving people with rheumatic and musculoskeletal diseases. International Journal of Integrated Care. 2023;**23**:14. DOI: 10.5334/ijic.6616

[114] Lunde A et al. Integrative nursing in Europe - a competency profile for nursing students validated in a Delphi-study. Nurse Education Today. 2023;**126**:105807. DOI: 10.1016/j.nedt.2023.105807

[115] Woolf AD, The European Union of Medical Specialists Section of Rheumatology/European Board of Rheumatology. Healthcare services for those with musculoskeletal conditions: A rheumatology service. Recommendations of the European Union of medical specialists section of rheumatology/European Board of Rheumatology 2006. Annals of the Rheumatic Diseases. 2007;**66**(3):293-301. DOI: 10.1136/ard.2006.061176

[116] Weinberg J. Integrative approaches to the testing and treatment of rheumatoid arthritis: A comprehensive review. Autoimmune. [Online]. Available from: https://www.rupahealth.com/post/integrative-approaches-to-the-testing-and-treatment-of-rheumatoid-arthritis-a-comprehensive-review [Accessed: March 15, 2025]

[117] Roseen EJ et al. Doctors of chiropractic working with or within integrated healthcare delivery systems: A scoping review protocol. BMJ Open. 2021;**11**(1):e043754. DOI: 10.1136/bmjopen-2020-043754

[118] Majnik J, Császár-Nagy N, Böcskei G, Bender T, Nagy G. Non-pharmacological treatment in difficult-to-treat rheumatoid arthritis. Frontiers in Medicine. 2022;**9**:991677. DOI: 10.3389/fmed.2022.991677

[119] Indridadottir O, Nisco-Madden J. Holistic physical assessment: A new framework for nursing practice Honoring the whole person. Journal of Holistic Nursing. 2024:08980101241261261. DOI: 10.1177/08980101241261261

[120] Jasemi M, Valizadeh L, Zamanzadeh V, Keogh B. A concept analysis of holistic care by hybrid model. Indian Journal of Palliative Care. 2017;**23**(1):71. DOI: 10.4103/0973-1075.197960

[121] Bett L. Nutritional Management of Rheumatoid Arthritis: An important role for nurses, degree [thesis] nursing degree programme. Arcada. 2020. [Online]. Available from: https://www.theseus.fi/bitstream/handle/10024/352720/Lenah%20Bett%20-%20Final%20Thesis.pdf?sequence=2

[122] Koithan M. Concepts and principles of integrative nursing. In: Integrative Nursing. Oxford University Press; 2014. pp. 3-16. (New York, 2014; online edn, Oxford Academic, 1 Feb. 2014). DOI: 10.1093/med/9780199860739.003.0001

[123] Jo Kreitzer M, Koithan M, Sullivan SD, Nunez M, Voss M. Integrative nursing and the ANA scope and standards of practice: Expanding the reach of nursing for families and society. Creative Nursing. 2022;**28**(4):228-233. DOI: 10.1891/CN-2022-0041

Section 4

Participation, Communication, and Patient-Centered Outcomes

Chapter 9

A New Outcome to Measure Community-Living Care Recipients and Their Informal Family Caregivers

Hiromi Nakamura-Thomas

Abstract

With a key goal of the long-term care system being to maintain the Quality of Life (QOL) of service users, this chapter introduces the Adult Social Care Outcomes Toolkit (ASCOT), a QOL outcome developed to measure Social Care-Related Quality of Life (SCRQoL), specifically for community-living adult care recipients and their informal family caregivers. This chapter explored whether the mutual interdependence of SCRQoL within cohabiting care recipient-caregiver dyads was associated with their overall satisfaction toward home-based rehabilitation services. This chapter revealed a significant positive actor effect of care recipients' SCRQoL on their own satisfaction, highlighting the crucial role of service satisfaction given the substantial impact of long-term care services on their home-based lives. Recognizing the vital supportive role of family caregivers in care recipients' community living, this chapter recommends that therapists providing home-based rehabilitation services utilize the ASCOT to capture SCRQoL in both care recipients and their family caregivers.

Keywords: social care-related quality of life, adult social care outcomes toolkit, community-living adult care recipients, informal family caregivers, home-based rehabilitation services

1. Introduction

Population aging is a global phenomenon. Among developed nations, Japan stands out with its exceptionally rapid rate of aging and the highest proportion of older adults globally, where 28% of the population is aged 65 years and older. In comparison, Germany's older adult population is 21%, France's is 20%, and the Netherlands' is 19% [1, 2].

In Asian countries, such as Japan, cultural norms rooted in Confucianism have traditionally positioned the care of frail or ill family members as a family matter, often undertaken by younger female relatives [3, 4]. This cultural backdrop contributes to the significant role of informal family care in Japan's long-term care system, which emphasizes community living. Since the system's inception in the year 2000 with 1.49 million users, the number of care recipients has steadily increased to 6.5 million by January 2025 [5], with 64% relying on co-residing family—mainly spouses and children—in addition to formal support [6]. This heavy reliance on family caregivers has led to substantial burdens, particularly for spouses, manifesting as limitations in social participation [7] and higher mortality rates [8]. Therefore, ensuring the sustainability of Japan's care systems necessitates careful consideration of the impact of services on these informal caregivers [9, 10].

A key goal of the long-term care system, as emphasized by the Ministry of Health, Labour and Welfare, is to maintain the Quality of Life (QOL) of service users [11]. Improving QOL has become a priority in policymaking at the international level. For instance, the Organization for Economic Co-operation and Development (OECD) proposed nine QOL indicators in 1976, encompassing health, education, work, leisure, income, individual environment, social environment, and safety [12]. This initiative spurred the integration of QOL considerations into policies across European countries. In contrast, health and medical contexts have historically focused primarily on physiological indicators. The concept of QOL gained significant attention in medicine during the 1970s, particularly through discussions at the Society for Medical Decision-Making regarding end-of-life care [13]. Driven by economic growth and advancements in medical technologies, there has been a growing emphasis on quality of life in addition to extending life expectancies.

Health-related QOL outcomes are prevalent in the health and medical fields. However, they may not fully capture the experiences of care recipients, who often face health decline, along with activity limitations and restricted social participation. Recognizing this, the World Health Organization (WHO) emphasizes a broader understanding of health as a state of complete physical, mental, and social well-being, extending beyond the mere absence of disease [14]. Moreover, WHO defines QOL as an individual's perception of their life situation within their cultural and value context, considering their aspirations, expectations, standards, and concerns [15, 16]. Consequently, these broader definitions highlight the limitations of solely relying on health-related QOL outcomes in social care settings, where a narrower conceptualization often prevails [17]. To overcome this inadequacy, the Adult Social Care Outcomes Toolkit (ASCOT) was developed in the United Kingdom to measure Social Care-related Quality of Life (SCRQoL), specifically for community-living adult care recipients [17] and their informal caregivers [18].

1.1 The adult social care outcomes toolkit (ASCOT)

The Adult Social Care Outcomes Toolkit (ASCOT) represents a suite of instruments developed to measure SCRQoL [17, 18]. SCRQoL refers to the aspects of quality of life that individuals accessing adult social care services deem valuable and important, and that are affected by these services. Adult social care services, often referred to as long-term care, encompass a diverse array of residential and community-based supports, including home care, day centers, and residential and care homes for adults across all age groups. To effectively measure SCRQoL in adults using these services, ASCOT includes several versions. Notably, a systematic review of 29 self-report instruments for assessing QOL in older adults receiving aged care services highlighted ASCOT's good validity, reliability, and responsiveness [19]. Among these self-report instruments within the ASCOT are the ASCOT-SCT4, a self-completion tool for community-dwelling adult care recipients with four response options [17], and the ASCOT-Carer SCT4, a similar self-completion instrument designed for informal caregivers [18].

ASCOT was initially developed for the economic evaluation of long-term care services. To facilitate this, its scores were designed to range from 0.00 (representing the worst possible state, equivalent to death) to 1.00 (representing the best possible state). Original scoring systems were developed specifically for the ASCOT-SCT4 [17] and the ASCOT-Carer SCT4 [20]. ASCOT has since been derecognized as suitable for economic evaluation [21, 22].

The landscape of informal caregiving varies across countries. For instance, some European countries offer financial support to individuals providing informal care, leading to the categorization of "informal paid caregivers" [23]. Additionally, the United Kingdom's definition of informal caregivers, relevant to the ASCOT-Carer SCT4, extends beyond family members to include friends and acquaintances [18]. This heterogeneity in defining informal care underscores the importance of studies employing the ASCOT-Carer SCT4 to clearly delineate between paid and unpaid caregivers, and between family caregivers and the wider group encompassing friends and acquaintances.

The ASCOT-SCT4 has been translated into several languages under the supervision of the original team, and its structural validity and reliability have been confirmed in these versions, including Japanese [24], Dutch [25], Finnish [26], and German [27]. Similarly, the ASCOT-Carer SCT4 has also been translated and validated in Japanese [28], Finnish [29], and German [30], also under the original team's guidance. Furthermore, for the economic evaluation of long-term care services, Japanese preference weights have been developed for both the Japanese ASCOT-SCT4 [31] and the Japanese ASCOT-Carer SCT4 [32]. Likewise, Finnish preference weights exist for the Finnish ASCOT-SCT4 [33] and the Finnish ASCOT-Carer SCT4 [29], and German preference weights have been developed for the German ASCOT-SCT4 [27] and the German ASCOT-Carer SCT4 [30].

1.2 Rehabilitation services in Japan

Two main types of rehabilitation services are available within the Japanese long-term care system: home-based and outpatient, including those provided at day service facilities [34, 35]. Home-based services involve physical and occupational therapists visiting patients' homes, with a 2019 nationwide survey reporting 115,000 recipients who typically used the service for 40 minutes, twice a week [36]. Outpatient rehabilitation services are often provided in conjunction with nursing care services like meals and bathing at day service facilities [36], serving a much larger population of 600,000 recipients in 2019, according to another nationwide survey [37]. These outpatient sessions generally occur once or twice a week and last for six to seven hours each time [37]. All services provided under the long-term care system in Japan are reviewed every six months [34–37]. Given that home-based rehabilitation services are typically more comprehensive and resource-intensive compared to outpatient rehabilitation services [34–37], it becomes particularly crucial to examine service users' satisfaction with home-based rehabilitation services.

2. Clarifying key concepts

The key concepts used in this chapter are clarified below to enhance understanding.

2.1 Social care-related quality of life (SCRQoL)

SCRQoL refers to the aspects of quality of life that individuals accessing adult social care services deem valuable and important, and that are affected by these services.

2.2 Adult social care outcomes toolkit (ASCOT)

The Adult Social Care Outcomes Toolkit (ASCOT) represents a suite of instruments to measure SCRQoL specifically for community-living adult care recipients and their family caregivers. Among the suite of instruments, the current chapter employs the ASCOT-SCT4 (a self-completion tool for community-dwelling adult care recipients with four response options) and the ASCOT-Carer SCT4 (a self-completion tool for informal caregivers).

3. Methods

3.1 Research approach

This chapter explored whether the mutual interdependence of SCRQoL within care recipient-caregiver dyads was associated with their overall satisfaction with home-based rehabilitation services.

3.2 Research design

To analyze the interdependence within care recipient-caregiver dyads, this chapter employed Actor-Partner Interdependence Modeling (APIM). **Figure 1** presents the hypothetical model for this chapter. In this model, overall satisfaction with home-based rehabilitation services was the predictor variable, and SCRQoL was the response variable. Actor effects are the predictor variable's effects on its own response variable. Partner effects are a predictor variable's effects on the response variable of the paired individual.

The hypotheses of this chapter were as follows: (1) A care recipient's SCRQoL, measured by the ASCOT-SCT4, would be associated with their own overall satisfaction with home-based rehabilitation services (an actor effect, path a_1). (2) A caregiver's

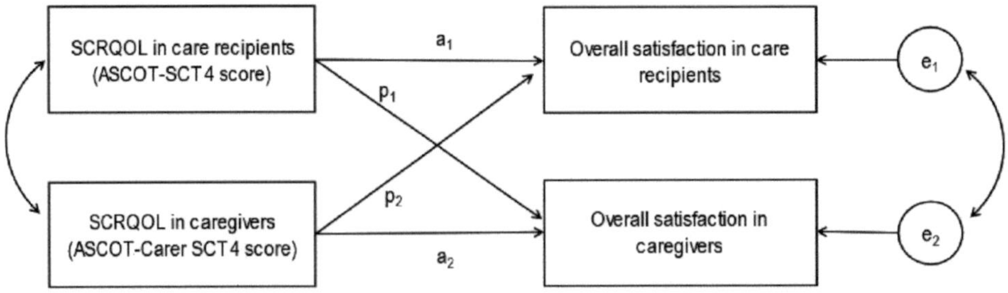

Figure 1.
A hypothetical model.

SCRQoL, measured by the ASCOT-Carer SCT4, would be associated with their own overall satisfaction with home-based rehabilitation services (an actor effect, path a_2). (3) A care recipient's SCRQoL, measured by the ASCOT-SCT4, would be associated with the caregiver's overall satisfaction with home-based rehabilitation services (a partner effect, path p_1). (4) A caregiver's SCRQoL, measured by the ASCOT-Carer SCT4, would be associated with the care recipient's overall satisfaction with home-based rehabilitation services (a partner effect, path p_2).

This modeling is considered the gold standard for analyzing pairwise data in dyadic relationships [38], making it well-suited for the care recipient-caregiver dyads in this chapter. This modeling has been successfully applied to various dyadic relationships, including child-parent relationships [39], friendships [40], romantic relationships [41, 42], couples [43, 44], and, importantly, patient-caregiver dyads [45].

3.3 Sampling

This chapter employed the following inclusion criteria for care recipients: (1) community-dwelling, (2) living together with their family caregivers, and (3) receiving home-based rehabilitation services for more than six months. Notably, these care recipients were newly registered in the Japanese social care system and had commenced home-based rehabilitation after undergoing inpatient rehabilitation to improve their independent living. For the caregivers, the inclusion criteria were: (1) acting as the primary caregiver for their family member, (2) providing primary care for more than six months, (3) living together with their care recipient, and (4) being unpaid family caregivers. The caregivers in this chapter were unpaid, reflecting the absence of a financial support system for family caregivers in Japan at that time.

3.4 Data collection

Data collection from the dyads in the greater capital area of Japan (Saitama and Chiba Prefectures) was conducted between August 2024 and February 2025, timed to align with the six-month intervals for the routine review of their services by their occupational or physical therapists.

The care recipients were asked to complete several questionnaires, including the Japanese version of the ASCOT-SCT4 (described below by Nakamura-Thomas et al. [24]) and a question assessing their overall satisfaction with home-based rehabilitation services. Additionally, they provided information on their sex, age, primary health issues necessitating care, and their care need levels, categorized into three tiers: low, moderate, and high, reflecting increasing levels of support required for independent living [34, 35].

The caregivers were also asked to complete several questionnaires, including the Japanese version of the ASCOT-Carer SCT4 (described below by Nakamura-Thomas et al. [28]) and a question assessing their overall satisfaction with home-based rehabilitation services. Additionally, they provided information on their sex, age, and relationship to the care recipients.

The Japanese version of the ASCOT-SCT4 [24] comprises eight attributes: control over daily life, social participation and involvement, occupation (doing things with value and enjoyment), personal cleanliness and comfort, food and drink, personal safety, accommodation cleanliness and comfort, and dignity. For each attribute, there are four possible response options representing a continuum of outcome states from best to worst: "ideal state," "no needs," "some needs," and "high-level needs." Care recipients were instructed to complete the questionnaire independently using a self-report paper-pencil format. However, if assistance was required, the therapists would read the questions, offer the response alternatives, and record the participant's choice accordingly.

The ASCOT-Carer SCT4 [28] comprises seven attributes: control over daily life, social participation and involvement, occupation (doing things with value and enjoyment), looking after oneself, personal safety, space and time to be oneself, and feeling supported and encouraged. For each attribute, there are four possible response options representing a continuum of outcome states from best to worst: "ideal state," "no needs," "some needs," and "high-level needs." The informal family caregivers were instructed to complete the questionnaire independently using a self-report paper-pencil format.

Overall satisfaction toward home-based rehabilitation services was assessed independently for both care recipients and caregivers using a 7-point Likert scale with the following response options: "extremely satisfied," "satisfied," "rather satisfied," "neither satisfied nor dissatisfied," "rather dissatisfied," "dissatisfied," and "extremely dissatisfied."

3.5 Data analysis

Data were analyzed using IBM Statistical Package for the Social Sciences (SPSS Statistics) version 29.0.0.0 and Analysis of Moment Structures (AMOS) 29.0 (IBM, Chicago, IL, USA) for Japanese. The participants' basic characteristics were summarized using descriptive statistics. For care recipients, this included valid data on sex, age, care need levels within the Japanese system, and their primary health issues. For caregivers, the summarized characteristics included sex, age, and their kinship with the care recipients.

Responses to the Japanese version of the ASCOT-SCT4 were scored using the utility weights, ranging from −0.38 to 1.00 [31], with scores below zero signifying a perception of social care-related quality of life worse than death [17]. Responses to the Japanese version of the ASCOT-Carer SCT4 were scored using the utility weights, ranging from 0.02 to 1.00 [32].

The 7-point Likert scale responses for overall satisfaction toward home-based rehabilitation services were converted to numerical values as follows: extremely satisfied = 7, satisfied = 6, rather satisfied = 5, neither satisfied nor dissatisfied = 4, rather dissatisfied = 3, dissatisfied = 2, and extremely dissatisfied = 1.

The model fit for the APIM was evaluated using the following goodness-of-fit indices: Goodness-of-Fit Index (GFI), Comparative Fit Index (CFI), and Root Mean Square Error of Approximation (RMSEA). For GFI and CFI, values of 0.90 and higher were considered indicative of a good fit, while a value below 0.05 was considered ideal for RMSEA [46]. Before conducting the APIM analysis, this chapter examined individual-level variance and group-level (pair-level variance in this chapter) variance [47]. Group homogeneity was identified with the interclass correlation coefficient (ICC). A high ICC results in a biased error variance in conventional regression models, overestimating the relationship between variables. An ICC of 0.25 or higher indicates that much of the variation in the dependent variables is due to the features of pairs rather than the individual characteristics [48, 49].

3.6 Ethical consideration

This chapter received ethical approval from an institutional review board (Saitama Prefectural University, 215006). Written informed consent was obtained from each participant directly before data collection commenced, ensuring their voluntary participation. Furthermore, given that the author had no role in the provision of their social care services, participants were assured that their decision to participate—or not—would not affect their access to care.

4. Results

4.1 Demographic characteristics of the participants

The data from 96 dyads with no missing data were analyzed for this chapter. **Table 1** shows the demographic characteristics of the participants. Among the 96 community-living care recipients receiving home-visit rehabilitation services, the frequencies

Variable		**%**
Care recipients		
Sex	Men	50.00
	Women	50.00
	Do not want to say	0
Age group (years old)		
	49–64	7.29
	65–74	15.63
	75–96	77.08
	Do not want to say	0
Care need level under the Japanese system		
	Low	9.38
	Moderate	47.92
	High	42.71
	Do not want to say	0
Primary health issue		
	Stroke	32.29
	Degenerative spine diseases	17.71
	Fractures	13.54
	Frailty	12.50
	Parkinson's disease	6.25
	Cancer	5.21
	Osteoarthritis	5.21
	Angina	4.17
	Others	3.12

Variable		%
	Do not want to say	0
Informal family caregivers		
Sex	Men	32.29
	Women	67.71
	Do not want to say	0
Age group (years old)		
	39–64	25.00
	65–74	30.21
	75–91	44.79
	Do not want to say	0
Taking care of		
	Husband	41.67
	Wife	22.92
	Own parent	29.17
	Parent-in-law	6.25
	Do not want to say	0

Table 1.
Participants' demographics (96 dyads).

of men and women were equivalent. Their ages ranged from 49 to 96 years. Among the age groups, 77% were aged 75 and older, followed by 16% aged from 65 to 74. Among the care need levels under the Japanese system, 48% of them were assessed to be moderate level, followed by 43% at a high level. Their primary health issues were stroke (32%), followed by degenerative spine diseases (18%), fractures (14%), and frailty (13%).

Among the 96 primary family caregivers who resided with the care recipients, 68% were women. Their ages ranged from 39 to 91 years. In the age groups, 45% were 75 years and older, followed by those aged 65 to 74 (30%). Forty-two percent of them took care of husbands, followed by their own parents (29%) and wives (23%).

4.2 Descriptive statistics of the measured variables

Table 2 shows the descriptive statistics of the measured variables (ASCOT-SCT4, ASCOT-Carer SCT4, and overall satisfaction toward home-based rehabilitation services). Among the care recipients, the ASCOT-SCT4 score ranged from 0.030 to 1.00. The mean score was 0.704 (standard deviation was 0.236). For the overall satisfaction toward home-based rehabilitation services, 41% of the care recipients indicated "satisfied," followed by "rather satisfied" (25%), "extremely satisfied" (21%), and "neither satisfied nor dissatisfied" (13%).

Among the caregivers, the ASCOT-Carer SCT4 score ranged from 0.327 to 1.000. The mean score was 0.824 (standard deviation was 0.163). For the overall satisfaction toward home-based rehabilitation services, 42% of the care recipients indicated "satisfied," followed by "rather satisfied" (20%), "extremely satisfied" (17%), and "neither satisfied nor dissatisfied" (16%).

Variable		
Care recipients		
ASCOT-SCT4 score		
	Range (the lowest; the highest)	0.030; 1.00
	Mean	0.704
	Standard deviation	0.236
	Skewness	0.038
	Kurtosis	−0.873
Overall satisfaction (%)		
	Extremely satisfied	20.83
	Satisfied	40.63
	Rather satisfied	25.00
	Neither satisfied nor dissatisfied	12.50
	Rather dissatisfied	1.04
	Dissatisfied	0
	Extremely dissatisfied	0
	Do not want to say	0
Caregivers		
ASCOT-Carer SCT4 score		
	Range (the lowest; the highest)	0.327;1.000
	Mean	0.824
	Standard deviation	0.163
	Skewness	0.338
	Kurtosis	−1.072
Overall satisfaction (%)		
	Extremely satisfied	16.67
	Satisfied	41.67
	Rather satisfied	19.79
	Neither satisfied nor dissatisfied	15.36
	Rather dissatisfied	4.17
	Dissatisfied	2.08
	Extremely dissatisfied	0
	Do not want to say	0

Note. ASCOT-SCT4 = Adult Social Care Outcomes Toolkit Self-Completion Tool with four response options, ASCOT-Carer SCT4 = Adult Social Care Outcomes Toolkit for Carer Self-Completion Tool with four response options.

Table 2.
Descriptive statistics of the measured variables (96 dyads).

4.3 Correlations among the measured variables

Table 3 displays the ICC values for the measured variables. Among these, the overall satisfaction with home-based rehabilitation services showed an ICC of 0.495 ($p < 0.001$), indicating a moderate level of homogeneity or similarity in satisfaction scores within the care recipient-caregiver pairs. This significant within-dyad

Variable	ICC			p-value
		95% CI Lower	95% CI Upper	
SCRQoL	0.002	—0.197	0.202	0.490
Overall satisfaction	0.495	0.328	0.632	< 0.001

Note. SCRQoL was measured using the Adult Social Care Outcomes Toolkit Self-Completion Tool with four response options (ASCOT-SCT4) in care recipients and the Adult Social Care Outcomes Toolkit for Carer Self-Completion Tool (ASCOT-Carer SCT4) with four response options in caregivers, ICC = Interclass correlation, CI = Confidence Interval.

Table 3.
Values in interclass correlation for measured variables.

correlation in satisfaction suggests that additional, more complex modeling approaches might be warranted to fully account for this interdependence.

4.4 Model examination

Figure 2 presents the results of the APIM. The model demonstrated a good fit to the data, as indicated by the following goodness-of-fit indices: GFI = 1.000, CFI = 1.000, and RMSEA = 0.000. The hypothesized model was partially supported, revealing a significant positive actor effect of care recipients' SCRQoL (measured by the ASCOT-SCT4) on their overall satisfaction toward home-based rehabilitation services (ß = 0.326, p < 0.01). In contrast, no significant actor effect was found for caregivers' SCRQoL (measured by the ASCOT-Carer SCT4) on their overall satisfaction toward home-based rehabilitation services (ß = 0.017, p = 0.865). Moreover, no significant partner effect was observed of care recipients' SCRQoL on their caregivers' overall satisfaction (ß = 0.026, p = 0.803), nor of caregivers' SCRQoL on their care recipients' overall satisfaction (ß = 0.029, p = 0.760). In addition, the initial model yielded an Akaike's Information Criterion (AIC) of 20.000 and a Bayesian Information Criterion (BIC) of 45.643. These values served as benchmarks for comparison with alternative models.

Additional analyses were conducted to explore the impact of the relationship type within the dyads, specifically examining pairs of wife (care recipient) and husband (caregiver), husband (care recipient) and wife (caregiver), parent (care recipient) and biological child (caregiver), and parent-in-law (care recipient) and child-in-law (caregiver). This additional model (Model 1), incorporating all relationship types, did not demonstrate a good fit to the data, as indicated by a CFI of 0.863, despite a GFI of 0.984 and an RMSEA of 0.000. Consequently, this model was rejected. A revised

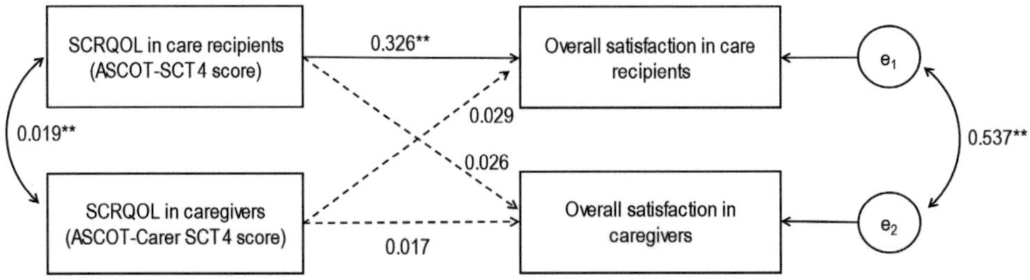

Figure 2.
The final model. Note. *Dashed arrows represent statistical non-significance,* p < 0.01.

model (Model 2), which excluded pairs of parent-in-law (care recipient) and child-in-law (caregiver), showed a good fit to the data, with the following goodness-of-fit indices: GFI = 0.998, CFI = 0.990, and RMSEA = 0.000. However, this model (Model 2) yielded AIC and BIC values (60.355 and 135.349, respectively) that were higher than those of the initial, more parsimonious model. Therefore, the initial model was sustained.

5. Discussion

This chapter explored the association between the mutual interdependence of SCRQoL within care recipient-caregiver dyads and their overall satisfaction toward home-based rehabilitation services. A key finding was the significant positive actor effect of care recipients' SCRQoL on their own satisfaction. This actor effect is particularly important as care recipients are the direct recipients of these home-based rehabilitation services. To ensure the continued uptake and effectiveness of these services, future studies should investigate the factors that contribute to care recipients' satisfaction. Supporting the importance of such factors, a previous survey of older care recipients found that care managers' 'explanation ability' and 'polite attitude and manners' significantly influenced satisfaction, with this association being stronger among those with higher long-term care literacy [50]. Moreover, the provision of long-term care services significantly impacts care recipients' home-based lives [51, 52], making higher levels of satisfaction with these services crucial, especially for older women. Indeed, a longitudinal chapter demonstrated that greater life satisfaction in older women was associated with a lower risk of functional decline or death over a 14-year period [53].

In contrast to care recipients, this chapter found no significant actor effect of family caregivers' SCRQoL on their own satisfaction. Furthermore, no significant partner effects were identified, meaning care recipients' SCRQoL did not significantly impact their caregivers' satisfaction, and vice versa. While caregivers did not directly receive home-based rehabilitation services, the correlation in satisfaction observed between the dyads suggests a potential interconnectedness. Individuals in close relationships are known to be interdependent [54], and this mutual influence may have led to similar levels of perceived satisfaction with the services, possibly due to emotional contagion. Additionally, the "explanation ability" and "polite attitude and manners" of care providers, identified as important factors in a previous chapter [50], might have also influenced family caregivers' satisfaction in this context. To better understand the factors driving caregivers' satisfaction and ensure service uptake by this group, future research should specifically investigate these aspects. Given the inevitable declines in health status and independent living often experienced by care recipients, home-based rehabilitation services remain crucial for maintaining SCRQoL in both care recipients and their family caregivers.

Given that the specific content, frequency, and duration of home-visit rehabilitation services are collaboratively determined by the care recipient, their family caregiver, and a case manager, considering their needs and home environment [55], the principles of decision-making, autonomy, and choice inherent in the ASCOT framework [17, 18] are highly relevant. This chapter, therefore, suggests that therapists providing home-based rehabilitation services employ the ASCOT to actively promote and assess decision-making, autonomy, and choice for both care recipients and their family caregivers. Moreover, considering the aim of home-visit rehabilitation services to improve both activities of daily living and social participation [56], utilizing the ASCOT can broaden therapists' understanding of the importance of addressing social participation for both care recipients and their family caregivers, moving beyond the traditional focus primarily on Activities of Daily Living (ADL) improvement in care recipients.

While this chapter provides valuable insights for therapists delivering home-visit rehabilitation services, several limitations should be considered. Firstly, the nonrandom selection of a solely Japanese participant limits the generalizability of the findings to other populations. Secondly, the focus on care recipients receiving home-visit rehabilitation within the Japanese long-term care system may restrict applicability to those with different service models, those not co-residing with family caregivers, or those receiving care in other countries. Similarly, the findings may not extend to caregivers who are not primary family members or those caring for unmarried partners, relatives, or friends. Lastly, this chapter examined care recipients already integrated within the long-term care system and having a certain level of service access. Future research could explore the experiences and outcomes of individuals with varying levels of access to long-term care, including those with more limited access or facing specific barriers to obtaining services.

6. Conclusion

This chapter revealed a significant positive actor effect of care recipients' SCRQoL on their own satisfaction, highlighting the crucial role of service satisfaction given the substantial impact of long-term care services on their home-based lives. In contrast, no significant actor effect of family caregivers' SCRQoL on their own satisfaction was found, nor were any significant partner effects observed between the SCRQoL of one dyad member and the satisfaction of the other. Recognizing the vital supportive role of family caregivers in care recipients' community living, this chapter recommends that therapists providing home-based rehabilitation services utilize the ASCOT to actively promote and assess decision-making, autonomy, and choice for both care recipients and their family caregivers.

Acknowledgements

The author expresses gratitude to all participants for their cooperation and to the therapists for their assistance in data collection.

Funding information

The author discloses receipt of the following financial support for the research, authorship, and/or publication of this article: This chapter was supported financially by a governmental grant in Japan (Japan Society for the Promotion of Science (JSPS), KAKENHI: Grants-in-Aid for Scientific Research): 20K02087.

Conflict of interest

The author declares no potential conflicts of interest with respect to the research, authorship, and/or publication of this article.

Author details

Hiromi Nakamura-Thomas
Graduate School of Health, Medicine and Welfare, School of Health, Medicine and Welfare, Saitama Prefectural University, Saitama, Japan

*Address all correspondence to: nakamura-hiromi@spu.ac.jp

References

[1] UN. Demographic statistics database. Available from: http://data.un.org/Data.aspx?d=POP&f=tableCode%3a22#POP [Accessed: February 13, 2020]

[2] OECD. Health at a glance 2019 OECD indicators. Available from: https://www.oecd-ilibrary.org/docserver/4dd50c09-en.pdf?expires=1582870884&id=id&accname=guest&checksum=AF50BFBCDBCF1277D2119C53F2722AA7 [Accessed: February 27, 2020]

[3] Hofstede G. Culture Consequences: Comparing Values, Behaviors, Institutions and Organizations across Nations. California: Sage; 2001

[4] Yoo WK. A research methodology for Korean neo-confucianism. Acta Koreana. 2013;**16**(1):177-197

[5] Ministry of Health, Labour and Welfare. A survey of circumstances of primary informal family caregivers. Tokyo: Ministry of Health, Labour and Welfare; 2022. (in Japanese). Available from: https://www.mhlw.go.jp/toukei/saikin/hw/k-tyosa/k-tyosa22/dl/05.pdf

[6] Ministry of Health, Labour and Welfare. The current state of the long-term care system and future contributions. Tokyo: Ministry of Health, Labour and Welfare; 2018. (in Japanese). Available from: https://www.mhlw.go.jp/file/06-Seisakujouhou-12300000-Roukenkyoku/0000213177.pdf

[7] Sone T, Nakaya N, Tomata Y, Tsuji I. Risk of psychological distress in partners with functional disability among older Japanese adults. Geriatrics & Gerontology International. 2018;**18**(5):775-782. DOI: 10.1111/ggi.13254

[8] Sone T, Nakaya N, Tomata Y, Nakaya K, Hoshi M, Tsuji I. Spouse's functional disability and mortality: The Ohsaki cohort 2006 study. Geriatrics & Gerontology International. 2019;**19**(8):774-779. DOI: 10.1111/ggi.13709

[9] Tamiya N, Noguchi H, Nishi A, Reich MR, Ikegami N, Hashimoto H, et al. Population ageing and wellbeing: Lessons from Japan's long-term care insurance policy. Lancet. 2011;**378**(9797):1183-1192. DOI: 10.1016/S0140-6736(11)61176-8

[10] Campbell JC. In: Campbell JC, Edvardsen U, Midford P, Saito Y, editors. Japan's long-term care insurance system in eldercare policies in Japan and Scandinavia: Aging Societies East and West. New York, NY: Palgrave Macmillan; 2014. pp. 9-30

[11] Ministry of Health, Labour and Welfare. A proposal for ideal systems for provision of medicine and long-term care after 2025. Tokyo: Ministry of Health, Labour and Welfare; 2023. (in Japanese). Available from: https://www.mhlw.go.jp/content/12403550/001059091.pdf

[12] OECD. Measuring social well-being: A progress report on the development of social indicators. OECD social indicator developing programme no 3. P213. Paris: OECD; 1976

[13] McNeil BJ, Keller E, Adelstein SJ. Primer on certain elements of medical decision making. The New England Journal of Medicine. 1975;**293**(5):211-215. DOI: 10.1056/NEJM 197507312930501

[14] WHO. Constitution: WHO remains firmly committed to the principles set out in the preamble to the constitution.

Available from: https://www.who.int/about/governance/constitution

[15] WHO. WHOQOL: Measuring quality of life. Available from: https://www.who.int/tools.whoqol

[16] WHO. World report on ageing and health. 2015. Available from: https://apps.who.int/iris/bitstream/handle/10665/186463/9789240694811_eng.pdf;jsessionid=5BB804E012659FC3.C72B8200.A0539E5C?sequence=1 [Accessed: October 30, 2019]

[17] Netten A, Burge P, Malley J, Potoglou D, Towers AM, Bzazier J, et al. Outcomes of social care for adults: Developing a preference-weighted measure. Health Technology Assessment. 2012;**16**:1-166. DOI: 10.3310/hta16160

[18] Rand S, Malley J, Netten A, Forder JE. Factor structure and construct validity of the adult social care outcomes toolkit for carers (ASCOT-Carer). Quality of Life Research. 2015;**24**:2601-2614. DOI: 10.1007/s11136-015-1011-x

[19] Siette J, Knaggs GT, Zurynski Y, Ratcliffe J, Dodds L, Westbrook J. Systematic review of 29 self-report instruments for assessing quality of life in older adults receiving aged care services. BMJ Open. 2021;**11**(11):e050892. DOI: 10.1136/bmjopen-2021-050892

[20] Batchelder L, Malley J, Burge P, Lu H, Saloniki EC, et al. Carer social care-related quality of life outcomes: Estimating English preference weights for the adult social care outcomes toolkit for carers. Value in Health. 2019;**22**(12):1427-1440. DOI: 10.1016/j.jval.2019.07.014

[21] Bulamu NB, Kaambwa B, Ratcliffe J. A systematic review of instruments for measuring outcomes in economic evaluation within aged care. Health and Quality of Life Outcomes. 2015;**13**:179. DOI: 10.1186/s12955-015-0372-8

[22] Dow J, Robinson J, Robalino S, Finch T, McColl E, Robinson L. How best to assess quality of life in informal carers of people with dementia; a systematic review of existing outcome measures. PLoS One. 2018;**13**:e0193398. DOI: 10.1371/journal.pone.0193398

[23] Rand S, Malley J, Vadean F, Forder J. Measuring the outcomes of long-term care for unpaid carers: Comparing the ASCOT-carer, carer experience scale and EQ-5D-3L. Health and Quality of Life Outcomes. 2019;**17**:1-12. DOI: 10.1186/s12955-019-1254-2

[24] Nakamura-Thomas H, Morikawa M, Moriyama Y, Shiroiwa T, Kyougoku M, Razik K, et al. Japanese translation and cross-cultural validation of the adult social care outcomes toolkit (ASCOT) in Japanese social service users. Health and Quality Life Outcomes. 2019;**17**(59):1-16. DOI: 10.1186/s12955-019-1128-7

[25] van Leeuwen KM, Bosmans JE, Jansen APD, Rand S, Towers AM, Smith N, et al. Dutch translation and cross-cultural validation of the adult social care outcomes toolkit (ASCOT). Health and Quality of Life Outcomes. 2015;**13**(56):1-13. DOI: 10.1186/s12955-015-0249-x

[26] Nguyen L, Linnosmaa I, Jokimäki H, Rand S, Malley J, Razik K, et al. Social care related outcomes in Finland. Construct validity and structural characteristics of the Finnish ASCOT measure with older home care users. Health and Social Care in the Community. 2021;**29**:712-728. DOI: 10.1111/hsc.13328

[27] Trukeschitz B, Litschauer J, Hajji A, Kieninger J, Schoch A, Malley J, et al. Cross-cultural adaptation and construct

validity of the German version of the adult social care outcomes toolkit for service users (German ASCOT). Health and Quality Life Outcomes. 2020;**18**(326):1-19. DOI: 10.1186/s12955-020-01533-7

[28] Nakamura-Thomas H, Yamaguchi M, Yamaguchi I, Rand S. Assessing the structural characteristics of the Japanese version of the adult social care outcomes toolkit for carers. Home Health Care Management & Practice. 2022;**34**:17-23. DOI: 10.1177/10848223211030269

[29] Nguyen L, Jokimäki H, Linnosmaa I, Saloniki EC, Batchelder L, et al. Valuing informal carers' quality of life using best-worst scaling—Finnish preference weights for the adult social care outcomes toolkit for carers (ASCOTCarer). European Journal of Health Economics. 2022;**23**:357-374. DOI: 10.1007/s10198-012-01356-3

[30] Trukeschitz B, Hajji A, Litschauer J, Malley J, Schoch A, Rand S, et al. Translation, cultural adaptation and construct validity of the German version of the adult social care outcomes toolkit for informal carers (German ASCOT-Carer). Quality of Life Research. 2021;**30**:905-920. DOI: 10.1007/s11136-020-02682-4

[31] Shiroiwa T, Moriyama Y, Nakamura-Thomas H, Morikawa M, Fukuda T, Batchelder L, et al. Development of Japanese utility weights for the adult social care outcomes toolkit (ASCOT) SCT4. Quality of Life Research. 2020;**29**:253-263. DOI: 10.1007/s11136-019-02287-6

[32] Shiroiwa T, Nakamura-Thomas H, Yamaguchi M, Morikawa M, Moriyama Y, Fukuda T, et al. Japanese preference weights of the adult social care outcomes toolkit for carers (ASCOT-carer). Quality of Life Research. 2022;**31**:2143-2151. DOI: 10.1007/s11136-021-03076-w

[33] Nguyen L, Jokimäki H, Linnosmaa I, Saloniki EC, Batchelder L, Malley J, et al. Do you prefer safety to social participation? Finnish population-based preference weights for the adult social care outcomes toolkit (ASCOT) for service users. MDM Policy & Practice. 2021;**6**(2):23814683211027904. DOI: 10.1177/23814683211027902

[34] Maruta M, Tabira T, Makizako H, Sagari A, Miyata H, Yoshimitsu K, et al. Impact of outpatient rehabilitation service in preventing the deterioration of the care-needs level among Japanese older adults availing long-term care insurance: A propensity score matched retrospective study. International Journal of Environmental Research and Public Health. 2019;**16**:1292. DOI: 10.3390/ijerph16071292

[35] Tsuchiya-Ito R, Ishizaki T, Mitsutake S, Hamada S, Yoshie S, Iijima K, et al. Association of household income with home-based rehabilitation and home help service utilization among long-term home care service users. BMC Geriatrics. 2020;**20**:314. DOI: 10.1186/s12877-020-01704-7

[36] Ministry of Health, Labour and Welfare. 182th social security council, long-term care benefit fee divisional meeting, home-based rehabilitation. 2020. (in Japanese). Available from: https://www.mhlw.go.jp/stf/newpage_13021.html [Accessed: April 3, 2025]

[37] Ministry of Health, Labour and Welfare. 180th social security council, long-term care benefit fee divisional meeting, outpatient (Day-Care) rehabilitation. 2020. (in Japanese). Available from: https://www.mhlw.go.jp/stf/newpage_12499.html [Accessed: April 3, 2025]

[38] Kenny DA, Kashy DA, Cook WL. Dyadic Data Analysis. New York: Guilford Press; 2006

[39] Cook WL, Kenny DA. The actor-partner interdependence model: A model of bidirectional effects in developmental studies. International Journal of Behavioral Development. 2005;**29**:101-109. DOI: 10.1080/01650250444000405

[40] Popp D, Laursen B, Kerr M, Stattin H, Burk WJ. Modeling homophily over time with an actor-partner interdependence model. Developmental Psychology. 2008;**44**:1028-1039. DOI: 10.1037/0012-1649.44.4.1028

[41] Asano R. Intrapersonal and interpersonal processes of salutogenesis model in romantic relationships: A dyadic data approach. The Japanese Journal of Experimental Social Psychology. 2011;**50**(2):158-167. DOI: 10.2130/jjesp.50.158

[42] Campbell L, Simpson JA, Kashy DA, Rholes WS. Attachment orientations, dependence, and behavior in a stressful situation. An application of the actor-partner interdependence model. Journal of Social and Personal Relationships. 2001;**18**:821-843. DOI: 10.1177/0265407501186005

[43] Chung ML, Moser DK, Lennie TA, Rayens MK. The effects of depressive symptoms and anxiety on quality of life in patients with heart failure and their spouses: Testing dyadic dynamics using actor-partner interdependence model. Journal of Psychosomatic Research. 2009;**67**:29-35. DOI: 10.1016/j.jpsychores.2009.01.009

[44] Böhlmann P, Mack JT, Weise V, Seefeld L, Bodenmann G, Zietlow AL, et al. The prospective impact of extradyadic stress on depressive symptoms and the mediating role of intradyadic stress in parents–an actor partner interdependence mediation model. PLoS One. 2024;**19**(11):e0311989. DOI: 10.1371/journal.pone.0311989

[45] Fan Y, Song M, Xu S, Tan Y, Li X. Subjective and objective effects of anxiety and fatigue on social function in patients with enterostomy and their family caregivers. PLoS One. 2024;**19**(11):e0309991. DOI: 10.1371/journal.pone.0309991

[46] Ledermann T, Rudaz M, Wu Q, Cui M. Determine power and sample size for the simple and mediation actor-partner interdependence model. Family Relations. 2022;**71**:1452-1469. DOI: 10.1111/fare.12644

[47] Byrne BM. Structural Equation Modeling with Mplus: Basic Concepts, Applications, and Programming. New York: NY; 2012

[48] Kim TK, Solomon P, Zurlo KA. Applying hierarchical linear modeling (HLM) to social work administration research. Administration in Social Work. 2009;**33**:262-277. DOI: 10.1080/03643100902987739

[49] Bosselut G, Boiché J, Salamé B, Fouquereau E, Guilbert L, Serrano OC. Transformational leadership and group cohesion in sports: Examining the mediating role of interactional justice using a within- and between-team approach. International Journal of Sports Science and Coaching. 2018;**13**:912-928. DOI: 10.1177/1747954118801156

[50] Wang Z, Fukayama K, Niu B. Does long-term care literacy matter in evaluating older care recipients' satisfaction with care managers? Empirical evidence from Japanese survey data. International Journal of Environmental Research and Public Health. 2023;**20**:2456. DOI: 10.3390/ijerph20032456

[51] Moriyama Y, Tamiya N, Kawamura A, Mayers TD, Noguchi H, Takahashi H. Effect of short-stay service use on stay-at-home duration for elderly with certified care needs: Analysis of long-term care insurance claims data in Japan. PLoS One. 2018;**13**(8):e0203112. DOI: 10.1371/journal.pone.0203112

[52] Hamada S, Takahashi H, Sakata N, Jeon B, Mori T, Iijima K, et al. Household income relationship with health services utilization and healthcare expenditures in people aged 75 years or older in Japan: A population-based study using medical and long-term care insurance claims data. Journal of Epidemiology. 2019;**29**(10):377-383. DOI: 10.2188/jea.JE20180055

[53] Shinohara N, Zhao W, Shan Y, Ukawa S, Ohira H, Kawamura T, et al. Temporal change in the association between life satisfaction and functional decline with gender differences: An age-specific prospective cohort study. Environmental Health and Preventive Medicine. 2023;**28**:42. DOI: 10.1265/ehpm.23-00019

[54] Fingerman KL, Bermann E. Applications of family systems theory to the study of adulthood. The International Journal of Aging and Human Development. 2000;**51**(1):5-29

[55] Ministry of Health, Labour and Welfare. An outline of the long-term care system. Tokyo: Ministry of Health, Labour and Welfare; 2022. (in Japanese). Available from: https://www.mhlw.go.jp/content/000801559.pdf

[56] Suzuki O. The meaning and issues of home visit habitation services in community medicine (in Japanese). El Hospital. 2021;**80**(6):521-525

Chapter 10

Life after Limb Loss: Addressing Activity Limitations through Rehabilitation

Peter Bredu-Darkwa

Abstract

Amputation represents a profound and life-altering event that significantly disrupts an individual's daily functioning and overall well-being. Increasing attention has been directed toward evaluating how individuals with amputations manage basic and complex daily tasks commonly referred to as Activities of Daily Living (ADLs) and Instrumental Activities of Daily Living (IADLs) to inform evidence-based rehabilitation strategies. This chapter explores the challenges amputees face in performing these activities, examines how such limitations influence their life satisfaction, and considers the critical role of rehabilitation in addressing these issues. A quantitative, cross-sectional survey involving 200 amputees was carried out at an Orthopedic Training Center in Ghana. Data collection utilized the Groningen Activity Restriction Scale and the Life Satisfaction Questionnaire-11. All statistical analyses were conducted using IBM SPSS version 23.0, with results presented in tabular form and figures. Multivariate analysis identified a notable negative correlation between functional limitations and life satisfaction. Participants reported difficulties in performing both ADLs and IADLs, with a mean activity limitation score of 36.57 ± 10.93. Their average life satisfaction was moderate, scoring 3.86 ± 1.15. The multivariate analysis confirmed a statistically significant inverse relationship between activity limitations and life satisfaction ($ß = -0.13$, $p < 0.001$). These findings underscore the need for rehabilitation professionals to thoroughly assess these challenges to inform effective program design, resource distribution, and policy development aimed at enhancing the quality of life for individuals living with limb loss.

Keywords: amputation, rehabilitation, satisfaction, wellbeing, activity, limitation

1. Introduction

Amputations occur globally for a wide range of reasons, including congenital limb abnormalities, poor vascular health, severe burns, cancer, and traumatic injuries. The global prevalence of limb amputation remains uncertain, with considerable disparities observed across different regions and countries. In the United States alone, estimates from 2005 indicated that approximately 1.6 million individuals were living with limb loss a figure projected to increase significantly, reaching an estimated 3.6

million by the year 2050 [1–2]. Among these amputations Bello and friends reported "90% are of the lower limbs and 75% of the Amputees are over 65 years of age". A significant variability exists in the number of acquired amputations across and within countries. Lower limb amputations are significantly more common than upper limb amputations, a trend consistently observed across various populations and clinical settings. Within the Navajo people of the United States, prevalence estimates, indicates a range from approximately 1.2 per 1000 among women and 4.4 per 1000 among men. Broadly, national date from the United States suggests that an estimated 30,000 to 40,000 amputation procedures are annually conducted. Mclarney et al. reports that "an analysis of data from commercially insured drivers under 18 years of age showed an annual incidence of major lower extremity amputations at approximately 38.5 cases per 100, 000 between 2009 and 2015" [1–6].

Amputation or Limb loss occurs when a limb or external body part is removed either entirely or partially through surgical interventions or due to spontaneous circumstances [7]. It may be one-sided or two-sided and can be performed at various levels of the body segment [8]. The most common are amputations of the knee, hip, or ankle followed by removal of the entire limb [9].

Individuals with amputation experience a disastrous change and alteration in their life regardless of the cause, and the effect on their quality of life and well-being is substantial [10]. The performance of personal, skilled, leisure, social and marital activities, including expression of sexual feelings between partners are greatly affected by amputation [11].

According to the International Classification of Functioning, Disability, and Health (ICF), activity limitations refer to "the difficulties an individual may experience in executing activities" [12]. Individuals' engagement in meaningful activities and their overall life satisfaction have been shown to be adversely affected by major limb amputations [13]. Fundamental routines, including Activities of Daily Living (ADLs) and instrumental Activities of Daily Living (IADLs), are a key component of everyday functioning and disruptions in these domains can significantly influence both quality of life and personal wellbeing [14–16]. These tasks constitute fundamental and essential components of a person's daily functioning. IADLs involve more cognitively demanding and multifaceted routines that encourage and support independent living such as managing transportation, preparing meals, shopping and performance of household chores [13, 17].

Following amputation, the capacity to perform ADLs upon discharge plays an important role in predicting a person's long-term satisfaction and quality of life [18]. Research indicates that individuals with amputation often face serious challenges in performing routine daily tasks post-surgery. Bello et al. reports that disability in individuals with amputations may result from restrictions and barriers which stem from the interplay between impairments in body structure and function as well as environmental factors that hinder participation and engagement [2]. Individuals living with limb loss often experience challenges in carrying out everyday tasks and may also encounter barriers in various aspects of social life, including forming relationships, pursuing education, and participating in community activities. Zunzunegui et al. defines activities of daily Living limitations as "requiring assistance and help in at least one of the following tasks: walking across a small room, bathing, toileting, transferring from bed and chair, using the toilet, dressing, or feeding oneself [19].

As reported by the World Health Organization, people with amputation often face limitations in carrying out daily activities which can adversely impact on their wellbeing, quality of life, satisfaction, and a sense of independence [20]. A report by

Wang et al. indicates that reliance on others for ADLs will decrease over time when individuals recognize the importance of these activities. A key indicator of progress during rehabilitation is the ability to perform ADLs. Additionally, life satisfaction is considered a critical outcome of the rehabilitation process [21]. Amputation can harmfully impact life satisfaction, often leading to reduced overall well-being and a more negative outlook when individuals assess their lives. These effects are basically attributed to instant physical limitations following the procedure and the lasting impact across various aspects of daily living [10, 22]. Additionally, amputations prevent successful reintegration into society due to the limitations placed on individuals with amputations and the restrictions to participation they experience in various life domains [23, 24].

Essentially, the rehabilitation and management of amputees should commence prior to the surgical procedure and be delivered by a multidisciplinary team with specialized expertise as reported by Esquenazi and DiGiacomo [25]. The rehabilitation, guided by holistic and multidisciplinary approach [26], typically comprises multiple stages of variable duration involving the pre-operative phase, the pre-prosthetic phase and when appropriate, prosthetic training [27].

The physician, occupational therapist, physiotherapist, prosthesis, social worker in a coordinated, team-based approach post amputation, and guided by effective rehabilitation strategies work together to effectively rehabilitate and manage the amputees to prevent complications and significantly improve health outcomes in patients [28, 29]. Evidence suggests that rehabilitation outcomes tend to be more favorable in individuals who undergo amputations due to traumatic injury compared to those whose limb loss resulted from disease-related causes [30].

This chapter examines the activity limitations encountered by individuals with limb loss and assesses the contribution of rehabilitation in mitigating these functional challenges. Special focus is placed on the difficulties amputees face in performing Activities of Daily Living (ADLs) and Instrumental Activities of Daily Living (IADLs), along with evaluating how effective rehabilitation efforts are in addressing these challenges.

2. Activity limitations, life satisfaction and amputee rehabilitation

2.1 Experiments

A quantitative, cross-sectional research design was adopted for this study, which was carried out at the Orthopedic Training Centre (OTC) in Ghana's Eastern Region. This facility primarily serves individuals with physical disabilities across Ghana and parts of West Africa, offering rehabilitation and related services. The OTC was selected as the research site due to its large and consistent population of amputees, many of whom either reside there temporarily or attend regularly for rehabilitation. A purposive sampling approach was used to choose the study location, while both purposive and simple random sampling techniques were employed to recruit participants. The random sampling method ensured that every eligible individual had an equal chance of being included, thereby enhancing the representativeness of the sample and allowing for efficient data collection. In total, 200 participants were selected for the study.

Eligibility criteria included adults (aged 18 and above) with either unilateral or bilateral amputations who were currently undergoing post-amputation rehabilitation whether they were using prostheses or not. Participants were also required to receive treatment or residing at the Centre for at least three months. This criterion ensured that respondents were stabilized and in a phase of adjustment post-amputation, making them better positioned to provide meaningful insights into the variables under study. The inclusion of both male and female participants allowed for the examination of gender-related perspectives on amputation and rehabilitation experiences.

Data collection was conducted using standardized, validated instruments. Respondents completed self-administered paper-based questionnaires under researcher's supervision to ensure accuracy and clarity. Two tools were used: the Groningen Activity Restriction Scale (GARS) and the Life Satisfaction Questionnaire-11 (LISAT-11). The GARS assesses the extent of difficulty individuals face in performing both ADLs and IADLs. It comprises 18 items rated on a 5-point Likert scale, where a score of '1' denotes independence and '5' indicates full dependence. Scores range from 18 (least limitation) to 72 (most limitation), with higher scores reflecting greater functional restrictions [31]. The GARS was chosen for its robust psychometric properties and its ability to measure limitations in ADLs and IADLs simultaneously, making it a valuable tool for comparative studies. It is flexible in administration and can be completed either independently or with the help of a researcher, depending on the literacy level of the respondent. The LISAT-11 was employed to explore the overall life satisfaction of amputees across multiple dimensions, such as physical and psychological health, social relationships, financial status, work, sexual life, and leisure. Each item is scored on a scale from 1 (very dissatisfied) to 6 (very satisfied). Rather than computing a total score, domain-specific mean scores were used to preserve detailed information across different aspects of life, which is more beneficial for clinical applications.

Before the main study commenced, the questionnaire was pilot-tested at the orthopedic unit of the Korle-Bu Teaching Hospital (KBTH) in Accra. Participants in the pre-test shared characteristics with the target population at OTC, providing a useful proxy for refining the survey instruments. The pilot helped identify ambiguities, estimate the time required for completion, and ensure the overall coherence of the questionnaire. Revisions were made based on feedback from this trial phase. Participants were thoroughly briefed on the study protocols, and informed consent was obtained in writing before data collection began. For respondents who encountered language barriers or difficulties understanding specific items, a translator was present to help. The research team remained on-site over multiple days to reach the target sample size, assigning each participant a unique identifier for follow-up and data verification. Completed questionnaires were reviewed for completeness and consistency before entry.

Data was analyzed using SPSS version 23.0. Descriptive statistics such as frequencies, means, standard deviations, and cross-tabulations were generated to summarize the findings. Results are presented in the accompanying tables and figures.

2.2 Data on activity limitations after limb loss

The study involved 200 participants with either upper or lower limb amputations. Of these, 107 individuals (54%) were male, and approximately 49 (24%) were aged between 31 and 40 years. The majority of respondents 174 (87%) had amputations of the lower limbs, while 179 participants (89%) had undergone unilateral amputation. Supporting these findings, research from Kano, Nigeria, reported that males represent the largest proportion of amputees in that region. Similarly, a study conducted among

Asian populations in the Navajo Nation, USA, indicated an amputation incidence rate of 1.2 per 10,000 women compared to 4.4 per 10,000 men [2]. Overall, the participants in this study were able to carry out Activities of Daily Living (ADLs) and Instrumental Activities of Daily Living (IADLs) but experienced some difficulties, reflected in a mean activity limitation score of 36.57 ± 10.93. This aligns with prior research among older Nigerian amputees aged 40 years and above, which showed elevated levels of activity limitations in this population [2, 5]. These findings indicate that advancing age, combined with amputation, tends to increase the severity of activity limitations and challenges in daily functioning. Regarding Activities of Daily Living (ADLs), the study revealed that participants encountered notable challenges, particularly in mobility-related tasks. Respondents reported some difficulty moving around within their homes (mean score: 2.07 ± 0.89) and walking outdoors (2.28 ± 0.91). More pronounced difficulty was observed in ascending and descending stairs, with a mean score of 2.69 ± 0.98. These findings align with expectations, as lower limb amputations are known to adversely affect physical functioning and overall health compared to non-amputee populations. Prior research has consistently demonstrated that amputees exhibit slower walking speeds and increased energy expenditure relative to individuals without disabilities, with approximately 60% of amputees identifying the inability to navigate uneven terrain as a significant barrier [32–34]. Furthermore, the literature indicates that amputation substantially restricts participation in a wide range of daily activities, limiting engagement in tasks formerly performed with ease [35]. The participants reported experiencing difficulties across nearly all Instrumental Activities of Daily Living (IADLs). Specifically, they indicated moderate limitations in preparing breakfast or lunch (2.24 ± 0.93), washing and ironing clothes (2.24 ± 0.94), and shopping (2.05 ± 1.18). Greater limitations were noted for preparing dinner (2.58 ± 0.92) and performing "light" household chores (2.71 ± 0.76). Notably, participants described "heavy" household tasks (3.53 ± 0.57) as nearly impossible to complete independently, often requiring assistance. These limitations can be attributed to the higher physical demands of such activities, consistent with existing literature that suggests that amputation results in a threefold reduction in functional capacity [10]. Supporting this, studies have found that major limb amputees generally experience decreased mobility, which adversely affects their ability to complete daily tasks and hampers successful reintegration into community life. Similarly, research focusing on upper limb amputees highlights how seemingly simple actions such as stabilizing a tomato to slice it or pouring water without spilling become problematic due to the loss of functional use of one hand [36, 37]. Detailed activity limitation scores for the study participants are presented in **Table 1** and **Figure 1**.

This table displays the mean values, standard deviations (SD), and score ranges reflecting the extent of activity limitations among respondents, as assessed by the Groningen Activity Restriction Scale. It includes overall limitation scores along with separate scores for Activities of Daily Living (ADLs) and Instrumental Activities of Daily Living (IADLs). Higher scores correspond to greater degrees of limitation. Participants' responses were recorded on a four-point scale, where a score of 1 denotes full independence and a score of 4 indicates total dependence. For enhanced clarity and ease of interpretation, these results are also depicted visually in **Figure 1**.

2.3 Impact of activity limitation and overall wellbeing and life satisfaction

To highlight the necessity for comprehensive rehabilitation among amputees, this study examined the influence of activity limitations on overall well-being and life

Activity category	Task description	Mean ± SD	Range (Min–Max)
Overall Score		36.57 ± 10.93	18–72
Activities of Daily Living (ADLs)			
	Dressing	1.29 ± 0.86	1–4
	Getting in and out of bed	1.61 ± 0.86	1–4
	Standing up from a chair	1.72 ± 0.96	1–4
	Washing face and hands	1.38 ± 0.78	1–4
	Washing and drying the body	1.63 ± 0.78	1–4
	Using the toilet	1.81 ± 0.84	1–4
	Feeding oneself	1.11 ± 0.46	1–4
	Moving around inside the house	2.07 ± 0.89	1–4
	Navigating stairs	2.69 ± 0.98	1–4
	Walking outdoors	2.28 ± 0.91	1–4
	Foot and toenail care	1.73 ± 1.01	1–4
Instrumental Activities of Daily Living (IADLs)			
	Preparing breakfast or lunch	2.24 ± 0.93	1–4
	Preparing dinner	2.58 ± 0.92	1–4
	Light household chores	2.71 ± 0.76	1–4
	Heavy household chores	3.53 ± 0.57	1–4
	Washing and ironing clothes	2.24 ± 0.94	1–4
	Making beds	1.96 ± 1.10	1–4
	Shopping	2.05 ± 1.18	1–4

Table 1.
Activity limitation scores of participants based on the Groningen activity restriction scale.

satisfaction. The Life Satisfaction Questionnaire-11 (LISAT-11), a tool that can be administered by either the client or the researcher, was employed to evaluate multiple dimensions of life satisfaction among participants. Responses on the LISAT-11 are rated on an ordinal scale from 1 (very dissatisfying) to 6 (very satisfying). Rather than aggregating total scores, mean domain scores were utilized to preserve the granularity of information across different life areas, which is crucial for tailored clinical interventions. The LISAT-11 was chosen due to its proven utility in delivering meaningful quality of life data for both clinical assessment and research contexts [38]. In the current sample, respondents reported a moderate overall life satisfaction, with a mean score of 3.86 ± 1.15. This aligns with findings from a Portuguese study where amputees similarly expressed moderate satisfaction with life, although it contrasts with Pereira et al.'s research, which documented lower levels of life satisfaction among amputees [39, 40]. Participants in this study generally expressed moderate contentment in domains such as self-care, partner relationships, physical health, and

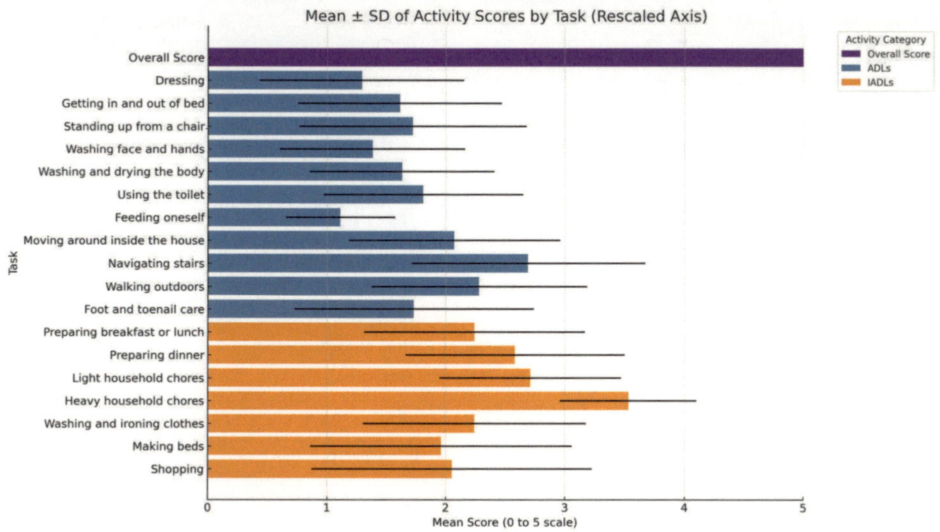

Figure 1.
Showing graphical presentation of activity limitation scores using the Groningen activity restriction scale.

family life. These results may reflect the consistent caregiving support many received from family members, which likely facilitates daily self-care activities. Additionally, satisfaction with physical health could be attributed to ongoing rehabilitation services provided at the facility, including medical treatment, physical and occupational therapy, and access to assistive devices such as orthotics, prosthetics, and wheelchairs, along with training in their use. The moderate satisfaction levels related to partner relationships and family life correspond with findings by Geertzen and Dijkstra, who noted that lower limb amputation can hinder marital and sexual expression between partners [11]. Conversely, participants expressed dissatisfaction with their vocational status, sexual life, financial situation, and psychological health. This pattern may indicate that the rehabilitation programs, while effective in addressing physical impairments, insufficiently target economic, emotional, and psychological challenges faced by amputees. This observation supports previous studies reporting psychological distress and employment loss following amputation [11, 41]. Moreover, lifestyle disruptions and compromised income sources due to disability have been documented, emphasizing the broader socio-economic impacts of limb loss [41]. The financial burden of amputation on individuals and healthcare systems has also been well recognized [42, 43]. Regarding sexual well-being, these findings concur with Williamson and Walters, who described difficulties amputees may face in achieving desired sexual positions, which may affect intimacy. Research further suggests that individuals with physical disabilities frequently encounter challenges in forming and sustaining intimate and romantic relationships [1, 44]. A summary of participants' life satisfaction scores is provided in **Table 2**.

To assess the direct influence of activity limitations on life satisfaction, the study employed logistic regression and correlation analyses. A multivariate regression model was utilized to examine the relationship while controlling potential confounding variables. The analysis revealed a strong, statistically significant negative association between activity limitations and life satisfaction ($ß = -0.13$, $p = 0.000$), indicating that greater activity limitations correspond to lower life satisfaction levels.

Life domain	Mean ± SD	Range (Min–Max)
Overall Life Satisfaction (Life as a whole)	3.86 ± 1.15	1–6
Vocational Situation	2.87 ± 0.96	1–6
Financial Situation	3.31 ± 1.06	1–6
Leisure Activities	3.31 ± 1.03	1–6
Social Contacts (Friends & Acquaintances)	3.57 ± 0.98	1–6
Sexual Life	2.87 ± 1.11	1–6
Ability to Manage Self-Care	3.75 ± 0.90	1–6
Family Life	4.21 ± 1.00	1–6
Partnership Relations	3.76 ± 1.47	1–6
Physical Health	3.74 ± 0.94	1–6
Psychological Health	2.97 ± 1.09	1–6
Overall LISAT-11 Score	38.22 ± 6.82	23–61

Table 2.
Satisfaction with life scores among respondents based on LISAT-11.

These results underscore the substantial impact that functional impairments have on the overall well-being of amputees. A detailed summary of these findings is presented in **Table 3**.

These findings indicate that increased difficulties in performing Activities of Daily Living (ADLs), and Instrumental Activities of Daily Living (IADLs) are associated with lower satisfaction across various aspects of life. In other words, activity limitations serve as significant predictors of life satisfaction levels. Supporting this, previous research has demonstrated a notable positive correlation between life satisfaction and health-related domains, including physical functioning among amputees [39]. Conversely, some studies focusing on older adults with physical disabilities, including amputees, have reported no statistically significant link between activity restrictions and life satisfaction. Nevertheless, evidence suggests that individuals experiencing greater mobility impairments tend to report diminished life satisfaction. Research specifically addressing amputees also highlights that mobility challenges can contribute to reduced overall life satisfaction, emphasizing the critical role of early rehabilitation interventions [40, 45, 46].

2.4 Addressing activity limitation through rehabilitation among amputees

Losing a limb significantly affects an individual's mobility and their capacity to carry out daily activities, which in turn hampers social participation, community integration, and overall quality of life. The primary aim of post-amputation rehabilitation is to equip the person with the skills needed to walk effectively, regain functional independence, and reintegrate socially. A major challenge faced by many amputees is the lack of adequate rehabilitation services and consistent follow-up care [29]. Ideally, rehabilitation and comprehensive management should commence prior to amputation and be delivered by a multidisciplinary team specialized in amputee care. Through a holistic and multidisciplinary approach, the rehabilitation process comprises several stages of varying length: preoperative phase; pre-prosthetic phase; and, if likely, prosthetic training [25–27]. Post amputation rehabilitation and management is a team

Variable	N	Univariate analysis			Multivariate analysis		
		Crude ß	95% CI	p-value	Adjusted ß	95% CI	p-value
Age (years)							
18–30	28	Ref.					
31–40	49	−2.45	−5.1-0.61	0.116	−2.66	−5.43-0.11	0.06
41–50	45	1.05	−2.05-4.17	0.505	−0.32	−3.22-2.57	0.825
51–60	47	−1.12	−4.21-1.96	0.473	−3.32	−6.26-(−0.37)	**0.027***
60+	31	−5.39	−8.7-(−2.02)	**0.002***	−5.37	−8.84-(1.92)	**0.003***
Sex							
Male	107	Ref.					
Female	93	.72	−1.19-2.63	0.456			
Marital status							
Single or divorced	82	Ref.					
Married	102	4.18	2.28–6.1	**0.000***	4.82	2.99–6.66	**0.000***
Widow or widower	16	−0.09	−3.60-3.43	0.962	1.9	−1.54-5.52	0.268
Education							
No formal Edu.	25	Ref.					
basic	48	2.91	−0.38-6.20	0.083			
Second cycle	78	0.34	−2.72-3.41	0.828			
Tertiary	49	2.22	−1.06-5.50	0.183			
Employment							
Employed	107	Ref.					
Unemployed	93	−2.33	−4.21-(−0.45)	**0.016***	−0.33	−2.25-1.59	0.735
Religion							
Christian	141	Ref.					
Muslim	45	−2.22	−4.50-0.06	0.056			
Others	14	−3.34	−7.18-0.27	0.069			
Amputation Location							
Upper Limb Amputation	26	Ref.					
Lower Limb Amputation	174	0.11	−2.72-2.95	0.08			
Form							
Unilateral	179	Ref.					
Bilateral	21	−8.91	−11.76-(−6.06)	**0.000***	−5.97	−9.05-(−2.90)	**0.000***

Variable	N	Univariate analysis			Multivariate analysis		
		Crude ß	95% CI	p-value	Adjusted ß	95% CI	p-value
Groningen score							
Activity limitation	200	−0.21	−0.29-(−0.13)	**0.000***	−0.13	−0.211-(−0.04)	**0.003***

Table 3.
Linear regression models (crude and adjusted) assessing the impact of activity limitation on life satisfaction with adjustment for confounders.

approach with a physician, occupational therapist, physiotherapist, prosthetist, social worker to prevent complications, method of walking with a prosthesis, application, removal, and pressure sores, etc. [29]. Mahesh and Yochitha also reported that with good rehabilitation methods patients can be managed effectively with prosthetic limbs [29]. The treatment team must consider the patient's physical and medical status, level of amputation, premorbid lifestyle, and cognition in providing this service, and will help the patient establish convincing short and long-term goals [25]. There is often a loss of economic power of the individual and his/her independence when they are not satisfactorily rehabilitated and integrated back into society [12], hence a multi-disciplinary team approach to rehabilitation and management offer the most effective means for effective re-integration of the patient with an amputated limb to their earlier lifestyle. The concern of rehabilitation specialists has long been the alterations and fluctuations that result from injury. To date, the restoration of mobility through proper shaping of the residuum, gait training, and proper selection and fit of prosthetic components of individuals with amputations have been the focus of rehabilitation [4]. Researchers have reported that psychological responses to amputation depend on several factors, which comprise expectations from the rehabilitation program [47–49]. There is a significant reduction in anxiety and depression scores following rehabilitation outcome in above-knee amputation than below-knee amputation [50]. The process of rehabilitation should be initiated before surgery, and post-operative rehabilitation should commence as soon as medically feasible to improve outcomes wherever possible among amputees [12]. In terms of outcomes, rehabilitation has been established to be better in amputees who had trauma as the cause of their amputations than those from disease [30]. Using functional independent measures to evaluate patients during rehabilitation in all the patients was reported to be good [12], but women were seen to be rehabilitated better and faster than men [51]. Furthermore, younger age group amputees responded better to rehabilitation than the elderly [12]. The rehabilitation provided can vary between individuals, but a core role is to provide training on the use of a prosthetic limb [52]. A prosthetic limb enables individuals with an amputation to engage in meaningful activities that may be too difficult to complete with their other limb [53] and it provides the ability for those with an amputation to prevent injury [37]. There is a protocol for providing training to individuals with an amputation of the upper limb that focuses on prosthetic use and describes characteristics of a successful training protocol for rehabilitation [52]. Interventions during rehabilitation aim to enhance a client's occupational performance; that is, the performance of everyday tasks and routines in real-world contexts to a level that is effective and satisfying [54]. In summary, rehabilitation for amputees involves a multidisciplinary approach aimed at restoring mobility, independence, and quality of life. Early interventions focus on wound healing, pain management including phantom limb pain, and psychological support to address emotional adjustment [54]. Physical therapy begins soon after surgery to maintain strength, flexibility, and balance in the residual limb and remaining body. Key strategies include the use of assistive devices, gait training, and desensitization techniques [55]. Occupational therapy helps patients relearn daily activities using adaptive methods or tools. Prosthetic training is a central component, involving custom fitting, functional use, and ongoing adjustments [54]. Mirror therapy and virtual reality are emerging techniques to reduce phantom pain and improve motor control. Peer support and vocational rehabilitation also play important roles in long-term adjustment. Overall, individualized, goal-oriented care is essential to maximize functional outcomes for amputees [53].

3. Conclusions

Amputation significantly affects both activity limitations and overall life satisfaction. Participants reported infrequent engagement in activities of daily living (ADLs) and instrumental activities of daily living (IADLs), especially those involving mobility and household tasks such as preparing meals. While they were able to perform these activities, it was often with difficulty and functional limitations, particularly in mobility-related ADLs and most IADLs. These challenges are largely due to the physical effort and energy demands associated with these tasks. Overall, respondents rated their life satisfaction as moderate, suggesting some positive outcomes from their ongoing rehabilitation. However, notable dissatisfaction was reported in areas such as vocational engagement, sexual activity, financial stability, and psychological well-being. In contrast, greater satisfaction was expressed regarding family life, partner relationships, and physical health. These disparities highlight how financial strain, difficulty returning to work, and challenges in intimate relationships can adversely impact psychological health. Activity limitation emerged as a key predictor of life satisfaction. Greater limitations in performing ADLs and IADLs were associated with lower levels of satisfaction. Therefore, effective rehabilitation plays a critical role in improving outcomes for amputees. The primary goal of post-amputation rehabilitation is to enable independent mobility, enhance functional ability, and support social reintegration. Ideally, rehabilitation should begin preceding the surgical procedure and be delivered by a specialized, multidisciplinary team. This team-based approach typically involves several phases: preoperative, pre-prosthetic, and prosthetic training if applicable. Core team members may include physicians, occupational therapists, physiotherapists, prosthetists, and social workers. A comprehensive plan must consider the individual's medical status, level of amputation, cognitive function, and pre-amputation lifestyle to establish realistic short- and long-term rehabilitation goals.

Acknowledgements

I wish to sincerely thank my supervisors, Mr. Isaac Owusu and Dr. Enoch Acheampong, for their invaluable guidance, unwavering support, and encouragement throughout this project. Their insightful feedback, constructive criticism, and dedication to high standards have significantly enhanced both my research and personal growth. Mr. Owusu's practical expertise and meticulous attention to detail, coupled with Dr. Acheampong's scholarly mentorship and rigor, created an ideal combination that shaped this work into its present form. I am deeply appreciative of their time, patience, and commitment. Additionally, I extend my gratitude to all the individuals and organizations who contributed their support during this journey. This accomplishment would not have been possible without your assistance.

Conflict of interest

The author hereby declares that there are no conflicts of interest related to this work.

Author details

Peter Bredu-Darkwa
School of Allied Health Professions and Midwifery, University of Bradford, Bradford, United-Kingdom

*Address all correspondence to: p.bredu-darkwa@bradford.ac.uk

References

[1] Williamson GM, Walters AS. Perceived impact of limb amputation on sexual activity: A study of adult amputees. Journal of Sex Research. 2010;**33**(3):221-230

[2] Bello B, Abdullahhi N, Abdulrahaman MA. Influence of socio-demographic characteristics on activity limitation, participation restriction and quality of life among amputees in Kano, Nigeria. Nigerian Journal of Physiotherapy and Rehabilitation. 2020;**1**:1

[3] Ziegler-Graham K, MacKenzie EJ, Epraim PL, Travison TG, Brookmeyer R. Estimating the prevalenmce of limb loss in the United States:2005 to 2050. Archives of Physical Medicine Rehabilitation. 2008;**89**(3):422-429

[4] Wetterhahn KA, Hanson C, Levy CE. Effect of participation in physical activity on body image of amputees. American Journal of Physical and Medical Rehabilitation. 2002;**81**:194-201

[5] Burger H, Marinček C. Return to work after lower limb amputation. Disability and Rehabilitation. 2007;**29**:17, 1323-1329. DOI: 10.1080/09638280701320797

[6] McLarney M, Pezzin LE, McGinley EL, Prosser L, Dillingham TR. The prevalence of lower limb loss in children and associated costs of prosthetic devices: A national study of commercial insurance claims. Prosthetics and Orthotics International. 2021;**45**(2):115-122

[7] Kohler F, Cieza A, Stucki G, Geertzen J, Burger H. Developing core sets for persons following amputation based on the international classification of functioning, disability and health as a way to specify functioning. Prosthetics and Orthotics International. 2009;**33**(2):117-129

[8] Wald J, Alvaro R. Psychological factors in work related amputation: Considerations for rehabilitation counselors. Journal of Rehabilitation. 2004;**70**(4):6-15

[9] Condie ME, Scott H, Crosse O. A survey of the lower limb amputee population in Scotland. In: Report Published by ReTIS: 2007. Glasgow, UK: University of Strathclyde; 2005

[10] Razak MMA, Tauhid MZ, Yasin NF, Hanapiah FA. Quality of life among lower limb amputees in Malaysia. Procedia - Social and Behavioral Sciences. 2016;**2016**(222):450-457

[11] Geertzen JHB, Van Es CG, Dijkstra PU. Sexuality and amputation: A systematic literature review. Disability and Rehabilitation. 2009;**31**(7):522-527

[12] Yilleng S, Dapap D. Evaluation of early psychological symptoms of major limb amputation in a tertiary hospital. Journal of BioMedical Research and Clinical Practice. 2020;**3**(3):389-395

[13] Fitzsimmons A. Mobility after amputation. Mobility Management. 2011

[14] Day A. Mortality rate and predictive factors in patients who undergo lower-limb amputations while hospitalized for other reasons [doctoral dissertation]. Vol. 165. TUI University; 2011

[15] Hamilton IS. An Intro to Gerontology, Ageing and Managing co-Morbidity and Disability. New York: Cambridge University Press; 2012. p. 94

[16] Pousada GT, Groba GB, Nieto RL, Pereira LJ. Exploring the psychosocial impact of wheelchair and contextual factors on quality of life of people with neuromuscular disorders. Assistive Technology. 2015;**27**:246-256

[17] Cahn-Weiner DA, Faris ST. Cognitive and neuroimaging predictors of instrumental activities of daily living. Journal of the International Neuropsychological Society. 2007;**18**:1-11

[18] Hoshino J, Ubara Y, Ohara K, Ohta E. Changes in the activities of daily living (ADL) in relation to the level of amputation of patients undergoing lower extremity amputation for arteriosclerosis obliterans (ASO). Circulation Journal. 2008;**72**:1495-1498

[19] Zunzunegui MV, Nunez O, Durban M, de Yébenes MJ, Otero Á. Decreasing prevalence of disability in activities of daily living, functional limitations and poor self-rated health: A 6-year follow-up study in Spain. Aging Clinical and Experimental Research. 2006;**18**(5):352-358

[20] Senra H, Oliveira RA, Leal I, Vieira C. Beyond the body image: A qualitative study on how adults experience lower limb amputation. Clinical Rehabilitation. Feb 2012;**26**(2):180-191

[21] Wang R, Zhang T, Langhammer B. Activities of daily living and life satisfaction of persons with stroke after rehabilitation in China: A longitudinal descriptive study. Topics in Stroke Rehabilitation. 2019;**26**(2):113-121

[22] Addabbo T, Sarti E, Sciulli D. Disability and life satisfaction in Italy. Applied Research in Quality of Life. 2015;**11**(3):925-954

[23] Kidmas AT, Nwadiaro CH, Igun GO. Lower limb amputation in Jos, Nigeria. East African Medical Journal. 2004;**81**(427):429

[24] Teichmann J, Sabo D. Epidemiology and classification of diabetic foot syndrome. Orthopade. 2009;**38**:1139-1148

[25] Esquenazi A, DiGiacomo R. Rehabilitation after amputation. Journal of the American Podiatric Medical Association. 2001;**91**(1):13-22

[26] Belussi L, Danza L. Method for the prediction of malfunctions of buildings through real energy consumption analysis: Holistic and multidisciplinary approach of energy signature. Energy and Buildings. 2012;**55**:715-720

[27] De-Rosende Celeiro I, Simon Sanjuan L, Santos-del-Riego S. Activities of daily living in people with lower limb amputation: Outcomes of an intervention to reduce dependence in pre-prosthetic phase. Disability and Rehabilitation. 2017;**39**(18):1799-1806

[28] Matsen SL, Malchow D, Matsen FA. Correlations with patients' perspectives of the result of lower-extremity amputation, 3rd. The Journal of Bone and Joint Surgery. American Volume. 2000;**82-A**(8):1089-1095

[29] Mahesh CH, Yochitha B. A clinical study on lower limb amputations. International Journal of Surgery Science. 2019;**3**(4):514-516

[30] Karmarkar AM, Graham JE, Reistetter TA, Kumar A, Mix JM, Niewczyk P, et al. Association between functional severity and amputation type with rehabilitation outcomes in patients with lower limb amputation. Rehabilitation Research and Practice. 2014;**1**:961798

[31] Suurmeijer TP, Doeglas DM, Moum T. Northern Centre for Health Care Research, University of Groningen, Netherlands. The Groningen activity restriction scale for measuring disability: it's utility in international comparisons. American Journal of Public Health. 1994;**84**(8):1270-1273

[32] Paysant J. Influence of terrain on metabolic and temporal gait characteristics of unilateral transtibial amputees. The Journal of Rehabilitation Research and Development. 2006;**43**(2):153

[33] Gates DH. Gait characteristics of individuals with transtibial amputations walking on a destabilizing rock surface. Gait & Posture. 2012;**36**(1):33-39

[34] Hagberg K, Branemark R. Consequences of non-vascular trans-femoral amputation: A survey of quality of life, prosthetic use and problems. Prosthetics and Orthotics International. 2001;**25**:186-194

[35] Kakooza SM, Nanyunja Z, Muwonge K, Kiyingi FP. The psychologıcal correlates of traumatic experıences and coping strategies of post amputation: A case study of Mulago Specıalızed Natıonal Hospıtal, Kampala-Uganda. Student's Journal of Health Research Africa. 2020;**1**(12):18-18. DOI: 10.51168/sjhrafrica.v1i11.9

[36] Cox PS, SKP W, Weaver SR. Life after lower extremity amputation in diabetics. West Indian Medical Journal. 2011:536-540

[37] Sproats M, Ranka J, Nott M. Addressing cognitive load in upper limb prosthetic training using perceive, recall, plan & perform (PRPP) intervention; a critical case study. Australian Occupational Therapy Journal. 2013;**60**(Supp 1):89

[38] Fugl-Meyer AR, Branholm IB, Fugl-Meyer KS. Life satisfaction in 18- to 64-year-old swedes: Concerning gender, age, partner, and immigrant status. Journal of Rehabilitation Medicine. 2002;**34**:239-246

[39] Dias MA. Health related quality of life and satisfaction with life: A study in patients with a lower limb amputation. In: Faculdade de Ci^encias do Desporto e de Educac ~ao Fısica da Universidade do Porto. Portugal: Faculty of Sport Sciences and Physical Education of the University of Porto; 2006

[40] Pereira MG, Ramos C, Lobarinhas A, Machado JC, Pedras S. Satisfaction with life in individuals with a lower limb amputation: The importance of active coping and acceptance. Scandinavian Journal of Psychology. 2018;**59**:414-421

[41] Mugo NN. The effect of amputation on body image and well-being: A systematic review. Available from: https://urn.fi/URN:NBN:fi:amk-201103283622

[42] Jindeel A, Narahara KA. Nontraumatic amputation: Incidence and cost analysis. The International Journal of Lower Extremity Wounds. 2012;**11**(3):177-179

[43] Joret MO, Dean A, Cao C, Stewart J, Bhamidipaty V. The financial burden of surgical and endovascular treatment of diabetic foot wounds. Journal of Vascular Surgery. 2016;**64**(3):648-655

[44] Taleporos G, McCabe MP. Physical disability and sexual esteem. Sexuality and Disability. 2001;**19**(2):131-148

[45] Jörgensen S, Iwarsson S, Lexell J. Secondary health conditions, activity limitations and life satisfaction in older adults with long-term spinal cord injury. PM. 2017;**9**(4):356-366

[46] Blace NP. Functional ability, participation in activities and life satisfaction of the older people. Asian Social Science. 2012;**8**:75-87

[47] Ghous M. Depression: Prevalence among amputees. Professional Medical Journal. 2015;**22**(2):263-266

[48] Manoj K, Dasika S. Assessment of anxiety and depression in patients who underwent amputation. Scholars Journal of Applied Medical Sciences. 2017;**5**(10A):3829-3835

[49] Ali Z, Khurshid L, Bhat T, Bhat AA, Vakil SM. Prevalence of psychiatric illnesses after major limb amputation and early recognition and treatment in economically lower income group patients. International Journal of Research in Orthopaedics. 2028;**4**:892-897

[50] Jane W, Tik SC, Greg B. Functional outcome of major limb amputation: A modern series. Journal of Prosthetics and Orthotics. 2010;**23**(30):152-156

[51] Smurr LM, Gulick K, Yancosek K, Ganz O. Managing the upper extremity amputee: A protocol for success. Journal of Hand Therapy. 2008;**21**(2):160-175

[52] Crepeau E, Cohn E, Schell BB. Willard and Spackman's Occupational Therapy. 10th ed. 2003. pp. 796-806

[53] Chapparo C, Ranka J. Occupation analysis: Cognition and acquired brain impairment. Occupation Analysis in Practice. 2011;**25**:147-162

[54] Keenan D. Upper limb amputations. In: Pendleton HM, Schultz-Krohn W, editors. Pedretti's Occupational Therapy: Practice Skills for Physical Dysfunction. 7th ed. St Louis, MO: Elsevier Health Sciences; 2011. pp. 1155-1183

[55] Mosby. Mosby's Field Guide to Occupational Therapy for Physical Dysfunction. Elsevier/Mosby; 2013

Chapter 11

Assessment and Therapy of Speech Sound Disorders Associated with Cleft Palate Using Electropalatography

Ichiro Yamamoto and Yuri Fujiwara

Abstract

Electropalatography (EPG) is a device that records and displays in real time the tongue and hard palate contact dynamics during speech. The clinical application of EPG has been underway since the 1970s. There have been many studies concerning assessment of speech sound disorders. Visual feedback training with EPG has been found to be effective in treating speech sound disorders. The authors have introduced the clinical use of EPG for the clients with cleft palate since 2004. EPG assessment has identified a variety of spatial distortions such as excessive, and more posterior tongue-palate contact or no contact for oral consonants in speakers with cleft palate. For these clients, EPG therapy was effective to become aware of their tongue movements. A synchronization system between EPG and endoscopy has also been introduced and is being used to discuss treatment strategies for difficult-to-cure cases. This chapter reviews how the authors have utilized EPG in their clinical practice in Japan. The significance of clinical use of EPG, including telepractice, is to be discussed.

Keywords: electropalatography, speech sound disorders, cleft palate, assessment, visual feedback therapy, telepractice

1. Introduction

Speech abnormalities associated with cleft palate include resonance, nasal airflow, and sound production errors [1]. Resonance and nasal airflow can be corrected with surgery or with speech aids to improve nasopharyngeal closure, but sound production errors cannot be corrected without articulation training. Sound production errors associated with cleft palate are called "cleft speech characteristics: CSCs" [2, 3]. John et al. [2] developed the cleft audit protocol for speech-augmented (CAPS-A) as an assessment tool for use in intercenter audit studies of cleft speech. Based on the CAPS-A, the Japanese speech outcome tool (CAPS-A-JP) was developed [4].

CAPS-A classifies CSCs as anterior oral, posterior oral, non-oral, and passive errors, while CAPS-A-JP classifies them into three groups: oral, non-oral, and passive errors. Oral CSCs include inter-dentalization, lateral misarticulation, palatal/

palatalization, double articulation (intraoral), posterior palatal or velarization with a raised tongue body, and backed to velar/uvula. Non-oral CSCs include active nasal/nasopharyngeal misarticulation, pharyngeal articulation, glottal articulation, and double articulation (oral and non-oral). Passive CSCs include weak pressure consonants and nasalized or nasal realization of pressure consonants. These sound production errors are basically assessed auditory. However, auditory assessments are subjective and may not agree among raters. The evaluation by electropalatography (EPG) provides objective support for auditory assessments.

2. Electropalatographic observation of cleft palate speech

2.1 Equipments

Electropalatography (EPG) is a tool that provides information on the location and timing of the tongue's contact with the hard palate during speech [5]. EPG requires that clients wear a custom-made artificial plate fit to their own palate. The EPG plate is embedded with 62 electrodes according to the anatomical landmarks and the wires from each electrode exit around the back of the rear molars to the corner of the mouth. The wires are connected to an EPG system, which shows real-time visual feedback of the tongue-palate contacts during speech. As synchronized recordings of the tongue-palate contact pattern and speech sounds are made, it is possible to analyze sound waves, sound spectrograms, and EPG patterns in synchronization. The authors started the clinical use of EPG in 2004. Initially, the Win-EPG system (Articulate Instruments Ltd., Edinburgh, UK) was imported and an artificial plate for each client was ordered to a dental technician's office in Edinburgh. However, this was time consuming and too expensive.

In order to reduce the time and cost, the authors have developed an artificial plate for EPG (McYam Plate; The EPG Research Center, Nishinomiya, Japan) [6]. McYam plate was created based on the same concept as the Reading type artificial plate. It is made of approved dental materials, embedded with 62 electrodes 1.4x 0.7 mm in size. The electrodes are arranged on the plate according to the same anatomical landmarks and special regulations as the Reading type plate; thus, data obtained using McYam plate can be compared with those recorded using the Reading plate. It is also possible to make inter-client comparisons of the EPG data. The cost was reduced to half by reducing the time required to create the EPG plate, by using thermoplastic vacuum resin instead of acrylic resin base plate and creation of a module with 4 electrodes of 12 different electrode widths.

A new EPG system (WinSTARS; Asahi Roentgen, Ltd., Kyoto, Japan) was developed as a Speech Training Aid and Recording System and patented in 2015 (Patent No. 5843894). The tongue-palate contact signal is transferred to a multiplexer through enamel wires and then by Bluetooth to a tablet-type personal computer. As there are no cables connecting the computer and multiplexer, client movement is not obstructed and a medical isolation transformer, which was necessary for WinEPG, is not required for clinical use of the plate (**Figure 1**). It is very convenient to operate and can be used at any place as needed. For EPG training, real-time visual feedback and delayed feedback are available. A model EPG pattern for a target sound can be displayed as necessary. The EPG recording setting is 100 Hz, and the audio settings are 22,050 Hz, 16 bits, and Mono. Video recording of the face is also possible, using a built-in web camera. When a client reads or names the prompted words or pictures

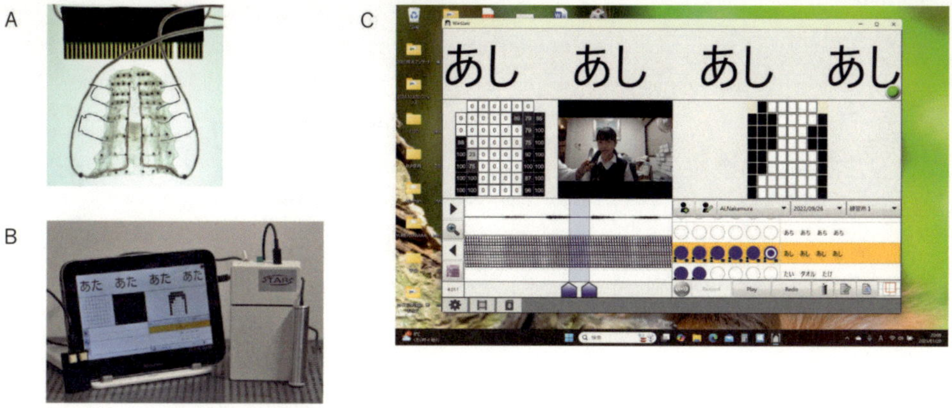

Figure 1.
EPG equipment. A: EPG artificial plate (McYam Plate) B: EPG system (WinSTARS). C: Screenshot of WinSTARS.

on the screen, his/her face is automatically recorded without the client's awareness (**Figure 1**). Data recording is so easy that even a client can do independently, which enables them to practice and make records at their home. In 2021, EPG and nasopharyngoscopy synchronization system was developed to see the relationship between nasopharyngeal closure function and articulation by replacing the face recording screen with a nasopharyngoscopy screen.

2.2 Typical tongue-palate contact patterns for Japanese alveolar and post-alveolar sounds

Visual feedback training with EPG requires a target pattern for each sound. There are several reports of typical adult EPG patterns for English lingual phoneme targets [5]. McLeod and Singh [7] presented comprehensive coverage of EPG patterns for typical English speakers. However, EPG patterns for Japanese phoneme are limited. Imai, Wakumoto, and Niu [8] reported the EPG patterns for only three sounds [ta], [sa], and [ɾa], using Dynamic Palatograph (DP-20, Rion Co., Ltd., Tokyo, Japan). The EPG artificial plate they used was made from a set of standard templates to fit the individual's palate. Therefore, the number of electrodes varied with each subject; furthermore, each electrode was placed at a different point within the hard palate. This made it difficult to compare lingual contact patterns among subjects and is probably a reason why there are limited EPG data regarding typical tongue/palate contact for Japanese sounds. Mochizuki, Yamagata, and Tokutomi [9] used the thin film type of palatography sensor, which has 96 electrode arrays covering the palate and maxillary teeth. Japanese consonants [s, t, n, ɾ, ʃ, k] in a short sentence were analyzed. The contact pattern of each sound was shown as the common contact area for 18 subjects. Although the number of consonants analyzed was greater than that of Imai et al. [8], EPG patterns of consonants were extracted during a short sentence reading, and the number of electrodes was different, making it difficult to use them as targets in our clinical practice with the Reading type McYam plate.

To create a targeted EPG pattern for visual feedback training, cumulative templates were generated from EPG data of 15 typical Japanese-speaking adults [10]. Nine alveolar and alveopalatal sounds [t, d, n, s, ɕ, ts, dz., tɕ, dʑ], which are often practiced, were recorded in vowel-consonant-vowel syllables, such as [ata], and

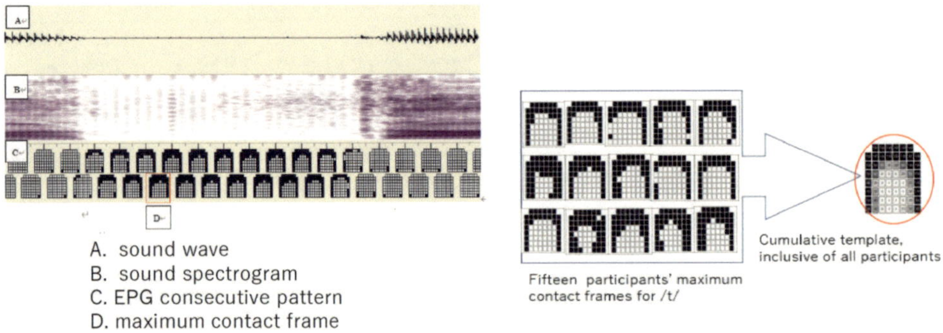

Figure 2.
The cumulative maximum contact frames of /t/ for 15 examples of typical Japanese speakers.

cumulative templates were generated from the maximum contact frame for each sound (**Figure 2**). EPG patterns varied from individual to individual, but the approximate patterns were consistent. The cumulative pattern of 15 individuals was considered a suitable target for visual feedback training (**Figure 3**).

However, it was questionable whether these target patterns are appropriate for clients with repaired cleft palate, as their dentopalatal morphology is different from that of normal subjects without cleft palate. To verify this question, cumulative EPG patterns were generated from data of 15 clients with repaired unilateral cleft lip and palate whose speech was perceptually adequate [11]. Although there was higher

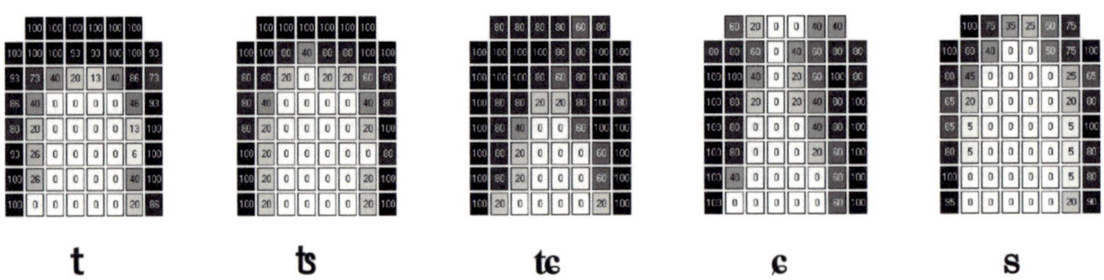

Figure 3.
Target patterns for Japanese sounds.

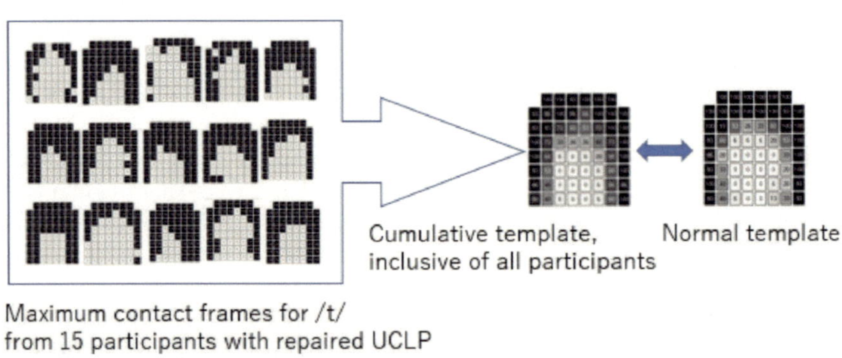

Figure 4.
Cumulative maximum contact frames of 15 post-operative cleft palate cases.

variability in tongue-palate contact patterns, the generated EPG patterns for each sound were largely similar to those of subjects without cleft palate (**Figure 4**).

2.3 EPG analysis of cleft speech characteristics

In this section, Cleft Speech Characteristics (CSCs) are analyzed using EPG. EPG videos (audio-visual information) are attached in appendices.

2.3.1 Lateral misarticulation

Tongue makes broad contact with the palate and does not form a midline groove for exhalation. Thus, airflow comes out from the side of the mouth and causes frictional noise. In Japanese, this misarticulation often occurs in high-front vowel [i] and syllables, such as [ɾʲi, nʲi, çi, tɕi, dʑi, kʲi, gʲi] (**Figure 5**) (Video 1 https://bit.ly/3Rocphb).

2.3.2 Palatal/palatalization

During alveolar sound production, the extensively raised tongue body makes contact with the anterior part of the hard palate (**Figure 6**) (Video 2 https://bit.ly/3Rocphb). Audibly, [ta] sounds like [tʲa].

2.3.3 Posterior palatal or velarization with a raised tongue body

During alveolar sound production, the tongue contact extends from the posterior part of the hard palate to the soft palate (**Figure 7**) (Video 3 https://bit.ly/3Rocphb). Alveolar sounds are distorted close to velar sounds.

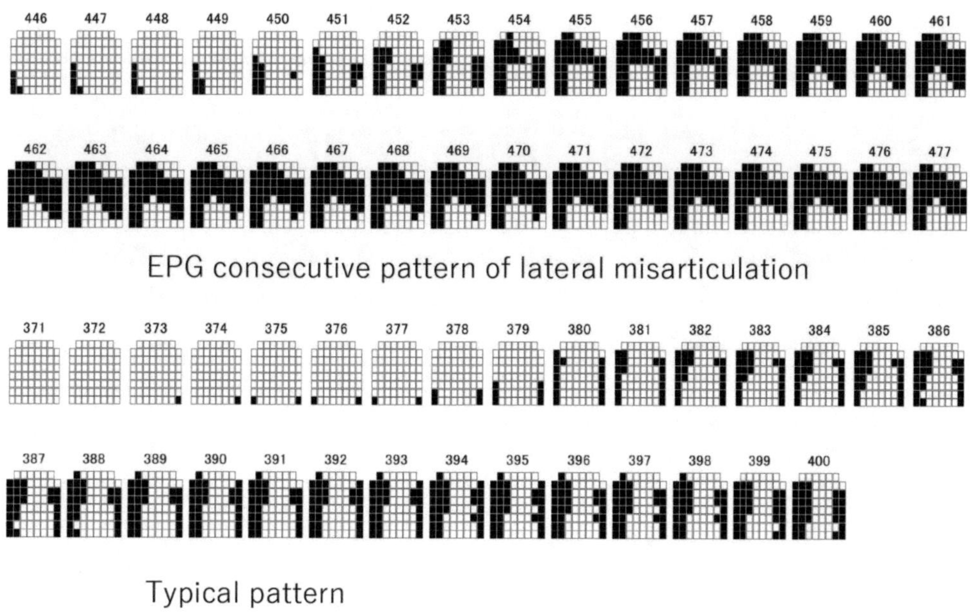

Figure 5.
Lateral misarticulation: [çi].

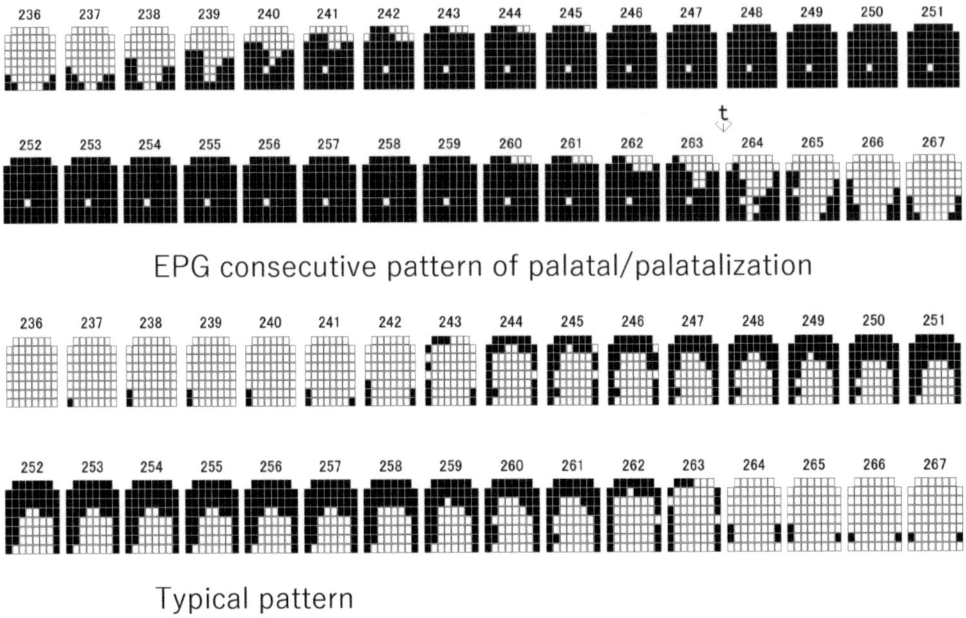

Figure 6.
Palatal/palatalization with raised tongue body: [ta].

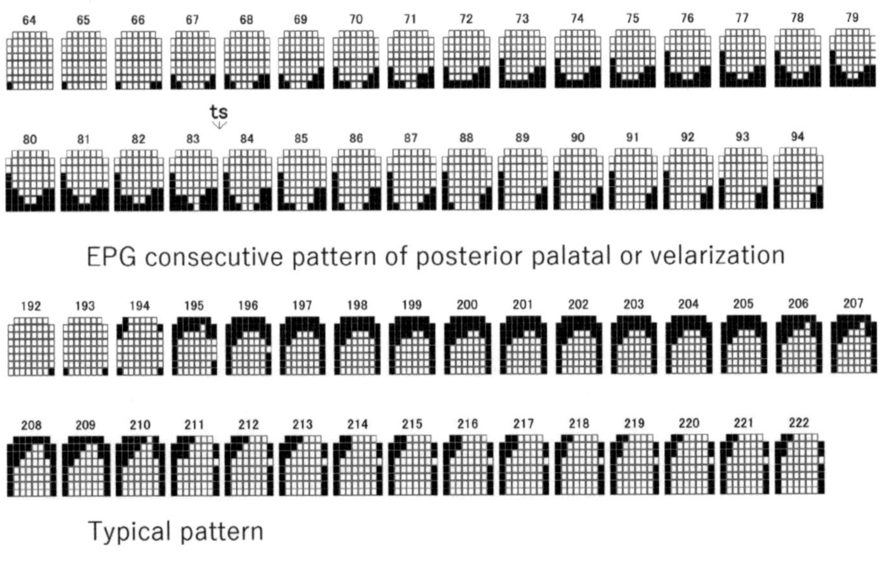

Figure 7.
Posterior palatal or velarization with a raised tongue body: [tsu].

2.3.4 Active nasal/nasopharyngeal misarticulation

This sound is mainly observed as a substitution of the consonants [s], [ts], and [dz] and syllables with the high-front vowel [i] and high-back vowel [u]. The tongue completely contacts the palate and prevents exhalation from the oral cavity, so the airflow is released from the nasal cavity through the nasopharynx (**Figure 8**) (Video 4 https://bit.ly/3Rocphb).

DOI: http://dx.doi.org/10.5772/intechopen.1010001

2.3.5 Double articulation (intraoral)

Double contact of the tongue with the alveolar area and hard palate, etc. It sounds neither [ta] nor [ka] (**Figure 9**) (Video 5 https://bit.ly/3Rocphb).

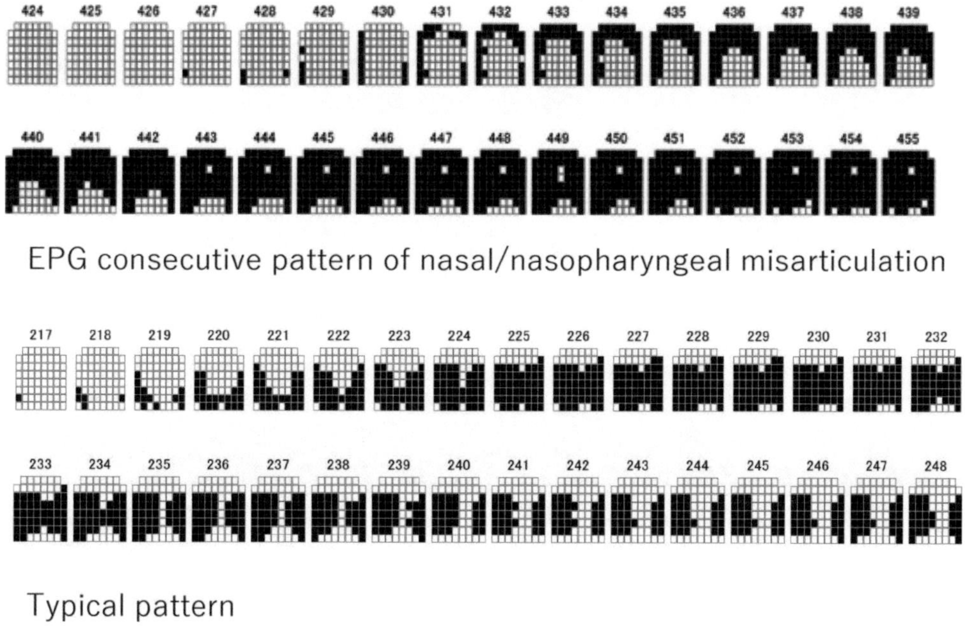

Figure 8.
Nasal/nasopharyngeal misarticulation: [çi].

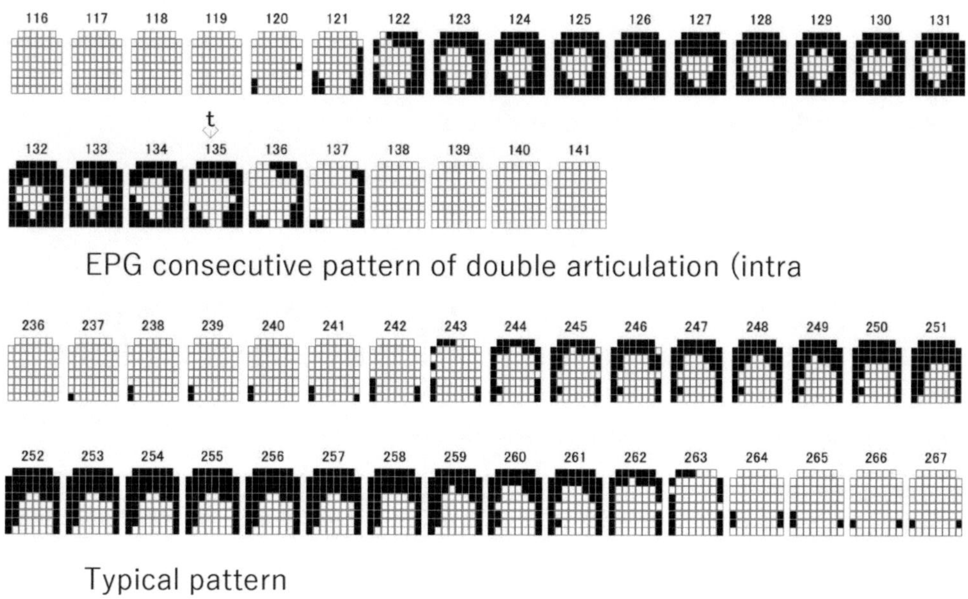

Figure 9.
Double articulation (intra-oral): [ata].

2.3.6 Pharyngeal articulation

Fricatives and affricatives originally produced in the oral cavity are produced in the pharynx. The oral cavity does not form a groove for the production of fricative sounds (**Figure 10**) (Video 6 https://bit.ly/3Rocphb).

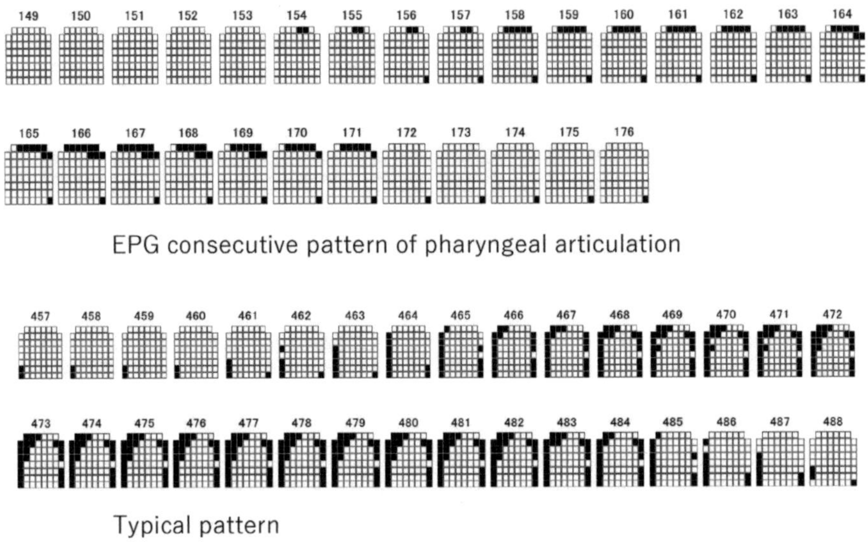

Figure 10.
Pharyngeal articulation: [sa].

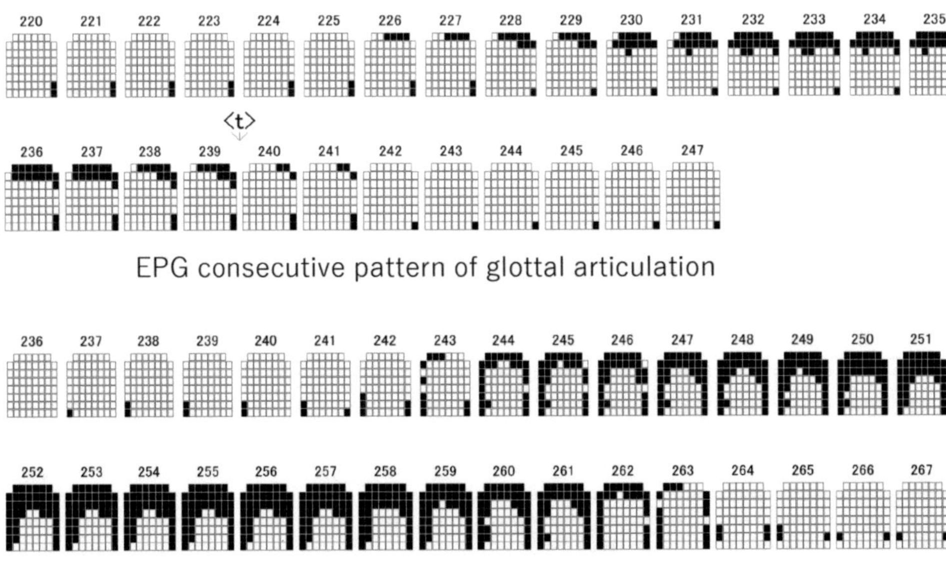

Figure 11.
Glottal articulation: [ta].

2.3.7 Glottal articulation

It is produced when the glottis is tightly closed and expiration is released in a single stroke. It is used compensatory when nasopharyngeal closure dysfunction makes it difficult to produce high-pressure consonants; plosives, fricatives, and affricatives. The oral cavity does not show the contact necessary for the production of each sound (**Figure 11**) (Video 7 https://bit.ly/3Rocphb).

3. Visual feedback therapy using EPG

Visual feedback training using EPG has been used in speech therapy in the last three decades. Compared with conventional speech therapy, it is reported that fewer therapy sessions are needed to achieve treatment goals [12, 13], and rapid improvement in articulation patterns has been observed during EPG therapy [14, 15]. It is also reported that this technique can improve clients' awareness of their articulation problems [16] and provide motivation for therapy [12]. From our experience, EPG therapy is effective for older clients with residual articulation problems that have not been improved by conventional speech therapy.

3.1 Articulation training in the clinic

Since the authors introduced visual feedback therapy for treating articulation errors in 2004, more than 200 clients have experienced EPG therapy. At the 13th International Cleft Congress (2017, Chennai), a retrospective study was presented to clarify the characteristics of the clients who benefited from EPG therapy [17]. Most of the clients started EPG therapy after 6 years of age. The average age at initiating EPG therapy was 11 years (**Figure 12**). The target speech sounds, most often practiced, were alveolar and alveolo-palatal consonants [t, d, ʦ, ʣ, s, ɕ, ʨ, n, ʥ, ɾ] in that order. The most prominent abnormal EPG pattern was "retraction", followed by "increased

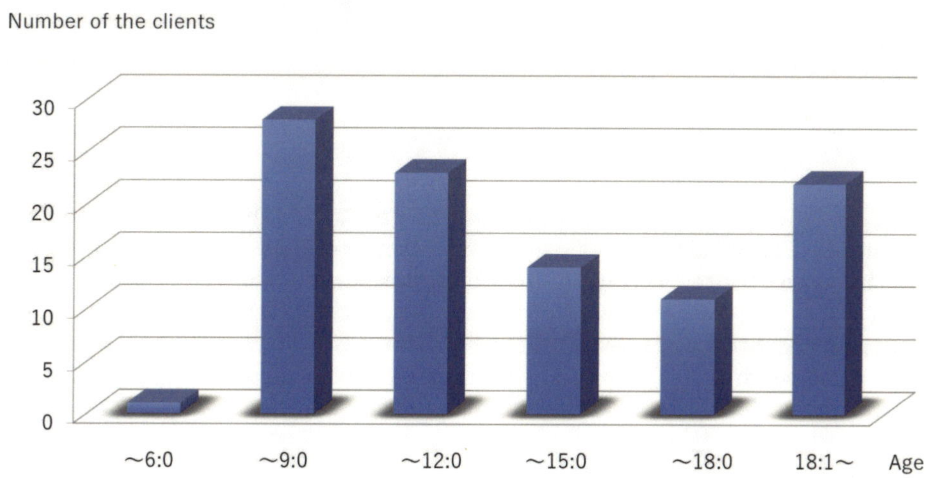

Figure 12.
The age at initiating EPG therapy.

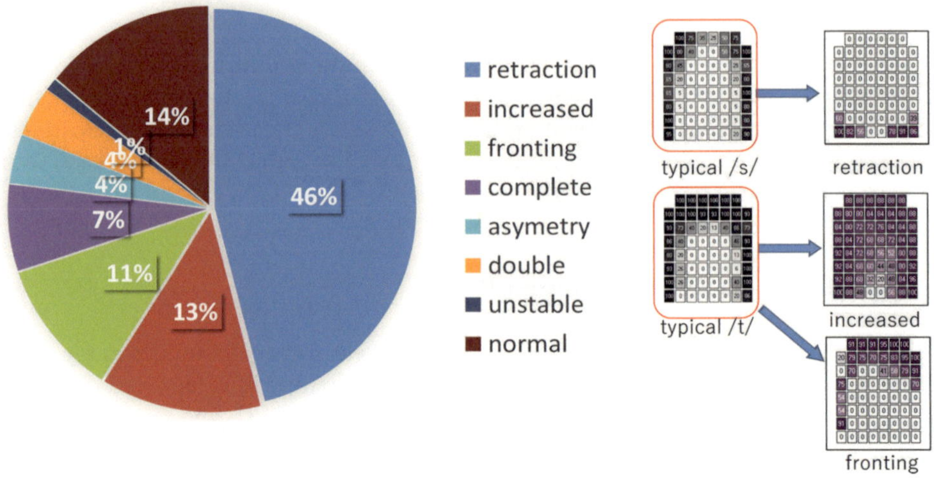

Figure 13.
Atypical EPG patterns at the first recording.

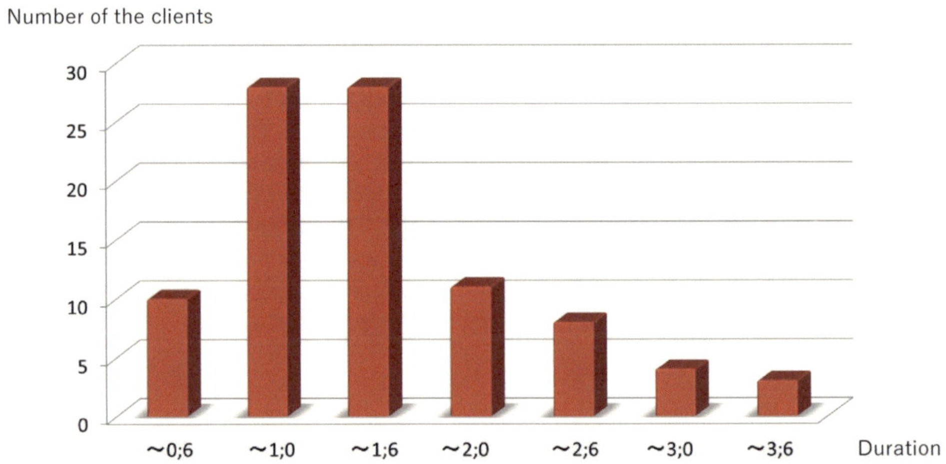

Figure 14.
Duration of EPG therapy.

contact", "fronting", "complete closure", "asymmetry", and "alveolar-velar double articulation" (**Figure 13**). The majority of the clients completed EPG treatment within 1 year and 6 months (**Figure 14**). In cases requiring a longer period of time, surgical and orthodontic intervention during the course interfered with EPG therapy.

This retrospective study revealed that EPG therapy is effective for school-aged clients with residual speech sound disorders, especially with alveolar and alveopalatal consonant errors. It is desirable to have done physical management before starting EPG therapy.

3.2 Articulation training at home

Although visual feedback training is effective in treating speech sound disorders, increasing the frequency of outpatient treatment was not easy, due to lack of manpower on the treatment side and the busy schedule of the caregivers. To increase training frequency, the authors started EPG home training using a portable training unit (PTU, Articulate Assistant Ltd., Edinburgh) and a tablet-type WinSTARS.

A preliminary study on the effectiveness of EPG home training was conducted on five patients with cleft palate [14]. They visited the clinic once a month and received visual feedback training by speech therapist and took PTU home to practice by themselves. Each participant practiced three to seven alveolar and alveopalatal sounds, which were perceptually judged as palatal/palatalization, posterior palatal or velarization, and lateral misarticulation. After 10 to 15 months of home training, they acquired perceptually acceptable realizations for all of the target sounds and were discharged from the EPG therapy. These participants had received conventional therapy for 3 to 8 years before they started EPG home training. Compared to this long duration, the EPG home training produced remarkable changes within a short period of time.

3.3 Telepractice using EPG

The 2019 Coronavirus pandemic (COVID-19) has had a serious impact on speech therapy. There was a period when the outpatient speech clinic was closed to prevent the spread of infection. Even after face-to-face therapy was resumed, it was required to wear a mask or face-shield and to keep physical distance. It was quite difficult to perform articulation therapy in this situation. In order to continue articulation training even with the COVID-19 pandemic, telepractice was introduced in many countries [18, 19]. Telepractice is a system that uses Internet-based telecommunications technology to provide specialized speech-language therapy, including evaluation, intervention, and consultation, remotely to patients or community speech-language pathologists. Even before the COVID-19 pandemic, telepractice has been incorporated into the field of speech-language pathology. Shprintzen and Golden-Kushner [20] reported on telepractice for speech disorders in Velocardiofacial Syndrome (VCFS). The symptoms presented by VCFS are diverse and require specialized knowledge to deal with, yet there is still a lack of understanding of VCFS in many areas. They are implementing remote video therapy to provide appropriate treatment for patients with VCFS in collaboration with speech therapists in other countries. Sweeney et al. [21, 22] proposed the program PLAT: Parent-led Articulation Therapy, which allows frequent practice at home with the help of parents, due to the significant lack of speech and language therapy (SLT) services for preschool or school-aged children after cleft palate surgery. This is a method of telepractice in which SLT provides an online articulation training program and checks the progress of the practice at home. All have implemented telemedicine to provide programs that meet the needs of underserved patients, inexperienced SLTs, and caregivers.

The authors started telepractice in 2020 and have done it for 37 patients so far. Initially targeted at patients who were unable to come to the clinic due to COVID-19, and subsequently targeted at patients who have difficulty making frequent visits for a variety of reasons. PTU (Articulate Assistant Ltd., Edinburgh) or a tablet-type WinSTARS (Asahi Roentgen Ltd., Kyoto) is loaned to most patients. Weekly online sessions used EPG to monitor the client's tongue-palate contact patterns remotely, and visual feedback was also utilized for self-practice at home. After 10- to 30-weekly 30-minute online sessions, their speech sound disorders resolved and speech intelligibility improved [23]. The combined use of EPG and telepractice seems to bring wider access to speech therapy for patients with speech sound disorders who have little opportunity to receive speech therapy for various reasons.

4. Relationship between articulation and nasopharyngeal closure function

The author has been organizing the Kobe Conference since 1994 [24]. This is a transdisciplinary team of plastic surgeons, dentists, otolaryngologists, and speech-language pathologists who meet approximately three times a year for joint consultations. Each time, 4–5 patients with residual speech sound disorders are invited. All participating professionals conduct perceptual assessment of speech, nasopharyngeal closure function tests (endoscopy, cephalometry, and nasometry) and listen to the needs of the patient and the family to determine a treatment plan. The most frequently consulted cases are those with nasopharyngeal closure dysfunction after primary cleft palate surgery, and some patients still have problems even after secondary surgery such as pharyngeal flap. Factors leading to nasopharyngeal closure dysfunction include residual organic problems, such as a short soft palate or fistula, or failure to use the closure function due to incorrect articulatory manipulation [25]. At the conference, the treatment plan takes into account organic problems, errors in articulatory manipulation, and the patient's overall development. To see the relationship between articulatory manipulation and nasopharyngeal closure function, a synchronization system between EPG and nasopharyngoscopy was implemented.

The idea for a synchronization system between EPG and nasopharyngoscopy came from the introduction of the software Articulate Assistant Advanced (AAA) provided by Articulate Instruments Ltd. (Edinburgh) [26]. This software is designed to record and analyze speech production data from instruments, such as ultrasound, video, electromagnetic articulography (EMA), VICON, magnetic resonance imaging (MRI), and EPG. It also controls the recording of ultrasound video and allows these to be synchronized with other instruments such as EPG.

In 2021, the authors started synchronizing EPG and nasopharyngoscopy using WinSTARS (**Figure 15**). Since then, synchronized EPG and nasopharyngoscopy were performed on 12 patients. This method was presented at the 68th Annual Meeting of the Japan Society of Logopedics and Phoniatrics, titled "Does articulatory manipulation alter nasopharyngeal closure function?" [27]. Videos showing the synchronization of EPG and nasopharyngoscopy can be viewed for one of these cases (Video 8

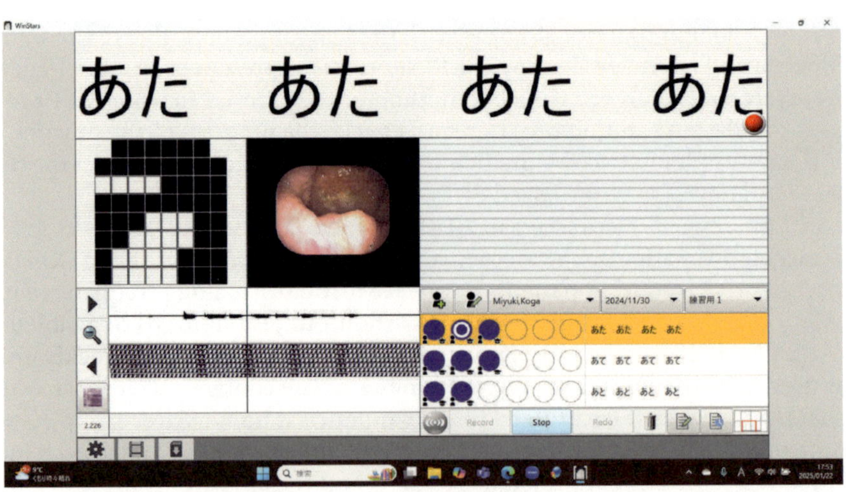

Figure 15.
Synchronized assessment: EPG and nasopharyngoscopy.

https://bit.ly/3Rocphb, Video 9 https://bit.ly/3Rocphb). In this case, as articulation improved, nasopharyngeal closure function also improved.

Henningsson & Isberg [28] reported the cases whose nasopharyngeal closure function altered between oral and glottal articulation. That is, good nasopharyngeal closure was observed when high-pressure consonants were produced orally, but not when glottal stops were produced. This is a good example of the relationship between articulatory manipulation and nasopharyngeal closure function. Golding-Kushner [29] recommended "that surgical management of velopharyngeal inadequacy be delayed until after speech therapy has eliminated abnormal compensatory articulation errors". Synchronized EPG and nasopharyngoscopy may be useful to confirm whether and when surgical treatment is indicated.

5. Future issues regarding the use of EPG

On the 24 January 2021, the 7th EPG Symposium was held online. At the invitation of the Japanese EPG Study Group, participants from several countries reported on the impact of the COVID-19 pandemic on research and clinical practice using EPG [30]. After the Symposium, Lee et al. summarized future developments regarding the use of EPG [31]. According to the report, EPG has been used extensively to investigate typical and atypical lingual articulation in dozens of languages [32]. In Japan, many studies were conducted with the DP (Rion Co., Ltd., Tokyo, Japan) in the 1980s, but they went downhill after DP production was discontinued in 1996 [33]. However, EPG studies using WinSTARS (Asahi Roentgen, Ltd., Kyoto, Japan) started to increase again from the 2000s. Recent studies in Japan have been conducted on a wide range of topics, not just cleft palate speech. For example, analysis of speech associated with jaw deformities [34], hearing impairment [35], lateral misarticulations [36], changes in tongue and palate contact dynamics due to speech rate control [37, 38], or research in the area of Japanese phonetics [39, 40]. International participants in the 7th EPG Symposium are also continuing their research using EPG and McYam plate [41, 42]. EPG is still the unique instrumental technique designed to capture the details of tongue and palate contact dynamics during speech.

Lee et al. [31] raised several areas where EPG hardware might improve further; thinner plates with better dental and palatal coverage, wireless connectivity, and new sensors for obtaining additional articulatory information. Various studies are being conducted on these issues, see Lee's paper for more information. Mat Zin et al. [43] also reviewed the EPG technology and stated "EPG can be upgraded and incorporates current technology, such as Bluetooth technology, telemedicine, and mobile application." Further improvements are expected to advance the research and clinical use of EPG in the future.

6. Conclusion

This chapter presents the clinical use of EPG, which provides detailed information on tongue-palate contact during speech. In the assessment, a variety of spatial distortions have been identified in speakers with cleft palate. EPG video in appendices would help to understand cleft speech characteristics (CSCs). Visual feedback training using EPG is particularly effective in school-age and older cases that are difficult to treat with regular training. EPG is also effective at home training and telepractice. The authors hope that the clinical use of EPG will expand as one of the tools of speech therapy.

Acknowledgements

We would like to thank Mr. Koichi Mizuno, a dental technician at Yamamoto Dental Clinic, who took on the task of creating the complicated EPG artificial plate and supported EPG's clinical and research work.

Conflict of interest

The authors declare no conflict of interest.

Appendices and nomenclature

EPG analysis of Cleft Speech Characteristics (CSCs) with EPG video (audio-visual information).

Author details

Ichiro Yamamoto[1*] and Yuri Fujiwara[2]

1 Yamamoto Dental Clinic, Nishinomiya, Japan

2 Osaka Health Science University, Osaka, Japan

*Address all correspondence to: yamamotomcyam@gmail.com

References

[1] Lohmander A, Olsson M. Methodology for perceptual assessment of speech in patients with cleft palate: A critical review of the literature. The Cleft Palate-Craniofacial Journal. 2004;**41**(1):64-70

[2] John A, Sell D, Sweeney T, Harding-Bell A, Williams A. The cleft audit protocol for speech-augmented: A validated and reliable measure for auditing cleft speech. The Cleft Palate-Craniofacial Journal. 2006;**43**(3):272-288

[3] Chapman KL, Baylis A, Trost-Cardamone J, et al. The Americleft speech project: A training and reliability study. The Cleft Palate-Craniofacial Journal. 2016;**53**(1):93-108

[4] Ogata Y, Tezuka M, Fujiwara Y, et al. Development and validation of a Japanese outcome tool for perceptual assessment of speech in patients with cleft palate. Folia Phoniatrica et Logopaedica. 2025. DOI: 10.1159/000544775

[5] Hardcastle WJ, Gibbon F. Electropalatography and its clinical applications. In: Ball MJ, Code C, editors. Instrumental Clinical Phonetics. London: Whurr Publishers; 1997. pp. 149-193

[6] Yamamoto I. A new EPG design for the client with cleft palate. In: Proceedings of the 5th International EPG Symposium; Queen Margaret University; Edinburgh. 2008

[7] McLeod S, Singh S. Speech Sounds: A Pictorial Guide to Typical and Atypical Speech. San Diego: Plural Publishing; 2009

[8] Imai S, Wakumoto M, Niu K. Assessment of articulation by use of palatography. The Japan Journal of Logopedics and Phoniatrics. 2000;**41**:159-169

[9] Mochizuki M, Yamagata K, Tokutomi K. Dynamic palatography including dental arch in sentence. Journal of Japan Prosthodontic Society. 1998;**42**:847-856

[10] Fujiwara Y, Yamamoto I. Typical adult speakers' tongue-palate contact patterns for Japanese alveolar and post-alveolar sounds. The Japan Journal of Logopedics and Phoniatrics. 2020;**61**:31-40. DOI: 10.5112/jjlp.61.31

[11] Yamamoto I. Tongue palate contact patterns for Japanese speakers with and without cleft lip and palate. International Journal of Speech-Language Pathology. 2020;**22**(1):70-77. DOI: 10.1080/17549507.2019.1593505

[12] Michi K, Yamashita Y, Imai S, Suzuki N, Yoshida H. Role of visual feedback treatment for defective /s/ sounds in patients with cleft palate. Journal of Speech, Language, and Hearing Research. 1993;**36**(2):277-285. DOI: 10.1044/jshr.3602.277

[13] Yamashita Y, Suzuki N, Imai S, Mori K, Takahashi K, Michi K. The efficacy of the speech training system for the treatment of articulation disorders in patients with cleft palate. Journal of Japanese Cleft Palate Association. 1999;**24**(1):52-60

[14] Fujiwara Y. Electropalatography home training using a portable training unit for Japanese children with cleft palate. Advances in Speech-Language Pathology. 2007;**9**(1):65-72. DOI: 10.1080/14417040601120904

[15] Whitehill TL, Strokes SF, Man YHY. Electropalatography treatment in an

adult with late repair of cleft palate. Cleft Palate-Craniofacial Journal. 1996;**33**(2):160-168

[16] Gibbon FE, Patterson L. A survey of speech and language therapists' views on electropalatography therapy outcomes in Scotland. Child Language Teaching and Therapy. 2006;**22**(3):275-2992

[17] Fujiwara Y, Yamamoto I. Who benefited from visual feedback therapy using electropalatography? In: Proceedings of the 13th International Congress of Cleft Lip and Palate and Related Craniofacial Anomalies; 8-11 February 2017; Tamil Nadu, India

[18] Fong R, Tsai CF, Yiu OY. The implementation of telepractice in speech language pathology in Hong Kong during the COVID-19 pandemic. Telemedicine Journal and e-health. 2021;**27**:30-38

[19] Kraljevic JK, Matic A, Dokoza KP. Telepractice as a reaction to the COVID-19 crisis: Insights from Croatian SLP settings. International Journal of Telerehabilitation. 2020;**12**:93-104. DOI: 10.5195/ijt.2020.6325

[20] Shprintzen RJ, Golding-Kushner KJ. The international use of teltepractice. Perspectives on Telepractice. 2012;**2**(1):16-25

[21] Sweeney T, Hegarty F, Powell K, et al. Randomized controlled trial comparing parent led therapist supervised articulation therapy (PLAT) with routine intervention for children with speech disorders associated with cleft palate. International Journal of Language and Communication Disorders. 2020;**55**:639-660. DOI: 10.1111/1460-6984.12542

[22] Sweeney T, Sell D, Hegarty F. Parent-led articulation therapy in cleft palate speech: A feasibility study. Journal of Clinical Speech and Language Studies. 2016;**23**:21-41

[23] Fujiwara Y, Yamamoto I, Kojima S, Kimura N. Telepractice using electropalatography for speech sound disorders –sustainable speech therapy under the pandemic of COVID-19. Journal of Japanese Cleft Palate Association. 2022;**47**:37-44

[24] Fujiwara Y, Yamamoto I, Ohsaki S. Transdisciplinary team approach to children with cleft lip and palate. The Japan Journal of Logopedics and Phoniatrics. 2021;**62**(1):7-13

[25] Peterson-Falzone S, Trost-Cardamone J, Karnell M, Hardin-Jones M. The Clinician's Guide to Treating Cleft Palate Speech. 1st ed. St. Louis: Mosby; 2006. pp. 17-19

[26] Articulate Instruments Ltd. Articulate Assistant Advanced User Guide: Version 2.13. Edinburgh: Articulate Instruments Ltd.; 2011

[27] Yamamoto I, Fujiwara Y, Koyama A. Does articulatory manipulation alter nasopharyngeal closure function? In: Proceedings of the 68th Annual Meeting of the Japan Society of Logopedics and Phoniatrics; 5-6 October 2023; Kurashiki, Japan. p. 86

[28] Henningsson G, Isberg A. Velopharyngeal movements in patients alternating between oral and glottal articulation: A clinical and cineradiographical study. Cleft Palate Journal. 1986;**23**:1-9

[29] Golding-Kushner KJ. Therapy Techniques for Cleft Palate Speech & Related Disorders. San Diego: Singular Thompson Learning; 2001. p. 6

[30] Lee A, Fujiwara Y, Liker M, Yamamoto I, Takei Y, Gibbon F.

Electropalatography (EPG) activities in Japan and the impact of the COVID-19 pandemic on EPG research and therapy: A report of presentations at the 7th EPG symposium. International Journal of Language & Communication Disorders. 2022;**57**:906-917

[31] Lee A, Liker M, Fujiwara Y, Yamamoto I, Takei Y, Gibbon F. EPG research and therapy: Further developments. Clinical Linguistics & Phonetics. 2023;**37**(8):701-721. DOI: 10.1080/02699206.2022.2080588

[32] Gibbon F. Bibliography of Electropalatographic (EPG) Studies in English. (1957-2013). Ireland: University College Coke; 2013

[33] Fujiwara Y, Yamamoto I. A review of electropalatographic studies written in Japanese. Journal of Japanese Cleft Palate Association. 2006;**31**(3):261-266

[34] Kojima S, Kaku M, Yamamoto I, Yasuhara Y, Sumi H, Yamamoto T, et al. Tongue-palatal contact changes in patients with skeletal mandibular prognathism after sagittal split ramus osteotomy: An electropalatography study. Journal of Oral Rehabilitation. 2017;**44**:673-682. DOI: 10.1111/joor.12530

[35] Uchiyama M, Nakamura H, Fujiwara Y, Kojima C, Hasegawa K. Articulation characteristics of a severely hearing-impaired speaker and trial therapy using electropalatography. Japanese Journal of Speech, Language, and Hearing Research. 2013;**10**(2):109-117

[36] Takei Y, Yamashita Y, Mori K, Tatara H, et al. Electropalatographic study of connected speech in lateral misarticulation. Oral Science International. 2023;**20**(1):18-27

[37] Uchiyama M, Fujiwara Y, Kojima C. Changes of articulatory movement accompanying speech rate control in normal subjects' tongue-palate contact analysis using electropalatography. The Japan Journal of Logopedics and Phoniatrics. 2016;**57**(4):382-390. DOI: 10.5112/jjlp.57.382

[38] Okumura S, Matsui M, Yamamoto I. The effect of the speech rates of the short sentences on the tongue-palate contact patterns – On the articulatory movements of the alveolar consonants. Bulletin of Osaka Health Science University. 2021;**4**:1-16

[39] Matsui M. On the input information of the C/D model for vowel devoicing in Japanese. Journal of the Phonetic Society of Japan. 2017;**21**(1):127-140

[40] Nakamura T, Fujiwara Y. A quantitative evaluation of coarticulatory effect of vowel environment on the consonants /s/, /t/, /k/. Journal of Rehabilitation Science. 2016;**12**:63-77

[41] Liker M, Zoric A. Speech errors and articulatory gestures: An electropalatographic investigation. Suvremena Lingvistika. 2020:247-264. DOI: 10.22210/suvlin.2020.090.02. UDK 811.163.42'342.22 Izvorni znanstveni članak Prihvaćeno za tisak: 16. listopada

[42] Patrick K, Fricke S, Rutter B, Cleland J. Clinical application of usage-based phonology: Treatment of cleft palate speech using usage-based electropalatography. International Journal of Speech-Language Pathology. 2024;**26**(4):595-610. DOI: 10.1080/17549507.2023.2238924

[43] Mat Zin S, Rasib S, Suhaimi F, Mariatti M. The technology of tongue and hard palate contact detection: A review. BioMedical Engineering OnLine. 2021;**20**:17. DOI: 10.1186/s12938-021-00854-y